Ophthalmology

EXAMINATION TECHNIQUES
QUESTIONS AND ANSWERS

**How to examine the eye and
revision for the FRCOphth, FRCS(Ophth)
MRCOphth and MRCP examinations**

DAVID C. BROADWAY MD BSc FRCOphth DO
*Consultant, Norfolk and Norwich Health Care Trust, Norwich, UK;
formerly Senior Registrar, Moorfields Eye Hospital, London, UK and
Clinical Research Fellow, University of British Columbia, Vancouver, Canada*

ADNAN TUFAIL FRCOphth
*Specialist Registrar, Moorfields Eye Hospital, London, UK;
formerly Research Fellow, Jules Stein Eye Institute, Los Angeles, USA*

PENG TEE KHAW PhD MRCP FRCS FRCOphth DO
*Professor, Moorfields Eye Hospital and Institute of
Ophthalmology, University College, London, UK*

D1354810

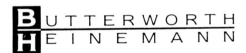

OXFORD AUCKLAND BOSTON JOHANNESBURG MELBOURNE NEW DELHI

Butterworth-Heinemann
An imprint of Elsevier Science Limited

First published 1999
  Reprinted 2002

British Library Cataloguing in Publication Data
A catalogue record for this book is available from the British Library

Library of Congress Cataloging in Publication Data
A catalog record for this book is available from the Library of Congress

0 7506 2500 7

Setting and colour origination by David Gregson Associates, Beccles, Suffolk
Printed in China by RDC Group Limited

Contents

Introduction

The main aim of this book is to help the exam candidate during the revision period leading up to postgraduate examinations and to help him/her develop a systematic approach when examining patients. The reader is encouraged to write in the book so as to personalize it. Additional notes written in the margin of a book are often easily remembered in the heat of an exam. If the reader feels that we have missed any critical areas, please write (or e-mail) and let us know (ophthexam@hotmail.com).

The first section aims to help the candidate develop a systematic method of examination. This is important since a common cause of exam failure is the inability of the candidate to competently examine patients and elicit physical signs. The crucial part of clinical exams is for the candidate to demonstrate to the examiners an ability to elicit physical signs and make sensible inferences, not to diagnose every rarity. If asked for causes, the candidate should give the common causes first, particularly those appropriate to the particular patient in question. For each system covered in the first section, an examination checklist is provided. The second, and main section, presents a series of 'medical' and 'surgical' conditions which involve the eye. In each case the disorder is defined and key clinical aspects are listed. A number of questions are then provided and for each of these an 'ideal' answer is offered. Most of the questions and answers are typical of those encountered in the clinical examination and viva situations, although some are more like those to be encountered in written examinations. We have attempted to pose questions and provide answers that comprehensively cover each condition to a level expected by the majority of postgraduate examiners. However, no book can cover everything – good luck!

David Broadway
Adnan Tufail
Peng Khaw

Section A
Clinical examination techniques

1.   Assessment of visual acuity

History

Patients (and/or parents) will usually be able to provide a certain amount of information about their vision and, in particular, if there is a history of amblyopia ('lazy-eye').

Reduced visual acuity in one eye should be suspected if there is constant unilateral strabismus, anisometropia or a history of occlusion therapy.

Clinical examination

Assessment of visual acuity (the resolving power of the eye) is the essential first part of any ocular examination. Accurate measurement of visual acuity may not be possible with infants, young children and those with learning difficulties. However, there are various methods by which estimates of visual function can be made.

The normal limit of resolution for the adult eye is one minute of a degree (1′). Where possible, visual acuity should be measured unaided and with any refractive error corrected. In the absence of appropriate spectacle correction, an estimate of corrected visual acuity can be made using a pinhole. Reduced visual acuity which is not correctable by refraction is due to an organic lesion, malingering or amblyopia. Near vision should also be tested in the same way. In certain cases (e.g. when a patient has very low vision or nystagmus) it is also useful to measure the VA with both eyes open, since it may be improved. Near vision is particularly relevant when assessing educational needs, and in such cases the patient should be allowed to hold the print at any distance (which is noted) and also adopt an abnormal head posture if this helps.

In practical terms it is not often possible to test near and distance vision with and without glasses in young children, as their concentration lapses. One should use tests that yield the most information in an order of priority.

Infants (mainly qualitative)

One should be aware that these methods of assessing vision have limitations.

1. *Fixing and following*:
   – best method for neonates
   – either to a light source or a human face.
2. *Startle reflex*:
   – a visually threatening provocation may induce the startle (Moro) reflex in a seeing baby
   – in practice it is difficult to isolate the threat to the visual system.
3. *Optokinetic nystagmus (OKN)*:
   – a drum with vertically painted stripes is rotated slowly in front of the infant, and the infant follows the stripes until they disappear from view and then refixates on a new stripe/target
   – providing there is some degree of visual acuity and no neurological abnormality, normal physiological OKN will be evident (the baby will follow the moving stripe, then refixate on the next stripe).
4. *Objection to occlusion*:
   – passive acceptance of occlusion is rare unless the vision of the occluded eye is poor
   – resistance to occlusion does not mean the vision is entirely normal
   – this is only a comparison of the two eyes and they may be equally good or equally bad!
5. *Cover testing* (see also p. 35):
   – infants with alternating squints usually have equal vision in each eye
   – if the child holds fixation with the squinting eye through a blink, the VA is probably nearly equal in the two eyes
   – infants with constant unilateral squints have amblyopia until proved otherwise

– infants with intermittent and latent squints usually (but not always) have equal vision.

6. *Visually directed reaching*:
   – requires careful observation of the child's behaviour
   – poor vision may be associated with semi-random exploratory hand movements towards an object of interest rather than the direct movement associated with normal vision.

7. *Picking up tiny objects (e.g. 100s and 1000s)*:
   – useful in infants over the age of nine months, once they have developed the necessary manual dexterity
   – not adversely affected by mild or moderate degrees of refractive error
   – a gross test, since blurred objects can still be located.

8. *Catford drum*:
   – a variation of OKN and thus subject to the same limitations
   – black dots on a drum with a white background are seen to oscillate. If seen, the dots draw a child's attention and an observer can see a corresponding series of oscillatory eye movements (OKN)
   – using dots of differing sizes an estimate of Snellen visual acuity can be made. The smaller the dot which elicits the nystagmus, the better the visual acuity
   – vision can be expressed in Snellen equivalents, but this is not a test of discrimination and the result should not be directly compared with Snellen acuity
   – a version using Vernier lines instead of dots is available, but is little used today.

9. *Stycar rolling balls*:
   – uses white polystyrene balls of differing size rolled on a darkly coloured background (e.g. a carpeted floor), while the child's reactions are observed.

10. *Preferential looking tests*:
    – require the use of Teller, Keeler or Cardiff acuity cards
    – the tests use the principle of forced choice preferential looking
    – a grating pattern is presented on one side of the card whilst the other side is plain. The child will look at the grating from preference

– the examiner views the child's eyes through a small hole in the card (or a TV monitor in the automated version) and notes in which direction the child looks. The examiner does not know on which side of the card the grating is positioned
– as the grating becomes finer a point is reached where the gratings can no longer be determined. The result can be expressed in Snellen's equivalents but is not really comparable and is better expressed in cycles/degree
– the method tends to over-estimate VA in amblyopes, but is probably the best method available in current clinical use for assessing VA in babies.

11. *Gratings and visual evoked responses (VEP)*:
    – an alternating square-wave grating, comprising black and white stripes of equal width, is presented electronically on a TV screen. The highest frequency grating which elicits a visually evoked potential (VEP) response correlates with the highest attainable visual acuity
    – a grating can be used as part of a forced choice preferential looking test, which is based on the fact that infants prefer to look at a patterned or striped image as opposed to a plain image.

12. *Spinning baby test*:
    – useful in the baby when the presence of vision is doubtful
    – the baby is held securely with the head supported and spun around the examiner
    – vestibular nystagmus is induced when the spinning stops, but soon disappears if there is vision. The nystagmus persists in the blind child.

Children

Distance vision

1. *Picture tests*:
   – useful in children over two years of age
   – a series of pictures (differing in size) is presented in a manner similar to a Snellen chart (see p. 7)
   – there are several charts available, the most commonly used being the Kay picture test

- the child is asked to name the object selected by the examiner
- the test is useful, but tests single optotypes only and can only be used in children who can speak and are not too shy.

2. *Sheridan Gardiner letter matching test*:
   - useful in children from three years of age
   - the child is positioned 6 m away from the examiner with a card on which several letters are printed. The examiner presents a card on which a letter is printed and the child points to the matching letter on his or her card
   - a disadvantage is that the test uses single optotypes, and thus can overestimate visual acuity in amblyopes
   - to avoid the 'crowding phenomenon', whereby visual acuity is better with single optotypes rather than linear (as seen in amblyopia), the test can be adapted by combining the matching card with the Snellen chart, or using the Cambridge crowding cards where a central letter is surrounded by four letters, above, below, to the right and to the left.

With children who have amblyopia it is better to use a linear test as soon as possible, since the degree of amblyopia can be underestimated with a single optotype test.

Near vision

1. *Sheridan Gardiner letter and Kay picture testing*:
   - reduced versions of the Sheridan Gardiner and Kay picture test cards are available.
2. *Maclure testing*:
   - a version of the 'Ladybird' children's reading scheme can be used for those children who cannot read at an adult level.

Adults

Distance vision

1. *Standard Snellen chart test*:
   - a test of minimum legible acuity based on the resolvable gap between the components of high contrast test-type letters

- the letters are presented so that gaps between letter components of different visual angles are on a decreasing scale as one reads down the chart
- each Snellen letter subtends an angle of five minutes of arc (5′) at the eye, and the gaps within the letter subtend an angle of 1′ when viewed from the specified distance (NB: 60′ = 1 degree)
- the smallest letter size which can be resolved by the patient is determined at a distance of 6 m
- the largest letter has a viewing distance of 60 m and the smaller ones viewing distances of 36, 24, 18, 12, 9, 6, 5 and 4 m.
- the normal eye can distinguish the 6 m letter at a distance of 6 m, and this is described as having 6/6 vision
- if the tested eye can only see the 24 m letter at a distance of 6 m, the visual acuity is recorded as 6/24
- the visual acuity should be determined unaided, with the subjects spectacle correction (if appropriate) and with a pinhole.

2. *Illiterate E and Landholt ring 'Snellen' chart test*:
   - can be used to diminish errors induced by the differences of the Snellen test-type letters
   - can be used for illiterate patients
   - Landholt broken rings consist of circles, each with a gap subtending 1′, the orientation of which varies and must be identified
   - illiterate E's are presented with the prongs of each E pointing in one of four directions, and this must be determined by the subject.

3. *Low vision testing*:
   - if patients have a visual acuity of less than 6/60, they may be positioned nearer the chart so that the largest letter is seen. If seen at 3 m the visual acuity is recorded as 3/60, if at 1 m, as 1/60
   - alternatively, the patient can be tested for an ability to count fingers held up, or to see hand movements at one or two metres
   - if a patient's visual acuity is such that hand movements cannot be seen, it should be determined whether there is any perception of light, and if so,

whether light can be seen in all four quadrants of the visual field.

4. *Contrast sensitivity testing*:
   - letters or gratings of similar size but decreasing contrast (relative to the background) are presented to the patient
   - various tests are available (e.g. Vistech and Pelli-Robson)
   - some conditions (e.g. optic neuritis) result in no measurable decrease in Snellen visual acuity, but a significant reduction in contrast sensitivity. Contrast sensitivity may also be reduced in amblyopia.
5. *Navigational vision*:
   - this can be assessed, and is often different (better or worse) to that implied by Snellen visual acuity and visual field assessments (also useful with children).
6. *Grating acuity chart testing*:
   - a test of visual acuity and contrast sensitivity
   - computer-generated gratings, reflecting light in a sine-wave pattern, are presented at various values of spatial frequency (e.g. varying on the horizontal axis) and contrast (e.g. varying on the vertical axis)
   - the subject has to select the highest resolvable frequency for the degree of contrast
   - this is used in research, but rarely clinically.

Near vision

1. *Reading vision testing*:
   - literate patients are tested using a special chart with paragraphs of differing sized print (Faculty of Ophthalmologists Test Type N chart) or, if this is unavailable, with newspaper print
   - tested at 30 cm with the appropriate refractive correction
   - patients with low vision tend to hold reading matter very close. In these cases their comfortable reading distances should be noted.

Checklist for assessment of visual acuity

History

1. Ask about known visual defects (especially refractive correction)
2. Remember the possibility of amblyopia.

Clinical examination

1. *Infants*
   - fixing and following
   - startle reflex
   - optokinetic nystagmus
   - objection to occlusion
   - cover testing
   - visually directed reaching
   - picking up tiny objects
   - Catford drum
   - Stycar rolling balls
   - preferential looking
   - gratings and VEP
   - spinning baby test
2. *Children*
   - picture tests (Kay chart)
   - Sheridan Gardiner matching letter chart testing
   - near vision tests (Kay, Sheridan Gardiner, Maclure)
3. *Adults*
   - standard Snellen chart testing
   - illiterate E and Landholt ring 'Snellen' chart testing
   - low vision testing
   - contrast sensitivity testing
   - navigational vision
   - grating acuity chart testing
   - reading vision testing.

2. Assessment of colour vision

History

The patient may report a change in colour appreciation or may report that he/she has a known congenital colour vision defect. Colour vision defects can be due to toxicity with certain drugs (see below) and a history of past and present use of medications is important.

Clinical examination

Testing can be subjective or objective.

Red desaturation:

- a quick, easy and sensitive test of optic nerve function
- useful in unilateral or asymmetrical disease
- the test involves observing a bright red object with one eye at a time and comparing the apparent brightness of the object between the eyes
- relative dimness of the object colour indicates red desaturation suggesting a possible optic nerve lesion
- may also occur in visual field quadrants as an early sign of disease (e.g. bitemporal red desaturation in the presence of a pituitary tumour).

Ishihara pseudo-isochromatic plate test:

- a commonly used, quick test for red-green confusion
- a visual acuity of about 6/18 or better is required to perform the test reliably
- the test is based on plates each consisting of a matrix of coloured dots arranged so that with normal colour vision a figure is visible
- the dots cover a large range of lightness values that will only allow recognition of the figure on the basis of colour discrimination rather than saturation or hue
- the full version contains 38 plates with the commonly used abridged version containing 14 plates
- each plate is viewed monocularly at a distance of 2/3 m under good illumination for 4 seconds
- the first plate is a control plate and should be read by complete achromats provided they have sufficient visual acuity, since the dots making the figure differ in contrast as well as colour from the surrounding dots (use of this plate may help to detect malingerers)
- most of the plates contain numerals but winding paths are also present in some plates to test illiterates or children
- lesions of the optic nerve result in a desaturation of all colours and a number of colours are confused including red and green
- an overall loss of hue discrimination resolves into a red-green defect as acuity improves
- the test is useful for both congenital and acquired red-green colour vision defects (protanopia and deuteranopia)
- certain drugs may affect colour vision such as digoxin, ethambutol, chloroquine and thioridazine
- one should always remember that about 5% of the population have defective colour vision and so the results of plate tests should not be taken in isolation.

Farnsworth–Munsell 100-hue test:

- this test allows grading of colour vision but is time consuming taking at least 20 minutes to perform
- the test was designed to test hue discrimination among persons with normal colour vision and chromatic discrimination loss

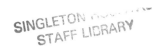

in those with congenital colour vision defects
- the test consists of 84 movable coloured tiles arranged in four boxes of 21
- the colours were chosen to represent perceptively equal steps in hue and are of approximately the same brightness
- the subject is given one tray at a time and allowed 2 minutes with each tray to arrange the colours in serial order according to their hue (chromatic order) between two reference tiles
- the total number of errors and their position suggest the diagnosis or the type of defect and also provide a measure of severity.

Anomaloscopes:

- anomaloscopes are used for reference testing against which other tests are judged
- the principle of the test involves the mixing of two colours, such as red and green, to match a third, such as yellow.
- impractical for routine clinical use.

Checklist for the assessment of colour vision

History

1. Congenital or acquired
2. Drug history.

Clinical examination

1. Red desaturation test
2. Ishihara pseudo-isochromatic plate test
3. Farnsworth–Munsell 100-hue test
4. Anomaloscopes.

3. Assessment of visual fields

Background

The normal visual field

- >90° temporally
- 60° nasally and superiorly
- 70° inferiorly
- due to greater sensitivity centrally and reduced sensitivity in the periphery, the field can be represented as a hill of vision, the peak relating to the fovea
- the hill of vision varies in height and shape with many factors including age, stimulus size or duration and the level of background light.

Visual field defects

- a visual field defect is a departure from normal of the shape and/or height of the normal hill of vision
- may be focal or general
- may be absolute or relative.

History

It is always worth asking the patient if they have noticed a visual field defect (e.g. 'Have you noticed if any part of your vision is missing?' or 'Have you noticed if any part of the world as you see it is missing?'), although it is common for visual defects to go unnoticed. It is also important to inquire about past medical and surgical history, additional neurological symptoms and dietary/drug/smoking history.

Clinical examination

In the exam situation a candidate is unlikely to be expected to detect very subtle visual field defects and in many cases it will be the technique by which one attempts to demonstrate a defect that will be examined. It is best to try and detect gross defects first. Each eye should be tested separately and the patient should be asked to cover one eye at a time with the palm (not fingers) of their hand. Bitemporal hemianopias and scotomata are easily missed if both eyes are tested together.

The following is a suggested routine:

1. The examiner should ask the patient to look at his/her face and inquire as to whether any part is missing.
2. Initially the examiner can check the patient's hemifields and quadrants by finger counting (i.e. by asking the patient how many fingers [either one or two] he/she is holding up). At first each eye is tested separately but it is important to check both hemifields simultaneously. This simple test may reveal gross field loss and make further confrontational analysis easier.
3. The candidate should then go on to examine the fields using a white-headed neurological pin for the peripheral field (beyond a central 30° radius) and a red-headed neurological pin for the central field (of a 30° radius). This is more accurate than finger-counting visual field analysis. Loss of red desaturation between quadrants is one of the earliest signs of a compressive optic nerve lesion.

To perform confrontation visual field testing (designed to detect gross defects and those with clear linear borders) the examiner must be positioned level with and facing the subject at a distance of about 1 metre. The examiner should then ask the patient to cover his/her right/left eye with the palm of his/her right/left hand and with the uncovered eye look at the centre of the examiner's left/right eye all the time. A comparison of examiner and patient fields is then made with an assumption that the examiner's fields are normal! By comparison of the mutually congruent fields a defect is detected by the absence of a patient response when the pin head is visible to the examiner.

4. If an homonymous hemianopia is present the site of the lesion may be further localized by looking for:
   - macular sparing
   - sparing of the temporal crescent
   - optokinetic nystagmus asymmetry
   - Wernicke's pupil
   - Macular sparing (central visual field of 5–10°) occurs with occipital lobe lesions because of collateral circulation to the occipital lobe pole by the middle cerebral artery in association with an occlusion in the posterior cerebral artery.
   - Sparing of an outer temporal crescent of visual field on the same side as the hemianopia is a feature of certain occipital lobe lesions. This occurs due to the unilateral representation of this part of the field by tissue deep in the calcarine fissure (very rare).
   - Optokinetic nystagmus (OKN) asymmetry indicates that a space occupying lesion resides in the parietal lobe. Such a lesion producing a right homonymous hemianopia is associated with loss of OKN to the right with its preservation to the left (NB: OKN asymmetry is not a feature of parietal lobe infarcts).
   - Wernicke's pupil (no pupil reaction with light stimulation from the side of the hemianopia, with normal responses from the contralateral side) or a contralateral relative afferent pupil defect in association with an incongruous homonymous hemianopia indicates an optic tract lesion (rare).

5. If a subtle central or paracentral scotoma is suspected a printed grid (Amsler chart) can be used to aid its detection. The patient should be asked to point out any areas of the grid that are missing or distorted.

6. Tangent screens can be used to detect possible central visual field defects (campimetry). Since the test surface is flat the value of testing beyond 30° is limited.

7. It is unlikely that a candidate would be asked to perform tangent screen campimetry (although standard in the old FRCS exam!) or bowl perimetry (manual or automated) but it is common to be provided with previously obtained visual fields (especially print-outs from computerized automated visual field analysers) and asked to comment on visual field defects.

Perimetry

The subject of perimetry cannot be covered comprehensively in this text but a few key points will be presented:

Types of perimetry:
- kinetic perimetry involves the detection of a moving target, the brightness of which is held constant (e.g. the Goldmann perimeter)
- static perimetry involves the detection of a stationary target, the brightness of which is increased (e.g. the Friedman analyser or the Henson, Allergan Humphrey or Octopus automated analysers)
- static perimetry is considered superior to kinetic perimetry in its ability to detect slopes and scotomata
- testing may be performed as a threshold or suprathreshold (the intensity of the stimulus is not reduced to the level of detection/non-detection) analysis
- a threshold analysis is more sensitive but takes longer to perform and is more at risk of detecting artefacts than a suprathreshold test
- a suprathreshold analysis is quicker to perform and particularly useful for screening.

Variable factors:
- the accuracy of a visual field plot depends on the patient's concentration and good fixation
- when testing the central 30°, refractive errors should be corrected
- pupil size should be taken into account.

Interpretation of automated visual field print-outs:
- check the patient details (name, age, eye, pupil size, refractive correction used)
- check the test parameters (i.e. type of test performed)
- check test reliability indices (test duration, fixation losses, number of false positive and false negative errors, fluctuation and the

computer assessment of reliability if available)

- check for any possible artefactual visual field defects (ptosis artefact, small pupil artefact or trial lens rim artefact)
- use the grey-scale plot of the visual field **but not in isolation** from the raw data to describe the defect.

Some computerized visual field analysers contain statistical software that is able to:

- flag suspicious areas
- compare the patient's field with normals data (i.e. taking age into account) on a point-by-point basis (to produce total deviation and pattern deviation plots). Generalized defects of the visual field (e.g. due to cataract) are demonstrated in the total deviation plot but not the pattern deviation plot. Specific focal defects are seen in both total and pattern deviation plots. An added value of the pattern deviation plot is that it may unmask a focal defect previously masked by generalized depression in the total deviation plot
- provide global indices (in dB) indicating how the height and shape of the patient's hill of vision deviates from normal:
  - mean deviation (the mean difference between the patient's overall visual field sensitivity in comparison with a normal, age-corrected, reference field)
  - pattern standard deviation (the standard deviation of the deviations and thus a measure of the degree to which the shape of a patient's field differs from a normal, age-corrected, reference field)
  - short-term fluctuation (an index of the patient's consistency during the test period determined by testing a number of points twice)
  - corrected pattern standard deviation (a measure of the degree to which the shape of the patient's hill of vision deviates from the shape of a normal, age-corrected, reference field)
- analyse changes in a patient's visual field with time
- perform the glaucoma hemifield test (a relatively crude test for detecting glaucomatous visual field defects based on the assumption that glaucoma frequently affects one hemifield more than the other).

Checklist for the assessment of visual fields

History

1. Awareness of field defect
2. Additional neurological symptoms
3. Past medical/surgical history
4. Dietary/drug/smoking history.

Clinical examination

1. Facial confrontation
2. Finger counting confrontation
3. White-pin peripheral field testing
4. Red-pin central field testing
5. Amsler grid
6. Tangent screen campimetry
7. Bowl perimetry
8. Automated perimetry.

Always keep likely visual field defects in mind, such as:

- a central scotoma
- a centrocaecal scotoma
- a paracentral scotoma
- an enlarged blind spot
- an altitudinal field defect
- a bitemporal hemianopia
- a homonymous hemianopia
- pie-in-the-sky quadrantinopia
- glaucomatous visual field defects (e.g. nasal steps and arcuate scotomata).

Don't forget to look for:

- congruity
- macular sparing

and, although very rare in both life and exams:

- sparing of an outer temporal crescent
- optokinetic nystagmus asymmetry.

4. Assessment of eye movements

Classification of eye movements

Saccade

- a fast conjugate eye movement (350–700° per second)
- voluntary
- to bring object images to the fovea
- mediated by fronto-mesencephalic/superior colliculus pathways
- contralateral control.

Quick phase of nystagmus

- a fast conjugate eye movement
- involuntary
- to direct the fovea to a potential object of interest during head/body rotation
- mediated by the paramedian-pontine reticular formation (PPRF)
- contralateral control.

Smooth pursuit

- a slow conjugate eye movement (25–50° per second)
- voluntary or involuntary
- to keep the image of a moving object at the fovea
- mediated by the parieto-occipito-temporal-mesencephalic pathway
- ipsilateral control.

Optokinetic

- a slow conjugate eye movement
- involuntary
- to keep retinal images fixed during prolonged head/body rotation
- unknown pathways
- response to acceleration
- fades with sustained constant speed of rotation.

Vestibular

- a slow conjugate eye movement
- involuntary
- to keep retinal images fixed during brief head/body rotation
- depends on vestibular motion receptors in the semicircular canals in each ear and the labyrinthine-pontine pathway
- stimulation of the horizontal canals results in horizontal nystagmus
- stimulation of the posterior canals results in vertical nystagmus
- stimulation of the anterior canals results in rotational nystagmus
- contralateral control.

Vergence

- a slow disconjugate eye movement
- voluntary or involuntary
- occurs with the accommodative response
- to move the eyes in opposite directions, in order to keep the images from an object at both foveae as it moves nearer or further away
- mediated by the occipito-mesencephalic pathway.

In an examination situation a candidate is most likely to be asked to examine the eye movements of a patient. The following scheme is suggested:

History

Specific points which should be addressed include the following.

Duration/age at onset

- includes determination as to whether the disorder is congenital (e.g. congenital ocular motor apraxia – very rare!) or acquired.

Causative factors

These may include:

- problems during pregnancy or at delivery
- trauma
- associated medical conditions (arterio-sclerosis, brainstem vascular disease, cerebrovascular accident [CVA], thyrotox-icosis, demyelination, myasthenia gravis)
- previous neurosurgery
- family history of strabismus.

Associated symptoms

These may include:

- diplopia – (3rd cranial nerve palsy or aberrant regeneration, trauma and the medical causes)
- fatigue – (myasthenia gravis, see p. 25)
- dysphagia – (oculopharyngeal muscular dystrophy)
- ophthalmoplegia – (Kearns–Sayre syndrome, see p. 233)
- additional neurological symptoms.

Drug history

- neostigmine – (myasthenia gravis)
- phenothiazine – (oculogyric crisis – unlikely to be seen in an examination setting!).

Clinical examination (See also 'Assessment of strabismus and cover tests')

1. The examiner should ask the patient to look straight ahead, and the eyes examined in their primary position. Certain abnormalities will be seen immediately (e.g. a complete 3rd cranial nerve palsy with ptosis). Some more subtle abnormalities may be detected by observing corneal reflexes from a pen-torch held in front of the patient. Asymmetry of the corneal reflex positions is indicative of a deviation.

   Paresis will result in a deviation in the direction opposite to the main action of the affected muscle (e.g. paresis of LR = poor abduction – eso – uncrossed diplopia; paresis of the right SR = poor elevation – L/R – vertical diplopia).

The deviation may be present:

1. only in the direction of the main action of the paralysed muscle
2. in the primary position and in the direction of the main action of the paralysed muscle
3. in all positions, but maximum separation is in the direction of the main action of the paralysed muscle.

2. The examiner should ask the patient to follow an object into the six cardinal positions of gaze, whilst keeping the head straight and still (versions):

	DEXTROELEVATION		LEVOELEVATION		
	RSR	CN3	LSR	CN3	
	LIO	CN3	RIO	CN3	
	RLR	CN6	LLR	CN6	
DEXTRO-VERSION	LMR	CN3	RMR	CN3	**LEVO-VERSION**
	RIR	CN3	LIR	CN3	
	LSO	CN4	RSO	CN4	
	DEXTRODEPRESSION		LEVODEPRESSION		

- dextroversion (to the right)
- dextroelevation (up and to the right)
- dextrodepression (down and to the right)
- levoversion (to the left)
- levoelevation (up and to the left)
- levodepression (down and to the left).

The six cardinal positions of gaze are useful in detecting single muscle or nerve problems. Muscle/nerve combinations for the positions of gaze are as shown below.

To aid recollection of the secondary actions of the vertical muscles remember 'RADSIN': 'Recti ADduct, Superior muscles INtort'.

Movements should be to the extreme position of gaze if subtle disorders are not to be missed (NB: with normal adduction the nasal cornea is buried by the caruncle to 1–2 mm, with normal abduction the temporal limbus (corneo-scleral junction) should almost reach the lateral canthus).

Elevation and depression of the eye in the central/vertical axis involve contributions from the vertical recti and oblique muscles and are not particularly useful in identifying single nerve problems but are useful in detecting gaze palsies (e.g. Parinaud's syndrome), A or V pattern strabismus or restrictive eye movement disorders.

3. Corneal reflexes should be observed, in both eyes, in each of the positions of gaze to aid the detection of any deviation.

4. The patient should be asked if there is any diplopia – again indicative of a deviation. The diplopia should correspond to the deviation. The candidate should remember that the higher eye will see the lower image, uncrossed diplopia in eso-deviation, crossed diplopia in exo-deviation (red and green glasses can be used if the patient is confused). When there is a vertical deviation ask where the greatest vertical separation occurs, since coincident A- or V-patterns may also cause a horizontal change in separation (e.g. right SR paresis = greatest vertical separation on dextroelevation – the increase in deviation may be confirmed by cover testing).

5. Cover tests can be performed and compared in both the primary position and the extreme positions of gaze (see p. 33). When the movements of an eye are tested separately with the other eye covered, ductions as opposed to versions are examined. With non-paralytic strabismus ductions are initially full, only becoming reduced with chronicity and secondary changes (consecutive squint).

6. Muscle sequelae occur following an extraocular muscle paresis. For example:

   a) paresis of muscle: LLR   RSO
   b) overaction of
        contralateral synergist   RMR   LIR
   c) contracture of the
        direct antagonist   LMR   RIO
   d) secondary inhibitional
        palsy of the contralateral
        antagonist   RLR   LSR

These changes are a result of Hering's and Sherrington's laws, and take place over a period of time. Overaction of the contralateral synergist is there from the start (providing the patient is fixing with the paretic eye), but the other stages take a variable amount of time to appear. Full sequelae indicates a long-standing condition.

Possible diagnoses to consider include:

- non-paralytic strabismus (perform cover tests – see p. 33)
- don't forget about A- and V-patterns, oblique muscle over- and underactions
- 3rd cranial nerve palsy (look for ptosis and check for pupil involvement – see p. 252)
- 4th cranial nerve palsy (use the Bielschowsky head tilt test – see p. 256)
- 6th cranial nerve palsy (see p. 258)
- don't forget about combined palsies or bilateral involvement (NB: With a complete 3rd cranial nerve palsy, the eye will not intort on attempted depression if there is an ipsilateral 4th cranial nerve palsy)
- restrictive eye movement disorders
- supranuclear eye movement disorders (see below).

NB: If the eye movements do not appear to fit an obvious neurological disorder or type of non-paralytic strabismus, consider dysthyroid eye disease, other types of orbital disease or myasthenia gravis.

7. To aid the diagnosis of supranuclear disorders, the testing of pursuits, saccades, convergence, doll's head eye movements, optokinetic nystagmus and caloric re-

sponses are useful. Don't forget to consider the diagnosis of internuclear ophthalmoplegia.

a) *Smooth pursuit eye movements.* The examiner should hold a visible target at about 1 m from the patient and ask the patient to follow it as it is moved slowly both horizontally and vertically. Any inability should be noted. In addition the velocity of movement should be observed. Abnormal pursuit velocity is compensated by occasional corrective saccades.

b) *Saccadic eye movements.* The examiner should hold two differing targets (A and B) in front of the patient, about 45° apart. Upon asking the patient to observe A followed by B and vice versa, the examiner observes the eyes moving rapidly from one stationary target to the other. Assessment of saccades is particularly useful in detecting internuclear ophthalmoplegia.

c) *Convergence.* The examiner should hold a target in front of the patient and progressively bring it nearer, whilst observing for convergence of the two eyes.

d) *Doll's head eye movements.* When a patient is unable to make a horizontal gaze movement to command and a horizontal gaze palsy is suspected, the examiner should attempt to induce doll's head eye movements. By holding the head of the patient and rotating it from side to side the examiner should observe whether the eyes deviate fully. If this occurs it indicates intact pontine reflexes, and the lesion is confirmed as supranuclear.

e) *Optokinetic nystagmus.* This normal physiological response is easily demonstrated using a rotating optokinetic drum (a white drum on which widely spaced, thinner black stripes have been painted). For diagnostic purposes it is useful in cases of suspected Parinaud's syndrome. Thus, if a patient has a vertical gaze palsy the candidate should determine whether there is associated convergence retraction nystagmus, which is best demonstrated using a downward rotating optokinetic drum. In addition, the candidate should look

for the light-near dissociation of Parinaud's syndrome.

f) *Caloric responses.* The candidate will not be asked to perform these in an examination setting, but may be asked about them. Caloric testing is dependent on endolymph convection currents, movement towards the ampulla resulting in stimulation. Thus, in order to exert maximum effects the horizontal semicircular canals are best positioned vertically (i.e. with the head inclined backwards by 60°), that is with the ampullae positioned superiorly. With warm water calorics the endolymph rises towards the ampulla and is stimulatory. The normal responses are such that warm water in the right ear produces a right-beating nystagmus whereas cold water would produce a left-beating nystagmus.

COWS: Cold – Opposite; Warm – Same

Caloric testing is useful in comatose patients to determine whether nuclear and internuclear brainstem pathways are functioning. Fronto-mesencephalic pathways do not function during coma, so warm water placed in a right ear produces the slow tonic vestibular movement to the left but no compensatory fast jerk movement to the right. The eyes remain deviated to the left for at least 30 seconds before returning to the primary position.

The candidate should constantly actively look for additional physical signs such as:

- ptosis (3rd cranial nerve palsy)
- pupil dilation (3rd cranial nerve palsy)
- variable pupil size (aberrant 3rd cranial nerve regeneration syndrome)
- light-near dissociation (Parinaud's syndrome)
- variable eyelid position (aberrant 3rd cranial nerve regeneration syndrome, Duane's syndrome)
- eyelid retraction – Collier's sign (Parinaud's syndrome) or Dalrymple's sign (dysthyroid)
- convergence retraction nystagmus (Parinaud's syndrome)
- head thrusting (congenital ocular motor apraxia)

- proptosis (orbital disease)
- features similar to those of Parkinson's disease, such as nuchal rigidity and seborrhoea (Steele–Richardson–Olszewski syndrome)
- neurological deficit (demyelination, cerebrovascular accident, trauma, tumour).

Checklist for the assessment of eye movements

History

1. Congenital/acquired
2. Cause (obstetric, traumatic, medical, surgical)
3. Associated symptoms (diplopia, fatigue, dysphagia, ophthalmoplegia)
4. Drug history.

Clinical examination

1. Primary position
2. Six cardinal positions of gaze (versions)
3. Convergence
4. Elevation and depression
5. Corneal reflections
6. Diplopia
7. Cover tests
8. Muscle sequelae
9. Smooth pursuit
10. Saccades
11. Doll's head eye movements
12. Optokinetic nystagmus
13. Caloric responses
14. Additional physical signs.

5. Assessment of the pupil

In order to understand pupil reactions and locate potential lesions, a knowledge of the neuro-anatomical basis of the light and near reflexes and the sympathetic/parasympathetic pathways is required. Furthermore, such an understanding aids selection of additional tests required to determine the aetiology of the pupil abnormality.

Neuro-anatomy

1. The iris sphincter is innervated by parasympathetic neurones originating from the Edinger–Westphal nucleus in the midbrain (part of the third cranial nerve [oculomotor] nucleus complex). The parasympathetic outflow travels with the third cranial nerve and its inferior division beyond the superior orbital fissure.
2. The iris dilator is innervated by sympathetic neurones in a three neurone pathway:
   - 1st order neurones: posterior hypothalamus via brainstem to cilio-spinal centre of Budge (T1 level of the spinal cord)
   - 2nd order (pre-ganglionic) neurones: spinal cord to para-vertebral sympathetic chain to superior cervical ganglion (base of skull)
   - 3rd order (post-ganglionic) neurones: enter the skull associated with the internal carotid artery, enter the cavernous sinus, join the ophthalmic nerve, enter the orbit via the superior orbital fissure, pass to the pupil dilator in the long ciliary nerves.

Reflexes

1. *The light reflex*
   - retinal ganglion cells – optic nerve afferent neurones – chiasm (~50% decussation) – optic tracts – superior colliculi – pretectal nuclei (synapse) – intercalated neurones – Edinger–Westphal nuclei (bilaterally) – parasympathetic outflow
   - light shone in one eye results in nerve impulses being transmitted to both iris sphincters equally.
2. *The near response*
   - consists of convergence, accommodation and miosis
   - may originate from area 19 of the cortex
   - outflow occurs with the third cranial nerve to the ciliary ganglion and finally the short posterior ciliary nerves
   - for every ciliary ganglion cell linked to the iris sphincter, 30 such cells are linked to the ciliary muscle
   - the response is bilateral and symmetrical
   - if a patient has normal pupillary reactions to light, there is no clinical indication to test the near response.
3. *The startle reflex*
   - pupil dilation which occurs following hearing an unexpected loud noise or with pain
   - occurs due to sympathetic outflow and inhibition of parasympathetic outflow.

It is quite common for a candidate to be told 'Examine this patient's pupils'. If possible this should be preceded by asking the patient a few questions.

History

After defining the main abnormality that has been perceived by the patient, such as a difference in pupil size, diplopia or poor vision, the candidate should proceed to ask specific questions to reduce the list of differential diagnoses.

Onset/duration of symptoms

This will help differentiate congenital disorders (e.g. congenital Horner's syndrome or third cranial nerve palsy) from acquired conditions. The onset of symptoms may help differentiate optic neuritis (rapid onset with symptoms at their worst about a week after onset) from compressive optic neuropathy (gradual onset with slowly progressive visual loss), for example.

Associated symptoms

Ask whether the patient has noticed any double vision (e.g. third cranial nerve palsy), a droopy eyelid (e.g. third cranial nerve palsy or Horner's syndrome), any decrease in vision (e.g. optic neuritis or ischaemic optic neuropathy but not papilloedema) or any pain with eye movements (e.g. optic neuritis).

Ask if there has been an associated headache (e.g. third cranial nerve palsy, herpes zoster ophthalmicus or temporal arteritis).

Causative factors

Ask about:

- use of topical eye medications (e.g. miotics or mydriatics)
- possible inadvertent topical administration of nose drops containing adrenaline or phenylephrine
- use of systemic drugs that can alter pupil size (constriction – opiates; dilation – anticholinergics, antidepressants, amphetamines)
- previous surgery, drugs or trauma which might have resulted in permanent change in pupil size or iris colour
- a family history
- a past medical history of diabetes mellitus or hypertension (risk factors for ischaemic optic neuropathy)
- dystrophia myotonica (a cause of light/near dissociation)
- NB: Don't forget the possibility of syphilis and Argyll–Robertson pupil.

Clinical examination

Observation

The candidate should ask the patient to fixate a distant point (to eliminate accommoda-

tion) and then look at both pupils noting the following:

1. Pupil size – normal pupil size, in typical indoor lighting conditions, is about 4–5 mm in diameter in young adults. Pupil size decreases slightly with age. The candidate should note if either or both pupils are abnormally large or small.
2. Anisocoria (asymmetry of pupil size) – it is important to decide which of the pupils is abnormal (see below). However, remember that both pupils may be abnormal with asymmetry. Furthermore, remember that simple/physiological anisocoria is a normal finding in 20% of the population.
3. Abnormal pupil shape, position (corectopia) and/or polycoria (multiple pupils) – causes include trauma, surgery, posterior synechiae, colobomata, aniridia, tumours, ICE syndrome, sphincter infarction and causes of iris atrophy such as Rieger's syndrome. If such a pupil abnormality is suspected a slit-lamp examination is required to differentiate the causes.
4. Ptosis – may accompany a third cranial nerve palsy or Horner's syndrome.
5. Other features of Horner's syndrome (see p. 76).
6. Features of Parinaud's syndrome – includes bilateral mid-dilated pupils (see p. 93).

Light reflexes

The candidate should use a torch with a collimated light source to test the pupil responses to light:

1. Direct/consensual light reflexes – the patient should be asked to maintain fixation on a distant object. The light should be shone into the eye from below and not directly in front, since this may result in loss of distant fixation with a resultant accommodation/near response leading to confusion. The direct response is noted and the fellow eye observed for the consensual response. The light is then shifted to the fellow eye and the observations repeated. If anisocoria is present the candidate should determine whether the anisocoria is greater in the dark, in the light or neither:

- if the anisocoria is greatest in the dark the smaller pupil is abnormal
- if the anisocoria is greatest in the light the larger pupil is abnormal
- if there is no difference in the degree of anisocoria between light and dark the anisocoria is either physiological or due to bilaterally fixed pupils (e.g. posterior synechiae formation secondary to uveitis).

The rapidity of response, magnitude of constriction and ability to maintain constriction should be noted. Remember that a degree of movement or 'pupil bounce' is normal, particularly in the young (hippus). An Adie's pupil has both slow constriction and slow dilation.

2. Relative afferent pupillary defect (RAPD, Marcus Gunn phenomenon) – the patient should be asked to fix on a distant object and a bright light, shone from below, should be moved alternately from one eye to the other, dwelling on the first eye for 3–5 seconds before swiftly moving on to the fellow eye. The test can be repeated until the result is certain (the swinging light test). The procedure tests for a difference in the afferent limb of the light reflex (in practical terms only to the optic chiasm) between the two eyes. Illumination of the (more) normal eye will cause both pupils to constrict. When the light is moved to the (more) abnormal eye, both pupils will dilate. Returning the light to the (more) normal eye again results in constriction of both pupils.

   The RAPD can be graded:
   - 3–4 +: immediate dilation occurs as the light is swung from the less affected or normal side to the more affected side
   - 1–2 +: no initial dilation occurs, but dilation does occur after a few seconds
   - subtle/trace: there is initial constriction, which occurs because the pupil dilates slightly while the light source is between the two eyes. However, this is followed by escape to a size that is larger than the initial size (i.e. the size when the light was shone in the less affected or normal eye).

An RAPD almost always implies pathology from the retina posteriorly (optic nerve, optic tract, brain) unless there is gross media (cornea, lens, vitreous) opacity, which would be visible clinically.

NB_1: Detection of an RAPD requires only one mobile pupil

NB_2: The candidate must be able to explain the principle behind the detection and aetiology of an RAPD since it is commonly asked.

The near response

If the light reflex is considered to be abnormal or sluggish, the candidate should examine the patient for a near response. The patient should be asked to fix on a distant target and the pupil sizes noted. The patient should then be asked to fix on a near target (15–20 cm from the eyes). The near target should not be a light, which would stimulate a light reflex! A normal response is constriction (with convergence).

If the near reaction is present but the light reaction is either absent or sluggish, then the causes of light/near dissociation should be considered:

- Argyll–Robertson pupil
- Parinaud's syndrome
- Holmes–Adie syndrome or Adie's pupil
- diabetes mellitus
- dystrophia myotonica
- aberrant third cranial nerve regeneration.

Ocular movements (see p. 14)

Eye movements should be examined if suspecting Parinaud's syndrome (impaired upgaze and convergence–retraction nystagmus), a third cranial nerve palsy or aberrant third cranial nerve regeneration.

Slit-lamp examination and fundoscopy

- if there is a fixed or irregular pupil, examination may reveal posterior synechiae, evidence of trauma, a coloboma, aniridia or iris atrophy as the cause of the abnormal pupil
- sectoral vermiform movements of the iris may be identified if an Adie's pupil is suspected. As the slit-beam is passed across the pupil, the characteristic sluggish movements occur secondary to segmental

palsy of the iris sphincter – this will be missed unless specifically looked for
- if Argyll–Robertson pupil is suspected there may be sectoral iris atrophy, evidence of syphilis or diabetes mellitus
- there may be evidence of diabetes mellitus, hypertension or dystrophia myotonica
- in the presence of an RAPD there may be unilateral/asymmetric optic atrophy, optic disc swelling or extensive retinal disease.

Extraocular examination

- in the presence of a Horner's syndrome a general medical examination may suggest a possible site or aetiology of the lesion
- a neurological examination should be performed if a third cranial nerve palsy is identified
- if an Adie's pupil is diagnosed the candidate should attempt to identify whether there is associated hyporeflexia of the tendon reflexes (Holmes–Adie syndrome).

Specific investigations

Pharmacological pupil tests

The candidate will not be asked to perform these tests, but may well be asked about them.

Pilocarpine (or methacholine)
- if the abnormal pupil is the larger (i.e. anisocoria is greater in the light) and slit-lamp examination has excluded traumatic iris damage, the 0.125% pilocarpine (or 2.5% methacholine) test should be considered. The pupil sizes are measured and a drop of the weak pilocarpine is instilled into both eyes. After 20–30 minutes under the same lighting conditions the pupil sizes are measured again. Marked constriction of the abnormal pupil is suggestive of the denervation hypersensitivity characteristic of Adie's pupil
- if no constriction occurs with the 0.125% pilocarpine, then 1% pilocarpine should be instilled into both eyes. Constriction of the larger pupil implies a third cranial nerve palsy, whereas an absence of response implies a sphincter tear or a pharmacological cause for pupil dilation.

Cocaine
- if the abnormal pupil is the smaller (i.e. anisocoria is greater in the dark) and slit-lamp examination has excluded the presence of posterior synechiae, then the cocaine test should be considered. 5–10% cocaine is instilled into each eye after pupil size has been recorded. Re-measurement is made under the same lighting conditions 30 minutes later. Cocaine blocks uptake of noradrenaline at nerve terminals causing dilation of normal pupils but no (or only slow) dilation of a miosed pupil associated with Horner's syndrome. The specific site of the lesion cannot be determined with the cocaine test.

Hydroxyamphetamine (or adrenaline/ phenylephrine)
- if the cocaine test is positive the 1% hydroxyamphetamine or 0.1% adrenaline (or 1% phenylephrine) test can be used to determine whether the lesion causing the Horner's syndrome is a preganglionic or postganglionic (third order neurone) lesion. The test should not be performed until 24 hours after performing the cocaine test
- 1% hydroxyamphetamine causes dilation of normal pupils and those with a preganglionic type of Horner's syndrome, but has no effect on the postganglionic type (i.e. a third order neurone lesion)
- conversely, 0.1% adrenaline (or 1% phenylephrine) has little, if any effect on pupil size unless there is a postganglionic type of Horner's syndrome, when it causes pupil dilation due to denervation hypersensitivity.

General medical investigations

Preganglionic Horner's syndrome
- Chest X-ray
- CT scan of chest with specific apex views
- CT/MRI scan of head and neck
- angiography, if carotid dissection is suspected.

Argyll–Robertson pupil
- FTA and VDRL
- lumbar puncture
- blood glucose.

Third cranial nerve palsy (see p. 252)

Parinaud's syndrome
- CT/MRI scan of head.

Checklist for the assessment of the pupil

Reflexes

1. The light reflex
2. The near response
3. The startle reflex.

History

1. Onset/duration of symptom(s)
2. Associated symptoms
3. Causative factors.

Clinical examination

1. *Observation*
   - pupil size
   - anisocoria
   - pupil shape, position and number
   - ptosis
   - Horner's syndrome
   - Parinaud's syndrome
2. *Light reflexes*
   - direct and consensual light reflexes
   - relative afferent pupillary defect
3. *The near response*
4. *Ocular movements*
5. *Slit-lamp examination and fundoscopy*
6. *Extraocular examination.*

Specific investigations

1. *Pharmacological pupil tests*
   - 0.125% pilocarpine (or 2.5% methacholine)
   - 5–10% cocaine
   - 1% hydroxyamphetamine (or 0.1% adrenaline or 1% phenylephrine)
2. *General medical investigations*
   - chest X-ray
   - CT/MRI scans
   - angiography
   - FTA/VDRL
   - lumbar puncture
   - blood glucose
   - blood pressure
   - haematological parameters, including ESR
   - biochemical parameters.

6.   Assessment of ptosis

History

Whenever possible obtaining a relevant history can be as useful diagnostically as performing a clinical examination or organizing specific investigations. Taking a history may confirm the complaint of ptosis, which in mild cases can be particularly useful. Specific points which should be addressed include:

Duration/age at onset

- includes determination as to whether the ptosis is congenital or acquired
- change in appearance (old photographs may be useful).

Family history

Of relevance in congenital cases since certain types of congenital ptosis, including that associated with blepharophimosis may run in families.

Causative factors

These may include:

- problems during pregnancy or at delivery (e.g. use of forceps)
- trauma
- eyelid tumour/swelling (mechanical ptosis)
- associated medical conditions (myasthenia, myotonia, myopathy, muscular dystrophy – the 4 m's).

It is also important not to forget the causes of pseudoptosis (see below) which may be elicited in a history.

Associated symptoms

These may include:

- diplopia (3rd nerve palsy or aberrant regeneration, trauma and the medical causes)
- jaw-winking (Marcus Gunn jaw-winking ptosis, see p. 118)
- fatigue (myasthenia gravis, see p. 25)
- dysphagia (oculopharyngeal muscular dystrophy)
- ophthalmoplegia (Kearns–Sayre syndrome, see p. 233)

Variability

An acquired ptosis which truly varies in degree with time and which in particular increases after sustained upgaze is classically due to myasthenia gravis. This symptom is also a feature of ptosis secondary to weakness or disinsertion of the aponeurosis since Muller's muscle fatigues. Many patients with other types of ptosis also complain that it tends to be worse at the end of the day or when tired.

Drug history

The patient may report taking an anticholinesterase drug such as Neostigmine if previously diagnosed as suffering from myasthenia gravis.

Clinical examination

General examination

The appearance of a patient with an apparent ptosis may help make the diagnosis:

- unilateral or bilateral (see below)
- age of patient (congenital causes are more likely in an infant, aponeurotic weakness in the elderly)

- signs of medical causes (e.g. the character-istic facies of dystrophia myotonica, see p. 117)
- signs of local trauma (eyelid or conjunctival scarring)
- frontalis overaction (which can mask the ptosis).

Ptosis or pseudoptosis?

An attempt should be made to exclude pseu-doptosis:

- ipsilateral:
  - small globe: microphthalmos
                  phthisis bulbi
                  cornea plana
  - hypertropia: (examine corneal light reflex)
- contralateral:
  - lid retraction
  - proptosis (see p. 28)
  - large globe hypotropia (examine corneal light reflex).

After this, to diagnose the presence of a true ptosis, the position of the lid level should be noted. The upper eyelid normally covers the superior limbus (corneo-scleral junction) by 2 mm. With a mild ptosis (of 2 mm) the upper eyelid margin thus lies 4 mm below the limbus. With a severe ptosis (of >4 mm) the upper eyelid margin thus lies >6 mm below the limbus.

Unilateral or bilateral?

Medical causes are bilateral, but the degree of ptosis may be either symmetrical or asym-metrical. Mild symmetrical ptosis can easily be missed on a casual examination.

Ptosis examination

The following need to be assessed:

Degree of ptosis
The normal adult cornea has an external ver-tical measurement of about 11 mm and the normal upper lid covers the upper 2 mm. The amount of ptosis can thus be measured by subtracting the interpalpebral distance from 9 mm (11–2 mm):
Amount of ptosis (mm) = 9 – Interpalpebral distance (mm).

Position and depth of the upper eyelid skin crease
These aspects are more readily appreciated in cases of unilateral ptosis.

- A crease that is higher than normal indi-cates an aponeurotic defect.
- The depth of the crease correlates to some extent with levator function (see below).

Levator function
Remember to inhibit the action of frontalis. This is achieved by applying pressure with the thumb on the brow above the ptotic eyelid. It is important since overaction of the frontalis muscle can mask a ptosis.
The amount of levator function is measured as the excursion made by the lid margin from full downgaze to full upgaze
A normal value is greater than 15 mm and a poor value is less than 4 mm.

The position of the eyelid during downgaze
This is useful in the diagnosis of levator muscle dystrophy (the commonest cause of a con-genital ptosis). Since the muscle is unable to relax (as well as contract) lid lag occurs on downgaze. In unilateral cases the affected lid thus remains higher on downgaze than the normal lid.

Fatigue and Cogan's twitch
These are both signs of myasthenia gravis.

- Fatigue is best demonstrated on asking the patient to sustain upgaze – the lid usually falls within 30 sec.
- Cogan's twitch is elicited by asking the patient to change gaze swiftly from down-gaze to the primary position (e.g. by follow-ing the examiners finger). If present the eyelid twitches. This may be associated with rapid eye movements (quivering) of 3–4° amplitude.

Aberrant eyelid movements
A variety of abnormal eyelid movements can occur with the Marcus Gunn jaw-winking syn-drome (with jaw movements) and in either Duane's syndrome or the aberrant third nerve regeneration syndrome (with eye movements).

Other eyelid signs

Patients with aponeurotic defects frequently have a deep upper lid sulcus and the eyelid skin is characteristically very thin. Patients with a ptosis due to blepharophimosis show palpebral phimosis, telecanthus, epicanthus inversus and often lower lid ectropion. Patients with a mechanical ptosis may show evidence of an eyelid mass or trauma. There may be signs of previous ptosis surgery.

Other ocular aspects

Eyelid closure and Bell's phenomenon

This is important in deciding subsequent ptosis management, since failure of eyelid closure or Bell's phenomenon (rotation of the globe upwards on lid closure) after corrective ptosis surgery may result in corneal exposure and its complications.

Eye movements (including saccades)

These may be abnormal or may alter the degree of ptosis. Abnormal eye movements occur with a third nerve palsy (or its aberrant regeneration), myasthenic ophthalmoplegia, ocular myopathy or oculopharyngeal muscular dystrophy. In one form of congenital ptosis there is an associated weakness of the superior rectus. Hypometric saccades are a feature of myasthenia gravis.

The degree of ptosis varies with eye movements in cases of aberrant third nerve regeneration.

Pupillary reactions

These are abnormal in patients with ptosis secondary to Horner's syndrome, third nerve palsy or aberrant third nerve regeneration.

Jaw-winking

This is a feature specific to the Marcus Gunn jaw-winking syndrome. The degree of a unilateral ptosis is altered by activation of the ipsilateral pterygoid musculature usually as a result of opening the mouth, chewing or sucking.

Corneal sensation and the presence of dry eye

Corneal anaesthesia and/or dry eye are relative contraindications to corrective ptosis surgery.

Fundus examination

This is required to identify the pigmentary retinopathy of Kearns–Sayre syndrome.

Specific investigations

'Tensilon' (Edrophonium) test for myasthenia gravis

Inhibition of the enzyme acetylcholinesterase prolongs the action of acetylcholine enhancing neuromuscular transmission in affected voluntary and involuntary muscle. Edrophonium is an anticholinesterase drug which has a swift, but brief, duration of action, making it useful in the diagnosis of myasthenia, but of no use in its treatment. If myasthenia is present a single intravenous dose usually improves ptosis, speech and general muscle strength within 1 min, the effect lasting 2–3 min. The extraocular muscles tend to be relatively resistant.

NOTE: Excessive dosage or administration of a normal dose to a susceptible individual can impair neuromuscular transmission (depolarizing block) and precipitate a 'cholinergic crisis' with the risk of bradycardia/heart block or severe bronchial obstruction. For this reason:

- a patient should receive a small test dose (2 mg) before the full dose (8 mg)
- atropine cover should be given or be readily available (0.4 mg)
- full resuscitation equipment and staff should be available
- children should receive a test dose of 20 µg/kg and full dose of 80 µg/kg.

Summary of method (for an adult):

1. Sit patient comfortably
2. Check that atropine and resuscitation equipment are available
3. Administer a small test dose (2 mg) of intravenous edrophonium
4. Wait 30 sec
5. If no adverse reaction occurs administer a further 8 mg of edrophonium
6. Observe the patient for 2–3 min. Look for any improvement and ask the patient if they notice any change (may be formally assessed with a Hess chart).

Other tests for myasthenia gravis

- single fibre nerve stimulation and electromyography
- anti-acetylcholine-receptor antibody titres
- CT scan of thymus.

For 3rd nerve palsy

(see p. 252)

For Horner's syndrome

(see p. 76)

Checklist for assessment of ptosis

History

1. Duration/age at onset
2. Family history
3. Causative factors
4. Associated symptoms
5. Variability
6. Drug history.

Clinical examination

1. General examination
2. Ptosis or pseudoptosis?
3. Unilateral or bilateral?
4. Ptosis examination
   a) Degree of ptosis
   b) Position and depth of the upper eyelid skin crease
   c) Levator function
   d) The position of the eyelid during downgaze
   e) Fatigue and Cogan's twitch
   f) Aberrant eyelid movements
   g) Other eyelid signs
5. Other ocular aspects
   a) Eyelid closure and Bell's phenomenon
   b) Eye movements (including saccades)
   c) Pupillary reactions
   d) Jaw-winking
   e) Corneal sensation and the presence of dry eye
   f) Fundus examination.

Specific investigations

1. 'Tensilon' (Edrophonium) test for myasthenia gravis
2. Other tests for myasthenia gravis
3. For 3rd nerve palsy
4. For Horner's syndrome.

7. Assessment of the orbit and proptosis

History

Due to lack of direct visualization of the pathology in orbital disease a precise history, particularly of symptoms and signs, is extremely helpful in the making of a differential diagnosis and in the determination of appropriate investigations.

Specific points which should be addressed include:

- speed of onset
- progression
- duration (old photographs may be useful)
- effect of head position/Valsalva manoeuvre
- associated symptoms (proptosis, diplopia, pain, loss of vision, symptoms of corneal exposure, altered lid position)
- past medical history and general state of health (sinus disease, malignancy, thyroid dysfunction, trauma)
- family history (e.g. neurofibromatosis).

Speed of onset/progression/duration

1. If proptosis develops within a few hours or even a few days it is suggestive of trauma, haemorrhage or infection.
2. Onset of proptosis over a few days or weeks is more suggestive of orbital myositis (pseudotumour) or certain types of malignancy (typically childhood rhabdomyosarcoma, neuroblastoma or leukaemia).
3. Slow onset of proptosis, over the period of about a year is characteristic of a pleomorphic adenoma of the lacrimal gland.
4. Intermittent/variable proptosis may occur with orbital varices, myositis, mucoceles or dermoid cysts.
5. Pulsatile proptosis may occur with a caroticocavernous fistula, neurofibromatosis, an arteriovenous malformation, a meningo-encephalocele or a frontal mucocele.
6. Dysthyroid eye disease can be associated with acute or chronic onset of proptosis.
7. Old photographs may help determine the duration of proptosis in chronic cases.

Effect of head position/Valsalva manoeuvre

Proptosis that varies with head position or the Valsalva manoeuvre is suggestive of orbital varices.

Pain

Orbital pain may be due to orbital pathology or referred pain. Lesions that cause orbital pain include:

- orbital infections
- posterior scleritis
- orbital haemorrhage
- orbital myositis (pseudotumour)
- some orbital tumours (typically malignant lacrimal gland tumours or metastatic tumours).

Common causes of referred pain include:

- tension or migrainous headache
- optic/retrobulbar neuritis
- sinusitis
- dental disease
- vascular disease (intracranial aneurysm, carotid artery disease or occipital thrombosis)
- trigeminal neuralgia
- cervical spondylosis.

Change in lid position

Patients with dysthyroid eye disease may have lid lag and/or retraction.

Change in vision

Visual impairment may occur due to optic nerve damage (compression or infiltration), choroidal folds or corneal exposure and by itself is a rather non-specific symptom. Some patients with an optic nerve meningioma complain of transient loss of vision on adduction of the eye. Hot baths or exercise may cause reduced vision in patients with optic neuritis.

Systemic symptoms

There may be symptoms suggestive of hyper- or hypo-thyroidism, trauma (remember CSF rhinorrhoea), sinus disease, migraine, disseminated malignancy or vasculitis.

Pseudoproptosis

The candidate should remember that if the patient has high myopia or buphthalmos the 'proptosis' may actually be pseudoproptosis. Other causes of pseudoproptosis include:

- asymmetry of orbital or other eye size
- abnormalities of palpebral apertures (e.g. ptosis, lid retraction, scarring, facial nerve palsy).

Clinical examination

General aspects

Initial examination of a patient with orbital disease should include corrected visual acuity (and preferably a refraction), colour vision, pupil reactions, visual fields, fundoscopy and eye movements. Ideally, the alternate cover test should be used when examining eye movements which may be affected by either a paralytic and/ or restrictive process (e.g. impaired upgaze in a blow-out fracture). The two processes may be differentiated by a forced duction test.

Specific aspects

It is important to view the entire face to provide an idea of symmetry. Facial asymmetry associated with orbital disease may result from trauma, neurofibromatosis, fibrous dysplasia, Sturge–Weber syndrome or Parry–Romberg syndrome. Determination of whether any proptosis is unilateral or bilateral or whether there is pseudoproptosis is important early in the ex-

amination. Specific features of the orbital examination include assessment of:

1. Globe displacement
2. Orbital margin and anterior orbit
3. Adnexae
4. Anterior segment (including intraocular pressure)
5. Posterior segment
6. Ocular movements
7. General systemic signs.

Globe proptosis and displacement

Assessment of proptosis should be combined with an assessment of additional horizontal and/or vertical displacement of the globe since masses outside the muscle cone can produce displacement in addition to proptosis, as opposed to masses within the muscle cone which produce axial proptosis.

Proptosis (the anterior movement of the globe within the bony orbit) can be assessed qualitatively and quantitatively. By standing behind and above a seated patient an examiner can raise their eyelids and observe the protrusion of each globe relative to each other. This can be of use in gross and asymmetrical disease but exophthalmometry is of more value. A crude measurement can be obtained by holding a transparent ruler in the coronal plane against the lateral orbital rim and measuring the distance to the corneal apex.

A more accurate measurement can be obtained using the Hertel exophthalmometer to determine the protrusion of each eye at a specified intercanthal distance. The candidate should ask the examiner for an exophthalmometer and should be familiar with its use. The instrument is held horizontally in front of the patient's eyes with the 45 mirrors uppermost. The base width is set so that the feet of the exophthalmometer lie on each of the lateral orbital rims at each lateral canthus. A note of the intercanthal distance should be made such that all subsequent measurements are made in a standard manner. Using the opposite eye to the eye of the patient that is being assessed, the candidate should align the red parallax lines, or the two appropriate vertical markers (depending on the exact model) in the mirror while the patient fixates on the candidates eye. A reading is made where the reflection of the corneal apex crosses the scale. Both sides are assessed and compared. The exophthalmometer is calibrated such that the measurement represents the distance from the lateral orbital rim to the apex of the cornea. The normal distance is <20 mm. In cases of unilateral proptosis a difference between the two eyes of more than 2 mm is considered significant. When the measurement is within normal limits, the candidate should not forget the causes of pseudo-proptosis:

- ipsilateral high axial myopia
- ipsilateral buphthalmos
- contralateral enophthalmos
- asymmetry of orbital size
- asymmetry of palpebral fissure size.

Displacement is assessed using a ruler placed in front of the patient's eyes (in the primary position) level with the canthi. One eye is covered to abolish the effect of any squint. Horizontal displacement is measured using the presumed midline of the face (bridge of nose) as a reference point. Measurement is made to either the nasal limbus or mid-pupillary point of each eye in turn. Vertical displacement is measured using a second ruler held at right angles to the first so as to measure from the ruler to the inferior limbus of each eye in turn.

Proptosis without displacement is referred to as 'axial' and is due to intraconal pathology, most commonly dysthyroid eye disease.

Proptosis with displacement is referred to as 'non-axial' and is due to extraconal pathology, most commonly tumours.

Dynamic properties of the proptosis/displacement should be assessed (i.e. whether there is an increase with the Valsalva manoeuvre or with each pulse).

Orbital margin and anterior orbit

A mass or erosion of the bony margin of the orbit may be felt with careful palpation. Masses should not be confused with normal anatomical landmarks. The orbital margin and anterior orbital contents should be gently palpated systematically in an anticlockwise or clockwise direction starting with the patient holding the eyes in the primary position fixing a distant target. The palpation can be performed by inserting the tip of a finger (e.g. the little finger) between the globe and the orbital margin. Normal anatomical landmarks include the anterior lacrimal crest (inferonasally), the zygomatic-maxillary suture (centrally on the inferior orbital margin), the lateral

orbital tubercle and lateral canthal tendon (laterally), the fronto-zygomatic suture (superio-laterally), the supraorbital notch (superiorly at the junction of the lateral and central thirds of the superior orbital margin) and the trochlea (superio-medially).

If a mass is palpated it should be further described on the basis of its:

- position
- shape and size
- surface
- edge (+ ability to get behind the mass or not)
- consistence/composition (hard, rubbery, spongy or soft)
- transillumination (fluid or air filled)
- pulsatility
- compressibility
- bruits
- tenderness
- state of local tissues (including colour, temperature and sensation)
- state of regional lymph nodes (pre-auricular, submandibular and cervical nodes).

It can help by asking the patient to look down when palpating a superior mass (although if the patient looks down too well it can tighten the orbital septum and make palpation more difficult) and up when palpating an inferior mass. A mass arising in the superio-nasal quadrant may be a:

- sinus mucocele
- dermoid cyst
- metastatic tumour
- encephalocele.

A mass arising in the supero-lateral quadrant is most likely to arise from the lacrimal gland. Dermoids often arise close to the fronto-zygomatic suture. A pulsatile mass is suggestive of an arterio-venous malformation or a defect in the bony orbital wall related to trauma, neurofibromatosis or an encephalocele. The candidate should be careful not to confuse a transmitted pulse with a true pulsatile mass.

The globes may be retropulsed (beware of possible reflex bradycardia), by placing fingers over both globes and gently pushing them in a posterior direction. A solid mass will resist retropulsation (e.g. dysthyroid eye disease, solid tumours or inflammatory masses).

Fullness in the temporal fossa may indicate a sphenoidal wing meningioma.

Sensation to light touch should be tested in the dermatomes supplied by the first and second divisions of the trigeminal nerve.

Adnexae

The candidate should note any lid or periocular changes, such as lid retraction, periorbital oedema, lid masses (and from which part of the orbital margin they appear to arise from), lid contour (classically S-shaped in neurofibromatosis) and colour changes (cafe-au-lait spots).

Anterior segment

Slit-lamp examination of the anterior segment may reveal signs of corneal exposure (interpalpebral punctate epithelial erosions or corneal ulcers), superior limbic keratoconjunctivitis (dysthyroid eye disease), a dilated single (sentinel) conjunctival vessel over a rectus muscle (dysthyroid eye disease) or epibulbar dark-red corkscrew vessels (arterio-venous malformation).

The candidate should lift the upper eyelid (and evert it if the examiner wishes) and retract the lower eyelid, looking particularly in the fornices for salmon-coloured masses (suggestive of lymphoma) or haemangiomas.

Intraocular pressure

If the candidate measures intraocular pressure (IOP), this should be measured with the eyes in the primary position and also on upgaze. Characteristically, there is a rise in IOP with upgaze in eyes with dysthyroid eye disease, but this can occur with other conditions associated with limitation of movement. A rise in IOP will occur when the eye is moved in a direction opposite to any limitation.

Posterior segment

At fundoscopy the candidate should carefully examine the optic discs for swelling, pallor and asymmetry. Choroidal folds, which are easily missed, are suggestive of orbital pathology. A myopic disc and/or staphyloma may suggest a large globe in a high myope giving rise to pseudoproptosis. Opticociliary shunt vessels at the optic disc are strongly suggestive of an optic sheath meningioma.

Ocular movements (see also p. 14)

Abnormal eye movements associated with orbital disease may occur with:

- trauma (e.g. blow-out fractures)
- restrictive myopathy (e.g. dysthyroid eye disease)
- neurological pathology.

If fibrosis results in contracture of an extra-ocular muscle the forced duction test will be positive.

General systemic

In many cases a full general medical examination is indicated. Some specific signs that should be looked for include:

- periorbital scars
- goitre
- thyroidectomy surgical scars
- nasal pathology
- signs of primary or secondary tumour.

Specific investigations

Imaging

Most of the specific investigations relating to orbital pathology are forms of imaging, including:

- Ultrasound
- X-ray
- CT scan (with or without contrast medium)
- MRI scan
- Venography/Angiography (rarely used)

Imaging may show:

- orbital enlargement (trauma, tumour)
- orbital wall erosion (benign pathology)
- orbital wall destruction (malignant pathology)
- calcification (phlebolith, meningioma, lacrimal gland carcinoma, retinoblastoma)
- hyperostosis (meningioma, Paget's disease, malignant osteoblastic secondary, fibrous dysplasia)
- enlargement of the optic foramen (optic nerve glioma, meningioma)

- enlargement of the superior orbital fissure (aneurysm or tumour with posterior extension)
- high ultrasound reflectivity (dysthyroid eye disease, blood – haemangioma or haemorrhage but not varices)
- low reflectivity (varices, mucocele, dermoid cyst, lymphoma).

Specific blood tests include:

- Full Blood Count (FBC)
- Erythrocyte Sedimentation Rate (ESR)
- Thyroid Function Tests (TFTs)
- Specific tumour markers.

Checklist for assessment of the orbit and proptosis

History

1. Speed of onset/progression/duration
2. Effect of head position/Valsalva manoeuvre
3. Pain
4. Change of vision
5. Systemic symptoms
6. Pseudoproptosis.

Clinical examination

1. *General aspects*
   - corrected visual acuity
   - refraction
   - colour vision
   - pupil reactions
   - visual fields
   - fundoscopy
   - eye movements (with alternate cover test)
   - forced duction test
2. *Specific aspects*
   - globe displacement
   - orbital margin and anterior orbit
   - adnexae
   - anterior segment (including intraocular pressure)
   - posterior segment
   - general systemic signs.

3. *Description of an orbital mass*
   - position
   - shape and size
   - surface
   - edge (+ ability to get behind the mass or not)
   - consistence/composition (hard, rubbery, spongy or soft)
   - transillumination
   - pulsatility
   - compressibility
   - bruits
   - tenderness
   - state of local tissues (including colour, temperature and sensation)
   - state of regional lymph nodes (preauricular, submandibular and cervical nodes).

Specific investigations

1. *Imaging*
   - ultrasound
   - X-ray
   - CT scan
   - MRI scan
   - Venography/Angiography
2. *Blood tests*
   - FBC
   - ESR
   - TFTs
   - Specific tumour markers.

8. Assessment of strabismus and cover tests

(written with advice provided by Bronia Unwin MPhil DBO(T), Department of Orthoptics, Moorfields Eye Hospital, London, UK)

History

Since strabismus commonly affects children, the history may only be available from the parents. A good history, however, can make the examination much easier to perform and the diagnosis easier to make. In addition to a history related to the eyes, the presence of other neurological symptoms should be determined. In relation to the strabismus, a number of specific questions need to be asked:

1. Has the patient or parent noticed an eye squinting or turning? If so, which one, or do both turn? In which direction has the eye turned (in/out/up/down)? Is there an inability to move the eye in a particular direction?
2. At what age was the squint first noticed?
3. Was the onset gradual or sudden? (NB_1: Acute onset deviations, especially in older children, may be associated with neurological abnormalities. Remember that a sudden onset esotropia at any age may be due to a sixth cranial nerve palsy. NB_2: In adults where a paralytic strabismus is suspected, the speed of onset, progression and time course of any symptom resolution should be asked. If there is a history of fatiguability, the candidate should think of myasthenia gravis).
4. Is the deviation constant or intermittent? Are the eyes ever straight? (NB: A variable constant deviation is easily confused with an intermittent deviation).
5. Is it always the same eye that deviates? Old photographs may be useful to assess this. If the same eye always deviates, then amblyopia should be suspected.
6. Does the patient have a compensatory head turn or tilt? Again, old photographs may help both in identifying this and in ascertaining its duration and/or progression.
7. Has the patient ever noticed double vision (diplopia)? If so, is the diplopia constant or intermittent, and is it worse when looking in a particular direction? It is also a good idea to ask whether the double vision disappears when one eye is covered. (NB: Increased clumsiness may be a sign of diplopia in the very young patient).
8. Has poor vision been noticed or documented in either eye?
9. Is there nystagmus ('dancing' or 'wobbling' of the eyes)?
10. Has the patient complained of photophobia, or does the patient close one eye in brightly lit environments? (NB: These symptoms are suggestive of intermittent exotropia).
11. Does the patient ever complain of eye ache/pain or headaches?
12. Has any previous treatment been instigated for the present condition, such as patching, orthoptic exercises, refractive correction, prisms or surgery? What were the results?
13. Is there a family history of refractive error or squint? (NB: Certain types of early onset strabismus tend to run in families).

A past medical history should also be ascertained, with specific questions tailored to the age and presenting symptoms of the patient.

With children, or when an early onset form of strabismus is suspected, the candidate should ask about any possible problems encountered during pregnancy or at birth, about prematurity, developmental problems and delays, difficulties at school and any systemic illnesses. Of particular importance is a history of hydrocephalus, cerebral palsy, Down's syndrome, cranial dysostosis or albinism.

With adults, particularly when a paralytic strabismus is suspected, the candidate should ask about a history of head trauma, diabetes, hypertension, shingles, demyelinating disease, thyroid disease, vasculitis, neurological disease (including myasthenia gravis) and any other systemic illnesses. In addition, a drug history should be taken since certain drugs such as penicillamine can induce myasthenic motility problems, although this is rare.

Clinical examination

Since many patients with strabismus are young children, the clinical examination can be fraught with all sorts of added difficulties and hazards! If confronted with a difficult child, the candidate should stay calm. Any reasonable(!) examiner will take this into account, and marks can be gained by an organized approach. Remember that involving the parents in the examination can be reassuring for a frightened child. If the patient is capable of understanding, the candidate should introduce himself as usual and explain what is to be done at each stage of the examination.

The clinical examination involves:

- inspection
- cover test
- examination of eye movements (see also p. 14)
- visual field analysis
- general ocular examination including visual acuity, colour vision, pupil reactions, slit-lamp examination, and fundoscopy.

Inspection

The candidate should note the following details.

Eyelid position
- a ptosis may indicate a third cranial nerve palsy, a congenital superior rectus palsy, or acquired myogenic disorders such as myasthenia gravis or ocular myopathy
- a pseudoptosis may arise from a vertical deviation of the globe
- upper lid retraction may be a feature of dysthyroid eye disease.

Epicanthic folds
- prominent epicanthic folds may give rise to the appearance of an eso-deviation when in fact there is only a pseudostrabismus
- the presence of mongoloid slants may indicate Down's syndrome
- both mongoloid and anti-mongoloid slants may be associated with A- or V-patterns as well as horizontal strabismus.

Facial asymmetry
- may create the impression of a vertical deviation when in fact there is only a pseudostrabismus
- may be associated with a long-standing congenital superior oblique palsy.

Globe position
- the candidate should note the positions of the corneal light reflections, which can help determine whether there is a true deviation
- any obvious fixation preference should be noted and an estimate as to whether this is constant should be made (this is more formally assessed as described below)
- there may be proptosis and/or globe displacement (e.g. with orbital tumours or trauma), which may occur with or without strabismus.

Nystagmus
- latent nystagmus may be a feature of an early onset esotropia and, less commonly, with an early onset exotropia
- the patient may have pendular nystagmus, compensatory head posture and head nodding (spasmus nutans)
- nystagmus blockage may occur in patients with congenital manifest nystagmus. The nystagmus is minimized by the development of a constant, non-accommodative esotropia (nystagmus blocking syndrome).

Compensatory head postures
Abnormal head postures are described when the patient is looking straight ahead. They are compensatory, and are a means by which the head and the eyes are held in a position other than the primary position in order to maintain a field of single vision lying straight ahead. There are three components of an abnormal head posture:

1. face turn
2. chin elevation or depression
3. head tilt.

The head posture is adopted by the patient so that the eyes are positioned, with minimal effort, away from the most troublesome position. The head posture may allow the patient to achieve binocular single vision, or may occasionally move the eyes into a position where deviation is maximum so that the two images seen by a patient with diplopia are separated, which may be more tolerable.

Compensatory head postures are most common in patients with paralytic strabismus, and are such that the face turns in the direction of the main action of the paralysed muscle (e.g. to the left with a left lateral rectus palsy, or to the right with a left superior oblique palsy). Chin elevation is most common with an elevator paresis, and chin depression with a depressor paresis. A head tilt usually occurs to the side of a hypotropic eye in order to reduce the vertical deviation, and probably to reduce the effects of torsion. A tilt towards the side of a hypotropic eye reduces torsion in oblique muscle pareses.

1. *Horizontal deviations*
   - A face turn may develop in a patient who is unable to look to one side (i.e. limited duction to one side due to nerve palsy, Duane's syndrome or muscle contracture). This may be in order to achieve binocular single vision (BSV), or because looking to one side maximizes visual acuity or avoids diplopia (e.g. with congenital nystagmus, early onset esotropia with nystagmus, or when the nose is used as an occluder to the adducting eye).
   - Simple face turns occur with horizontal palsies. A face turn to the left may be a feature of a mild left lateral rectus palsy, enabling the maintenance of BSV. However, a face turn to the left may also be a feature of a severe right lateral rectus palsy, when BSV cannot be achieved, but the diplopia can be separated to make it more tolerable (rare).

2. *Vertical deviations*
   In cases of strabismus that do not just involve the horizontal muscles, the adopted abnormal head posture is more complex. In the case of a vertical muscle palsy:
   - the chin elevation or depression compensates for the primary action of the defective muscle
   - the face turn avoids the position in which the primary action of the defective muscle exerts its maximum effect
   - the head tilt compensates for the secondary torsional action of the defective muscle and vertical effects of the palsy (NB: the torsional power of the oblique muscles is greater than of the vertical

recti). If the head is tilted to the right, the right eye becomes intorted and elevated, the left eye extorted and depressed
   - with a left superior rectus palsy, for example, there will be chin elevation, a face turn to the left and a head tilt to the left shoulder
   - with a symmetrical, bilateral fourth cranial nerve palsy there will be chin depression
   - with an asymmetrical, bilateral fourth cranial nerve palsy there will be chin depression and a head tilt (and slight turn) away from the side of the most affected eye
   - remember the Bielschowsky head tilt test (see p. 257)
   - a head tilt that disappears regardless of which eye is patched implies the presence of a cyclovertical strabismus.

The candidate should remember that apparent compensatory head postures may be due to:

- non-ocular torticollis
- deafness or disorders of balance
- disorders of the spine
- neurological disease.

Cover tests

- cover tests are simple tests, based on dissociation of the two eyes, that can both reveal and assess the degree of any ocular muscle imbalance
- performing a cover test is essential in order to classify a squint
- before performing a cover test, one should examine the corneal reflexes (using a pen-torch held at $\frac{1}{3}$ m) to detect any obvious deviation
- if a patient has spectacles, the tests should be performed both with and without them (preferably after a reliable recent refraction)
- if a patient has a compensatory head posture, the cover test should be performed with the head in both the abnormal and normal positions
- in some instances it is ideal to perform cover tests in all nine cardinal positions of gaze. However, this is usually considered too lengthy in an exam setting!

- beware of the exam case, where an older child has been taught to relax their accommodation to control a squint. Do not be afraid to ask them if they have been taught to do this, since they will often accommodate and squint for you.

The targets

- a cover test should always be carried out for both distant (6 m) and near ($\frac{1}{3}$ m) targets. In suspected distance exotropia (divergence excess), it should also be carried out beyond 6m. In addition an accommodative target and a light should be used because some squints will change when accommodation is exerted
- the smallest acuity symbol/letter on a Snellen chart (seen by the eye with the lowest VA) should be used for the distant target
- a small and detailed object should be used as a near target (be sure to have some interesting pictures and small toys to show children)
- light from a pen-torch should also be used as a target (the light does not induce accommodation but one has to be careful that the torch itself is not doing so) and this has the advantage of producing corneal reflections. Furthermore, a light source may be the only way the candidate will achieve fixation with an infant (NB the normal reflection is slightly nasal of the mid-pupillary position due to the slight temporal position of the fovea). Remember that some accommodative squints will appear 'straight' to a light and can be missed if only a light is used.

The occluder

- a commercially available occluder or piece of opaque card, large enough to completely occlude one eye at a time should be used. Since an occluder may frighten young children, a hand may be used, but make sure that they do not peep between your fingers.

The cover/uncover test

- performed first and is used:
  a) *To detect a manifest deviation (heterotropia)*
     - the patient fixates the required target and the occluder is placed over one of the eyes (if there is an obvious tropia, cover the fixing eye first). As this is done the fellow (non-occluded) eye is observed for movement. If the non-occluded eye moves to take up fixation then this eye has a manifest deviation. If the non-occluded eye remains still then this eye does not have a manifest deviation. The test is then repeated for the other eye. If on covering one eye, the uncovered eye moves out (temporal) to fix, the deviation is convergent (eso); if it moves inwards (nasal), the deviation is divergent (exo); if it moves down, the deviation is hyper and if it moves up the deviation is hypo.
     - the candidate should take care to pause between uncovering the first eye and covering the second eye. The occluder should cover an eye for at least 2–3 seconds before removal
     - with a unilateral squint, the squinting eye takes up fixation when the fellow eye is covered, but returns to the deviated position as the cover is removed
     - with an alternating squint, the squinting eye takes up fixation when the fellow eye is covered, but retains fixation when uncovered, the previously fixing eye assuming the deviated position
     - if no eye movement occurs in the non-occluded eye or upon uncovering the occluded eye the test implies that there is no manifest deviation. However, the test does not detect latent deviations and a further cover test, examining the reactions of the covered eye, is required to make such a differentiation.
  b) *To detect a latent deviation (heterophoria)*
     - performed after elimination of a manifest squint to reveal a latent deviation in the absence of a manifest deviation or a combined deviation (i.e. a manifest deviation with a latent element)
     - the aim of the test is to break down fusion and so reveal any heterophoria
     - the test is performed with the patient fixing a near and distant target, with

and without spectacles and in the presence/absence of any abnormal head posture

- the test is performed by transferring the occluder from one eye to the other without pause between each transfer. The occluder should be left covering each eye for several seconds after each transfer, since this is most disruptive to fusion, allowing sufficient time for the eyes to dissociate. Repeating the test is more dissociating to fusion than performing the test once. After this dissociation the eye being uncovered is observed for movement as it regains BSV. There may be diplopia prior to recovery.
- the candidate should note:
    the rate of recovery (an indicator of fusion amplitude; if slow, the fusion amplitude is poor and decompensation is probable)
    the magnitude of movement (slight, moderate, marked)
    the direction of movement of the uncovered eye
- if the movement of the uncovered eye is in a temporal direction then an esophoria exists (the eye having converged undercover and moved outwards to regain BSV). If the movement of the uncovered eye is in a nasal direction then an exophoria exists. If there is a vertical movement of an eye on uncovering it, there is a vertical phoria. Downward movement indicates hyperphoria and upward movement, hypophoria. When either eye elevates under cover suspect a dissociated vertical deviation (DVD).

The alternate cover test

- involves covering each eye in turn so that either one or the other eye is always covered (practice on yourself to get the speed right)
- the test is used as part of the cover test to identify a latent squint and is also used in the prism cover test.

Remember

- it is possible to have a combined manifest (heterotropia) and latent (heterophoria) deviation (e.g. a microtropia with associated heterophoria)
- most people have a slight heterophoria under certain circumstances and true orthophoria (no manifest or latent deviation) is uncommon
- cover tests may not reveal some microtropias.

Measurement of ocular deviations

Prism cover test

If a deviation is present it can be quantified by neutralizing the movement with prisms. Providing the patient can co-operate and has adequate visual acuity and central fixation, this test is the most accurate way of measuring the angle of deviation. It can be carried out at any distance and in any direction of gaze. It is a free space test, and thus representative of normal everyday conditions.

First, the patient fixates a target and a standard cover test is performed in order to determine the direction of the deviation. After this, a prism bar (or one of a series of single prisms) is held in the opposite hand to the occluder and an alternate cover test is performed. The prism bar is held in front of the non-fixing eye and moved up or down whilst the movement of the eye is observed. Holding the prism before the same (non-fixing) eye, the cover is alternated so that one eye is always occluded, producing full dissociation. The prism power is adjusted until there is no movement with the alternate cover test. The prism power is increased again until reversal of the movement occurs, and the angle of deviation is taken at the value of the prism immediately before this happens.

The base of the prism is placed in the opposite direction to the deviation so as to neutralize the movement. Thus, for an exo-deviation a base-in prism should be used, for a hyper-deviation a base-down prism should be used. Another way to remember this, is that the prism-apex should be where the eye is. Single prisms have to be used if the deviation is large and exceeds the power of the prism bar. It should be noted that large angles are less accurately measured than small angles with this test. A combination of back-to-back prisms may have to be used if there is a combined vertical and horizontal deviation. Although in theory one eye fixes in the primary position and the prisms are placed before the other eye, in practice it is difficult for the patient to see through two prisms. It can be easier to use a prism bar in front of each eye, with the patient holding one of them.

Hirschberg's test

This is a useful technique when the deviated eye has poor visual acuity, for very young patients, or for the patient with a very large angle squint where the angle is too big to measure with prisms. It is not as accurate as the prism cover test. A pen-torch is held in front of the patient and the position of the corneal reflections is noted. A light reflection from a deviated eye which is located at the pupil margin represents a deviation of about 10–15° for average sized pupils, and at the limbus, a deviation of about 45°. Approximately 1 mm of displacement of the light reflection from the centre is equivalent to 7° of deviation.)

The Krimsky prism reflection test

This is a method of quantifying the degree of strabismus by placing prisms in front of one of the eyes until the corneal reflections of the examining light are similarly positioned relative to the iris/pupil in both eyes. The test is less accurate than the prism cover test, but it is useful when a patient's visual acuity is too low or co-operation is inadequate for the prism cover test. The procedure is usually done for near. The patient fixates a light and the position of the corneal reflexes is noted. The prisms are placed in the same direction as for the prism cover test, but there are two ways to perform the test:

1. The prism is placed before the squinting eye and its power is increased until the reflexes are symmetrical in each eye
2. The prism is placed before the fixing eye, which moves the image off the fovea. The fixing eye will move to compensate for this and the other eye will move the same amount due to Hering's law. Eventually the reflexes will become symmetrical as the squinting eye moves into a central position. This method cannot be used for patients with gross mechanical restrictions,

where the squinting eye is unable to take up a central position.

The above tests are all objective tests. Other, subjective tests (see under Specific Investigations) used to measure deviations are available and include:

- the major amblyoscope (synoptophore)
- Maddox rod (for distance)
- Maddox wing (for near)
- Two Maddox rods test (for torsion).

Eye movements (see also p. 14)

The diagnostic positions are:

- up and right (RSR + LIO)
- right (RLR + LMR)
- down and right (RIR + LSO)
- straight down (RIR + LIR)
- down and left (LIR + RSO)
- left (LLR + RMR)
- up and left (LSR + RIO)
- straight up (LSR + RSR).

When assessing versions (binocular eye movements – cf. ductions, which are uniocular eye movements, i.e. assessed with the fellow eye occluded) in patients with strabismus, the candidate should look for:

- limitation of movement of a muscle which may be due to a paresis or mechanical restriction (look for operation scars)
- upshoots or downshoots of the eyes on horizontal versions
- overaction of a muscle, which is usually due to underaction of its fellow yoke muscle in the opposite eye, or occasionally due to a primary overaction. Bilateral inferior oblique overaction is relatively common in early onset esotropia (20%) and partially accommodative esotropia. Movements may be graded as overactions (+1 to +4) or underactions (−1 to −4), with 0 being normal
- A- and V-patterns (changes in the horizontal deviation of the eyes between 30° of downgaze and 30° of upgaze, which have to be >10D for an A-pattern and >15D for a V-pattern). V-patterns are more common than A-patterns.
- secondary changes (sequelae) in neurogenic paralytic strabismus.

Visual field analysis (see also p. 11)

Ocular motility disorders may be associated with visual field defects, either as a cause (i.e. secondary to reduced binocular single vision) or as two features of a particular neurological disease or trauma:

- cerebral tumours
- head injuries
- demyelinating disorders
- pituitary tumours
- orbital pathology.

General ophthalmic examination

This is important in all cases, but particularly so in patients with non-paralytic esotropia or exotropia which may have resulted from ocular disease (especially if unilateral or asymmetrical) or pathology affecting the afferent visual system. Furthermore, in adults with paralytic strabismus, examination of the eyes may provide clues as to the possible aetiology (e.g. hypertensive or diabetic retinopathy).

Specific syndromes

The candidate should always (and especially during exams!) be on the lookout for specific ocular motility syndromes such as:

- Duane's syndrome
- Brown's syndrome
- Mobius syndrome
- double elevator palsy.

Specific investigations

Investigation of binocular function

Most ophthalmology units have an orthoptist who carries out the assessment of squints; however, it is important that the candidate understands an orthoptic report. A general knowledge of the principles of orthoptic investigation is required, but it is unlikely that candidates will be asked to perform specific orthoptic examinations in an exam. It is a good idea to visit the orthoptic department fairly early on in your career to see the various tests performed; it will then make more sense when you read the reports. Furthermore, it will also save the embarrassment of going along to the orthoptic department just before the exam and confessing that orthoptics is a total enigma to you, and that you only have an hour in which to be taught it all!

Assessment of binocular function

It is important to investigate binocular function and determine its degree, since management depends on this. The most important thing is determining the presence or absence of fusion (see below for definition). If fusion is absent, no matter how accurately the eyes are aligned by surgery or by prisms, they will not function as a pair, and if the patient has diplopia it will not be possible to join it.

Definitions

Retinal correspondence
This is the physiological relationship between the retinal elements, both anatomically and functionally, of both eyes.

1. *Normal retinal correspondence (NRC)*:
   - Retinal correspondence is considered normal when the foveae of each eye have a common visual direction, and the nasal retina of one eye corresponds to the temporal retina in the other.
   - Retinal correspondence is normal in intermittent strabismus.

2. *Abnormal retinal correspondence (ARC)*:
   - The fovea of the fixing eye corresponds with and has a common visual direction with a point other than the fovea in the deviating eye. Thus, points nasal to this 'pseudo fovea' correspond with points temporal to the true fovea in the fixing eye, and points temporal to the 'pseudo fovea' in the squinting eye correspond to points nasal to the true fovea in the fixing eye. This means that there is an area of nasal retina in the squinting eye that projects as if it were temporal retina. The important factor to remember about ARC is that it is a binocular condition, and can only be diagnosed with both eyes open; once the fixing eye is covered, the deviating eye will take up foveal fixation. The candidate should not confuse ARC with eccentric

fixation, which is a uniocular condition in which a point other than the fovea is used for fixation and can only be detected uniocularly.

- Retinal correspondence may be abnormal in patients with constant esotropia (rare in exotropia), particularly if of early onset and of small angle.

Binocular vision (BV)
- the simultaneous perception of two images, one from each eye
- diplopia is a form of BV
- may be anomalous when the visual direction of the foveae are abnormal.

Binocular single vision (BSV)
- the ideal form of binocular vision
- the simultaneous perception of two images, one from each eye, giving rise to the perception of a single image. This occurs under everyday viewing conditions without the aid of instruments (i.e. can only be diagnosed with 'free space' tests)
- normally bifoveal without strabismus (i.e. normal BSV with bifoveal fixation and NRC)
- may be anomalous when extra-foveal in one eye and associated with strabismus (i.e. abnormal BSV with a small angle squint and ARC)
- may be anomalous with abnormal BSV with monofoveal fixation and peripheral fusion (NRC).

Worth's grades of binocular vision
1. *Simultaneous perception (SP)*:
   - the ability to perceive an image on each retina simultaneously, whether or not they are superimposed
   - not always possible, since some patients with strabismus suppress either eye alternately
   - if patients can superimpose the images from each eye (i.e. get the lion into the cage on the synoptophore – see below) they are said to have simultaneous foveal (SFP), macular (SMP) or paramacular (SPMP) perception (depending on size of targets)
   - patients with a lack of retinal correspondence are unable to superimpose

the images, which appear not to relate to each other at all.
2. *Fusion*:
   - sensory – the ability to join, or mentally blend, two similar images, one in the left eye and one in the right, and see them as one
   - motor – the ability to perform vergence movements (convergence, divergence, vertical and torsional vergences) and keep the two similar images joined
   - some patients have superimposition only; the images appear to join but split as soon as the eyes are moved, and there is no vergence. If one image is seen to 'bob', the prognosis for fusion is poor
   - as for SP, fusion may be foveal, macular or peripheral, according to the size of slides used. The candidate should not be tempted to think that peripheral fusion is unimportant – it plays a significant role in keeping eyes straight. Hence, patients with very restricted visual fields have great difficulty trying to control diplopia.
3. *Stereopsis*:
   - the binocular appreciation of depth, dependent on the ability to fuse and perceive two slightly differing images, one formed on each retina
   - may be detailed or gross.

Suppression
- the cortical inhibition of unwanted stimuli, resulting in the abolishment of the perception of one retinal image (an active cortical process)
- occurs under binocular conditions
- physiological suppression occurs to prevent the awareness of physiological diplopia
- pathological suppression may occur in patients with manifest strabismus to avoid the symptoms of diplopia, confusion with a manifest squint or of incompatible images
- suppression may be constant or intermittent, and can vary in area (peripheral or central) density.

Assessment of retinal correspondence

The state of retinal correspondence should be investigated in all cases of constant strabismus.

The candidate should first ensure that the patient is capable of simultaneous perception. Tests determine either (1) the relationship between the fixing eye fovea and the corresponding retinal area of the non-fixing eye which receives the same image as the fixing eye, or (2) the visual directions of the two foveae.

1.
   a) Worth's four lights test
   b) Bagolini glasses test
   c) Vertical prism diplopia test (with or without red and green glasses)
   d) Major amblyoscope (synoptophore)
   e) Lang two pencil test (can be useful in the young patient as a gross test for ARC)
   f) Prism adaptation test.
2.
   a) After image test
   b) Binocular visuscopy (fovea–foveolar test).

NB: BSV responses to tests in the presence of a manifest squint indicates ARC.

Assessment of suppression

It is important to determine the type and degree of suppression so that anti-suppression exercises can be instigated when indicated.

Tests of peripheral suppression
1. Worth's four lights test (6 m, $\frac{1}{3}$ m and macular – for central suppression)
2. Bagolini glasses
3. Major amblyoscope (synoptophore)

Tests of central suppression
1. Four dioptre prism test
2. Worth's four lights test (see above).

Tests for density of suppression
1. Bagolini filter bar
2. Testing the ease with which the suppression may be overcome or diplopia noticed.

NB: Sometimes a patient will suppress when fixing with the usually fixing eye, but appreciate diplopia when fixing with the usually squinting eye; this is called 'fixation switch diplopia'.

Assessment of fusion

Fusion (or its absence) is important in determining both the type of strabismus management and the prognosis. If fusion is absent the prognosis for restoration of BSV is poor, orthoptic exercises are contraindicated, and surgery should only be performed on cosmetic grounds (having excluded the chance of post-operative diplopia). It is most important that suppression is not overcome in these cases, since intractable diplopia may result.

Normal amplitudes of fusion (prism dioptres)

Convergence	near: 35–40	distance: 15
Divergence	near: 15	distance: 5–7
Vertical:		
– supra	near: 3	distance: 3
– infra	near: 3	distance: 3
Torsional (degrees):		
– incyclo	near: 3–5	distance: 3–5
– excyclo	near: 3–5	distance: 3–5

There is in fact a wide variation among normals, and a convergence range of 20 prism dioptres and over should be considered satisfactory in a normal individual. Vergences, especially convergence, can be greatly improved with training.

Use of prisms to assess fusion
- convergence: base-out
- divergence: base-in
- supravergence: base-down
- infravergence: base-up.

1. *Tests of fusion:*
   a) 20 dioptre base-out prism test
   b) red/green filter tests with prisms
   c) Worth's four lights test with prisms
   d) Bagolini glasses test with prisms
   e) Major amblyoscope (synoptophore)
2. Measurement of fusion amplitude in patients with BSV (i.e. determination of the prism fusion range (PFR).

Assessment of stereopsis

Tests may be qualitative or quantitative. Quantitative tests measure stereoacuity in seconds of arc.

Qualitative tests
1. Lang two pencil test
2. Major amblyoscope (synoptophore), except Braddick slides.

Quantitative tests
1. Random dot stereogram tests (TNO, Lang, Frisby, Randot)
2. Polarization tests (Titmus – Wirt: fly, animals, circles).

Orthoptic tests

Worth's four dot test (Worth's lights)
This is a test of partial dissociation based on complementary colours, using red and green glasses. The test can be used to test for (1) sensory fusion (or possibly superimposition alone), (2) abnormal retinal correspondence (ARC), (3) suppression and (4) diplopia. The patient wears a pair of red–green goggles (red = right eye) and gazes at four lights, two green, one red and one white, positioned at 6 m followed by 0.3 m. A macular version of the test (adapted from a Foster torch) is available, and is more discriminating. If all four lights are seen, either (a) there is normal BSV, or (b) (if the patient has a manifest squint) there is ARC. If two red lights are seen (the red and white), the patient has right suppression. If three green lights are seen (the two green and the single white) the patient has right suppression, and if two red lights alternating with two green lights are seen then the suppression is alternating. If two red and three green lights are seen the patient has a diplopia response, which may be horizontal, crossed or uncrossed (exo- or eso-), or vertical. The diplopia can be corrected with prisms and the fusion range can be measured using this test.
NB: As a test of fusion Worth's lights is fairly gross, and it provides little information about the quality of fusion, unless combined with the prism fusion range test.

Bagolini glasses test
The test spectacles consist of two striated lenses, either loose or mounted as an easier-to-use lorgnette. One lens is set at 45°, the other at 135°. The patient looks at a point source of light, and the striated lenses produce two lines at 90° to the striations and to each other (i.e. dissimilar images, one to each eye). The test employs minimal dissociation and is probably the most 'natural' of orthoptic tests, since the background of the room is still clearly visible. The test is usually carried out for near, but it can be performed at 6 m. The problem with the

6 m test is that artefacts are produced from other lights in the room, but if these are dimmed it alters everyday conditions and abolishes one of the strong points of the test. With normality (BSV) or a manifest squint with ARC, a cross (centred at the point source of light) will be seen. With an exo- or eso-tropia (with diplopia) the cross will be perceived to cross either above (exo-) or below (eso-) the point source of light. With suppression just one line will be seen, or if the suppression is only central, a gap at the intersection may be reported. With microtropia, for example, a small gap in one line around the fixation light is commonly reported; this indicates a small central suppression scotoma.
The glasses can be used in conjunction with prisms to test for fusion using perceived diplopia, but as with Worth's lights alone it provides little information about the quality of fusion.

Lang two pencil test
This simple test primarily for stereopsis can be used in young children as a gross test for ARC and for gross stereopsis. The patient (with both eyes open) is asked to oppose the tip of a pencil with the tip of a second pencil held by the examiner. The test is then repeated with the squinting eye covered. If the cover makes no difference there is suppression, no BSV and poor stereopsis. If the cover makes the task more difficult, it can be presumed that the squinting eye is contributing to the appreciation of BSV and stereopsis and that there is probably ARC.

Prism adaptation test
This test uses prisms to overcorrect the deviation, thus placing images on unsuppressed retina and producing diplopia, and this is used to stimulate fusion. It is used in patients with virtually equal visual acuity in the two eyes, a deviation of less than 40 dioptres, and a similar deviation for near and far. The deviation is measured by the prism cover test. Fresnel prisms (divided between both eyes) are used for about two weeks and the patient's motor response is observed. The long duration of the test improves accuracy and reliability, but a disadvantage of the test is that use of the prisms degrades the images. If the visual axes converge to the same angle of deviation, there is ARC. If there is divergence, there is lack of

BSV. If a residual microtropia remains or if the eyes take up the primary position, BSV should be confirmed.

The drawback to this test is that the visual acuity is degraded by the prisms, which are usually divided equally between the eyes. The test is not in widespread use but is of value, as a predictive test, in patients who repeatedly reconverge after surgery.

Vertical prism diplopia test

This is a test to assess the state of retinal correspondence. A 10-dioptre prism is held base-up or base-down in front of one eye so as to displace images on to unsuppressed retina, producing diplopia. The diplopia is vertical, or both vertical and horizontal, if there is a horizontal deviation. The horizontal element is corrected with prisms until the two images lie directly above each other (i.e. they are aligned, not superimposed). The test can be performed with red–green glasses, which sometimes makes it easier. If the images can be aligned with the same strength prism as the prism cover test measurement there is normal retinal correspondence (NRC), but if the images are aligned with a prism of weaker strength than the prism cover test measurement, there is ARC.

After-image test

Another test which can be used to identify ARC involves stimulating one fovea with a flash of vertical light and the other fovea with a flash of horizontal light. This can be carried out with a flash unit or on most synoptophores; the principal is the same whichever method is used, but using the flash unit is easier. The squinting eye is occluded and a horizontal after-image is given to the fixing eye; the fixing eye is then occluded and a vertical after-image given to the squinting eye. The patient is asked to look at a blank wall and/or blink their eyes and describe the after-image that they see. If a cross is seen this indicates NRC, or if a displaced cross is seen this indicates ARC.

NB: The interpretation is opposite to that of the Bagolini glasses test because the after-image test is a test of fovea/foveolar projection, whereas the Bagolini glasses test is a test of fovea/extrafoveal projection. For this reason, the after-image test cannot be used in patients with eccentric fixation.

The bifoveal (or fovea–foveolar) test (also called binocular visuscopy)

This test is performed to assess retinal correspondence using a piece of apparatus called a visuscope (an adapted ophthalmoscope), which projects a star on to the fovea of the squinting eye whilst the patient fixates a target (e.g. a spotlight) with the normally fixing eye. The patient states the position of the star relative to the spot. If the images coincide there is NRC, whereas if they are separate there is ARC. If ARC is identified, the patient can be asked to guide the star onto the spot to show the examiner the area of the retina in the squinting eye which corresponds to the fovea of the fixing eye. The test is difficult to perform and is rarely used. However, the visuscope is a useful instrument for examining a patient's fixation in amblyopia.

Four dioptre prism test

The test is used to test for (1) normal bifoveal BSV and (2) central or paracentral suppression in patients with possible microtropia. The patient fixates a small Snellen chart letter (for near and/or distance), and a 4D prism is used base-out in front of the eye with better visual acuity. The examiner observes the other eye for movement. With normality the eye behind the prism moves inwards, and the observed eye makes an equal outward movement (Hering's law) followed by a rapid corrective inward movement to regain foveal fixation. If there is central or paracentral suppression, the corrective movement does not occur.

Using a right micro*eso*tropia as an example, the patient fixates a small target and the 4D base-out prism is introduced in front of the other (left) eye. The left eye will make a nasal movement (to the right) to continue target fixation. The right eye also moves to the right (Hering's law), with resultant diplopia. Finally, the right eye will make a convergent movement to overcome the diplopia. If there is bifoveal fixation, the same response in reverse will be obtained if the prism is placed before the left eye. If, however, there is a small central suppression scotoma in the right eye when the prism is put before the left eye, the movement of the left eye will again be nasal (to the right) and the right eye will move to the right due to Hering's law. This time, however, there will be no diplopia produced because of the suppression scotoma, so no correcting converging movement of the right eye occurs. If the prism is placed before the right eye again no movement occurs because there is no diplopia produced, as the image lies within the suppression scotoma.

NB: A base-in prism is used for patients with a micro*exo*tropia.

Bagolini filter bar test

This test can be used to determine the density of suppression, which is useful in patients undergoing occlusion therapy where there is a risk of developing diplopia. The filter bar consists of a series of red filters of increasing density, which is used in conjunction with a point source of light. The patient fixates a light and the bar is placed before the dominant eye. The patient will see the light as red. The intensity of the filter is increased until the patient sees two lights, or the light is seen as white, and the strength of the filter is recorded. Easily elicited, diplopia indicates that there is a risk with occlusion.

Prism fusion range (PFR)

For the assessment of fusion, measurement of the PFR is probably the method of choice for patients with latent squints. A prism bar is introduced in front of one eye while the patient fixates a target at near or distance. The strength of the prism is increased until diplopia is appreciated (subjective response). At this point one eye will be seen to deviate, and often fixation is changed from one eye to the other as the patient looks at the diplopic images – this provides an objective assessment. If there is a tendency to suppress, then a 'control' such as the Worth's lights test or Bagolini glasses test can be used so that single vision due to fusion can be differentiated from single vision due to suppression. There are different responses to the diplopia within the test; patients may be able to rejoin the diplopia easily or with difficulty, they may be able to rejoin it if the prism strength is slightly reduced, or may have to go right back to a very weak prism to obtain single vision. Obviously if single vision is obtained only momentarily, or with difficulty, the quality of motor fusion is not good. The presence of blurred vision while testing convergence indicates that accommodative convergence is being used – this may mean that the patient will experience blurred vision on exerting conver-

gence (e.g. to control an intermittent exo-deviation).

Measurement of the PFR is also suitable for intermittent squints, used at the distance where the deviation is latent. However, the method is not so good for manifest squints, since they are often associated with suppression; thus the use of a control is necessary and the manifest squint should be corrected before the fusion range is tested.

Twenty dioptre base-out prism test

A 20 dioptre base-out prism is introduced in front of one eye. This produces diplopia, and a subsequent fusional movement occurs to join it. When the prism is removed, diplopia occurs again and the eye diverges to join it. This movement is easily seen, and provides an objective assessment of the presence of BSV. The test is most often used for babies with suspected pseudo-squint, since the response can be reliably elicited at about the age of six months. A 15 or 10 dioptre prism can also be used – these are easier to overcome, but the response is not so easily seen.

The major amblyoscope (synoptophore)

The candidate should make the effort to look at a synoptophore, which is much easier to understand once it has been seen. The synoptophore is an instrument that may be used to measure deviations and assess binocular vision, retinal correspondence, suppression, fusion and/or stereopsis. The instrument has two independent mobile tubes each consisting of an eyepiece (+6.50DS) and a mirrored right-angled bend with a slide carrier at the end. Thus, the slides presented to each eye can be moved separately and in relation to each other. The eyes are completely dissociated, since each looks down a separate tube; thus it is not possible to diagnose BSV on the synoptophore, only the grades of BV. The relative positions of the two slides can be assessed on a graduated scale. It is a distance instrument, but patients often interpret its use as a test of near vision, which results in proximal convergence. Thus, eso-deviations tend to measure more, and exo-deviations less, than with free space tests such as the prism cover test.

Simultaneous perception is tested using dissimilar pictures in front of each eye (e.g. a lion and a cage). If both objects are seen at the same time, simultaneous perception exists and the patient is asked to place the lion in the cage by moving the two tubes.

If the patient cannot see the two dissimilar pictures simultaneously, then there is suppression.

Abnormal retinal correspondence can be detected using the synoptophore to measure and compare the objective and subjective angles of a deviation.

The objective angle is measured by presenting each eye alternately with a small target (e.g. simultaneous perception slides) and moving the tubes until no movement of the eyes occurs when each eye is covered. The fixing eye is set at 0 and the patient is made to look from the lion to the cage by extinguishing the lights in front of each eye alternately. The observer watches the eye movements, and gradually moves the tube in front of the non-fixing eye until the movement stops. Both horizontal and vertical elements can be corrected. The objective angle is read off the scale, and is traditionally recorded in degrees (horizontal) or dioptres (vertical). If visual acuity is low or a child does not co-operate, the tube in front of the squinting eye can be moved until the corneal reflections (CR) are symmetrical – this is recorded as the objective angle by CR.

The subjective angle is measured by asking the patient to superimpose the two simultaneous perception slides (e.g. lion and cage). The fixing eye is set at 0 and the patient is asked to move the tube horizontally until the pictures are superimposed. The examiner moves the vertical control (measured in dioptres). If the patient sees one image tilted, the torsion can be corrected (measured in degrees). There is a special slide for this, but any with obvious linear features can be used.

- If the objective angle = the subjective angle there is NRC.
- If the objective angle > the subjective angle by more than a few degrees there is ARC.

NB: Some patients will not be able to demonstrate a subjective angle due to suppression or lack of retinal correspondence.

Fusion is tested using two similar pictures, differing in only one or two small differences, such that the two slides joined together complete the picture. An example is a rabbit with a bunch of flowers (no tail) on one slide, and a rabbit with a tail (no flowers) on the other. Each picture can be moved independently, and the patient is asked to join the two pictures to make a single rabbit with a tail and a bunch of flowers. The pictures may join, but split as soon as the tubes are moved; this is superimposition and not true fusion. Once the slides have been joined, the range of motor fusion is tested by converging and diverging the tubes until the patient notices diplopia or suppression (one of the controls disappears). If there is ARC, the patient will fuse at the anomalous angle.

The synoptophore is the best method of assessing cases where fusion is doubtful, especially if the deviation is complex and has horizontal, vertical and perhaps torsional components; it is also very useful for measuring such complex cases and for measuring the deviation in nine positions of gaze in incomitant squint.

Stereopsis is tested, qualitatively, using two pictures of the same object (e.g. a bucket with a handle) observed from a slightly different angle. If the patient appreciates depth (e.g. of the bucket), then stereopsis is present. Use of the synoptophore provides only a gross assessment of stereopsis, unless the Braddick slides (a form of random dot stereogram) are used.

The synoptophore can also be used for orthoptic exercises.

Maddox wing test

This subjective test is designed to quantify heterophoria for near vision. The instrument dissociates the two eyes for near vision by means of two septa, so that the right eye sees only a white vertical arrow and a red horizontal arrow, whereas the left eye sees only a vertical and horizontal scale of numbers. Horizontal deviation is determined by asking the patient to which number (dioptres) the white arrow points (even numbers – exo, odd numbers – eso). Vertical deviation is determined by asking the patient to which number the red arrow points. Cyclophoria is assessed by asking the patient to place the red arrow parallel to the horizontal scale, and the measurement of torsion is read from a scale on the side (degrees). The test is useful for the measurement (and even detection) of small angle squints which are difficult to see, and is popular because it requires little skill and is quick.

Maddox rod test

This test may be used to measure subjectively small manifest deviations (providing there is no ARC) or heterophoria. The test is best for distance but can be used for near. The eyes are dissociated by presenting a white light to the fixing eye and a red line to the other eye. The rod, positioned in front of one eye, consists of a series of red glass rods (i.e. strong cylinders) which convert a white spotlight into a red streak at 90° to the axis of the rods. The rod (mounted in a trial 'frame') can be rotated so that a vertical line can be produced to measure horizontal deviations, whereas for vertical deviations a horizontal line is used. The test is carried out in a darkened room, and because the two images are dissimilar and cannot be fused, the eyes become dissociated and will deviate to the fusion free position. The patient is asked about the position of the line (same side as rod, uncrossed, eso; opposite, exo; below, hyper of the eye behind the rod; above, hypo). Measurement of deviation is achieved using a series of prisms placed with the base of the prism opposite to the direction of deviation. The power of the prism is adjusted until the patient superimposes the red line and the white dot.

Hess (or Lees') chart testing

Hess (or Lees') charts are used to aid in making a diagnosis of incomitant ocular motility disorders (showing both underaction of affected muscles and overaction of yoke muscles), and also to quantify any degree of change over a period of time (e.g. with dysthyroid eye disease, or to document recovery following nerve palsies or a blow-out fracture).

The Hess screen is a grey board marked with a grid on which small red lights are individually illuminated. The patient holds a green torch and directs the green light onto the illuminated red spot. The patient wears red and green goggles, and is only able to see the red light through the red glass and green light through the green glass (the eyes are therefore dissociated by colour).

The Lees' screen consists of two illuminated screens at right angles to each other, each marked with dots. The eyes are dissociated by a mirror at 45° which bisects the screens, one of which is illuminated. The patient sits facing the blank screen and sees the illuminated screen through the mirror. The dots are judged to be on the screen ahead, and the patient points with a pointer to the dot indicated by the examiner. The tests are carried out without glasses and the patient must have NRC and no suppression.

The same type of recording chart is used for both tests and is interpreted in the same way. A candidate will not be asked to produce a Hess/Lees' chart, but may well be asked to interpret one. The chart provides a visual display of the eyes' deviation, having been dissociated by means of either complementary colours or a mirror. The principle of the method is based on foveal projection, normal retinal correspondence and both Hering's and Sherrington's laws of innervation, and is performed with each eye fixing in turn. Each screen consists of a central dot, an inner square of 8 dots and an outer square of 16 dots. The examiner points at the dots in turn and the patient indicates with a second pointer where the dot is perceived to be. In normality, the indicated and perceived dots will be superimposed in all positions of gaze. With a right lateral rectus palsy (as an example of abnormality), when the patient fixes with the right eye the normal left medial rectus will be excessively innervated and the patient will indicate points beyond the screen's medial point. Conversely when fixing with the left eye, the poorly innervated right lateral rectus will result in the patient indicating points short of the correct lateral points.

Notes on interpretation

- each chart is marked:
  - green before RE (i.e. fixing LE)
  - green before LE (i.e. fixing RE)
- the dots which indicate the main actions of the muscles are labelled with the names of the muscles
- when looking at the completed charts the deviation of the RE (fixing LE) is on the right side, and vice versa. The plot is displaced in the direction of the deviation, so is easy to interpret.
- the affected eye has the smallest field
- the affected muscle shows the greatest shrinkage from the normal
- the plots demonstrate the extent of muscle sequelae (i.e. spread of concomitance), can show A- and V-patterns and can also be used to measure the size of deviation, since each small square = 5°.

The field of binocular single vision

A perimeter can be used to map out areas of field where BSV is maintained and areas where there is diplopia in patients who are able to fuse images in part of their binocular visual field. The field is plotted on a perimeter (usually an arc or a Goldmann type). The target is placed in an area where it is fused, and moved until diplopia occurs or facial contours block off the second image – these limits are recorded. The test is particularly useful for patients with incomitant squint, both diagnostically and in the management. The test can be used to assess change over a period of time, and to provide the clinician with an idea of how symptomatic a patient is likely to be. The test is especially useful for patients with blow-out fractures, neurogenic palsies or dysthyroid eye disease.

A field of uniocular fixation can also be plotted. The test is a uniocular test in which the patient follows a target until foveal fixation cannot be maintained. It is useful in patients with gross limitations (e.g. dysthyroid eye disease).

Stereopsis tests

1. *Random dot stereogram tests*
   a) The TNO test: Computer-generated red and green dots (with varying degrees of disparity up to 15 seconds of arc) are positioned so that shapes may be seen when the plates are viewed through red–green glasses, providing the patient has a degree of stereopsis. The test has no monocular clues.
   b) The Frisby test: Test plates consist of perspex sheets of differing thickness with a series of identical shapes (a circle within a square) printed on one side of the perspex, and one where the circle is printed on the other side. The patient is positioned with the face parallel to the sheet (so as to avoid parallax), and has to identify the odd man out (i.e. the circle that appears to be deep to the square or to float above the square). The disparity (15–600 seconds of arc) is varied by altered thickness of perspex or viewing distance.
   c) The Randot test: Test plates made with random dots are viewed with polarized spectacles, which produce the dissociation. The test has no monocular clues.

2. *Polarization test for stereopsis*
   The Titmus vectograph test relies on the presentation to one eye of an image polarized at 90° to an image to the other eye. The patient, wearing polarized spectacles, is asked to view sets of circles, one in each set being disparate from the others (up to 40 seconds of arc). If the patient fails the test the housefly image (3000 seconds of arc disparity) can be used, although there are monocular clues with the gross plates.

All the above stereopsis tests are free space tests, and they are suitable for heterophoria and small angle squints with ARC. Larger angle squints should first be corrected with prisms. (See also Lang two pencil test p. 42.)

Measurement of the AC/A ratio

The AC/A ratio is the amount of accommodative convergence (measured in prism dioptres) that occurs in association with each dioptre sphere of accommodation exerted. A normal ratio is 3–5 : 1. A high ratio is associated with excessive convergence and a low ratio with convergence insufficiency. An abnormal ratio may be associated with strabismus, and it is more important when high, when there is a significant increase in an eso-deviation (or decrease in an exo-deviation) at near fixation compared to distance. It may result in a convergence excess type of esotropia. In an intermittent exotropia it may enable the deviation to be controlled for near. Management of strabismus depends to some extent on the level of the AC/A ratio.

Methods of measurement involve changing the stimulus to accommodation and assessing how much accommodative convergence occurs by:

1. Using spherical lenses to alter the degree of accommodation required to fixate on a target (usually at 6 m), and then measuring the change in angle induced by each dioptre change in accommodation (gradient technique)
2. Changing the distance of the fixation target from infinity to $\frac{1}{3}$ m (heterophoria technique).

With either technique, the deviation is measured using the prism cover test. The gradient method is considered the best and can be performed as follows:

- measure angle for distance = N (no accommodation) (e.g. 10)
- measure angle for distance with −3.00DS lenses = A (accommodation) (e.g. 40)
- use the formula (A − N)/3DS = (40 − 10)/3 = 10 : 1.

This can also be done with + 3.00DS lenses, but only for near, since the patient will not be able to see for distance through them. Other strengths of lenses can be used, and the power of the lens used becomes the denominator of the formula.

Presurgical, post-operative diplopia assessment

Prior to cosmetic squint surgery, an assessment of possible post-operative diplopia should be performed. The test is carried out in patients over the age of eight years (occasionally younger) who do not have fusion and are at risk of experiencing diplopia if their angle of squint is reduced such that they move out of their suppression scotoma. It is really an assessment of the size of the area of suppression.

Visual acuity should be measured, although dense amblyopia does not always prevent diplopia. The patient fixates a light (or target) and a prism is placed before the squinting eye to simulate the post-operative state (base-out prism for convergent squint, etc.). The strength of prism is gradually increased and the patient asked to report if diplopia is experienced. If diplopia is appreciated, the patient is asked if it is obvious or if it can be ignored. The prism strength should be increased until the deviation is overcorrected (and then reduced in an attempt to place the image within a suppression scotoma). If surgery is subsequently performed, the amount of correction should be adjusted to correspond with the prism power in an attempt to avoid post-operative diplopia. It can also be carried out using a fixation target.

Some examples:

1. 40 dioptre esotropia – no diplopia even if overcorrected – postoperative diplopia unlikely
2. 40 dioptre esotropia – diplopia at 45 dioptres – diplopia likely if deviation overcorrected (this is quite a common response)
3. 40 dioptre esotropia – diplopia at 30 dioptres – diplopia likely if deviation reduced by 30 dioptres. However, the patient could still have a significant reduction in squint without any problems
4. 40 dioptre esotropia – diplopia at 10 dioptres – a high-risk patient; there would be no significant improvement in appearance without a high risk of diplopia
5. 40 dioptre esotropia – constant diplopia, no fusion – diplopia may be worse if the images are closer together, or may be better! It is for the patient to decide individually.

The post-operative diplopia test is not appropriate in intermittent squint or in cases of constant squint with demonstrable fusion.

Botulinum toxin is a useful method of assessing the likelihood of post-operative diplopia in certain cases (e.g. example 5).

Checklist for the assessment of strabismus

History

1. Presence of squint
2. Age of onset
3. Acute/sudden onset
4. Constant/intermittent
5. Alternating
6. Abnormal head position
7. Diplopia
8. Visual acuity
9. Nystagmus
10. Photophobia
11. Headache/eye ache
12. Previous therapy
13. Family history
14. Obstetric and perinatal history
15. Past medical history.

Clinical examination

1. *Inspection*
   - eyelid position
   - epicanthic folds
   - facial asymmetry
   - globe position
   - nystagmus
   - compensatory head posture
2. *Cover tests*
   - cover/uncover test
   - alternate cover test
3. *Measurement of ocular deviations*
   - prism alternate cover test
   - corneal reflections and Hirschberg's test
   - Krimsky prism reflection test
4. *Eye movements*
5. *Visual fields*
6. *General ophthalmic examination*
7. *Specific syndromes.*

Specific investigations

1. *Assessment of binocular function*
   - retinal correspondence
   - suppression
   - fusion
   - stereopsis
2. *Measurement of the AC/A ratio*
3. *Post-operative diplopia assessment.*

9. Slit-lamp examination of the anterior segment

History

Symptoms relating to anterior segment pathology include:

- red eye
- swelling of the conjunctiva (oedema or chemosis)
- foreign body sensation
- discomfort or pain
- burning
- itchiness
- discharge
- dryness
- reduced visual acuity
- haloes
- photophobia
- lacrimation
- epiphora
- lymphadenopathy.

The symptoms are not always very specific and can be out of proportion to the degree of pathology (especially with blepharitis, as anyone who has worked in an ophthalmic accident and emergency department will know!).

Conjunctival injection (hyperaemia) occurs with most types of ocular inflammation but has a tendency to be most intense in the fornices with conjunctivitis and at the limbus with uveitis or acute glaucoma. Generalized conjunctival hyperaemia is also a feature of corneal abrasion/erosion, surface foreign bodies, episcleritis, scleritis or orbital cellulitis. The hyperaemia of pingueculitis, marginal keratitis, episcleritis or scleritis may be localized to one specific area.

Chemosis may occur with any type of conjunctivitis but is particularly prominent with allergic eye disease or viral infection.

A description from the patient of any discharge can be helpful. A watery/serous discharge is most common with viral or toxic inflammation whereas a mucoid discharge is more indicative of allergic/vernal conjunctivitis or keratoconjunctivitis sicca. The associated complaint of itchiness rather than foreign body sensation is more indicative of allergy than dry eye or infection. A purulent discharge occurs with bacterial infection and a mucopurulent discharge with early bacterial or chlamydial infection. In severe bacterial membranous conjunctivitis the discharge may be partly haemorrhagic.

Pre-auricular lymphadenopathy is occasionally reported by the patient and is most common with viral or chlamydial infections.

The symptom of seeing haloes around point sources of light is classic of acute angle closure glaucoma due to corneal epithelial oedema but can occur with other types of epithelial disturbance or corneal opacification.

Photophobia (hypersensitivity to light) is a common symptom of anterior segment inflammation but is most intense with iritis, since light induced miosis of an inflamed iris is painful. Uveitis may also give rise to pain with accommodation, whereas this is less likely with other forms of anterior segment inflammation. Photophobia is also a symptom of migraine.

Lacrimation is excessive production of tears due to irritation of corneal and conjunctival nerves and reflex stimulation of the lacrimal gland. Lacrimation should not be confused with epiphora which is overflow of the normal amount of tears due to eyelid malposition or lacrimal drainage failure.

Clinical examination

A candidate may be instructed to:

- 'Examine the anterior segment of this patient'
- 'Examine this patient's cornea'
- 'Use the slit lamp to examine the eye of this patient'.

It is often useful to look at the patient in general before examining the eye in isolation – extra clues are always helpful!

With the slit-lamp examination an attempt to be systematic, working in an anterior–posterior fashion is advised. Do not carry out invasive procedures (evert a patient's eyelid, measure IOP, perform gonioscopy, use topical fluorescein or Rose Bengal stains or perform Schirmer's test) without the permission of the examiner and the patient.

General inspection

- skin disease (rosacea, eczema, haemangioma, rash)
- specific facial appearances.

Eyelids

- blepharitis (crusts, Meibomian gland plugging, meibomitis, margin notching, rosettes)
- entropion/ectropion
- punctal position and patency
- abnormal lashes (trichiasis, madarosis, poliosis)
- lid retraction
- swellings/masses
- ptosis (see p. 24).

Precorneal tear film

- debris
- size of tear meniscus (usually about 0.2 mm high)
- tear film break up time (see below).

Conjunctiva

- dilated conjunctiva vessels (hyperaemia/injection)
- subconjunctival haemorrhage
- papillae
- follicles
- infiltrate
- oedema (chemosis)
- pigmentation/naevi
- foreign body
- membranes and pseudomembranes
- granulomas

- cicatrization (check fornices and caruncle, look for symblepharon)
- surgical scarring (e.g. post-conjunctival, strabismus or retinal detachment surgery)
- filtration bleb.

Cornea

The candidate is advised to examine the cornea by direct illumination, scleral scatter and retro-illumination. It is suggested that one should start with an overall view of the cornea and its morphology followed by an organized progression from epithelium to endothelium. The depth of a lesion should be noted (i.e. epithelial, sub-epithelial, Bowman's layer, anterior stroma, mid-stroma, deep stroma, Descemet's membrane, endothelial). In addition to its depth a corneal lesion should be described with respect to its position (e.g. superior, interpalpebral, inferior or central). Specific features to look for include:

1. *overall morphology*:
   - evidence of previous surgery (e.g. sutures, wound, wound leaks)
   - presence of contact lenses
   - peripheral melts/ulcerations
        dellen
        phlycten
        Terrien's marginal degeneration
        Mooren's ulceration
        rheumatoid or other systemic disease
   - keratoconus
   - keratoglobus
   - pellucid marginal degeneration
2. *foreign body*:
   - metallic (ferrous, non-ferrous)
   - non-metallic
3. *epithelium*:
   - abrasion
   - infective keratitis
        infiltrate
        dendritic ulcer(s)
        microdendrites
   - (macro-) erosion(s)
   - punctate epithelial erosions
   - punctate epithelial keratitis
   - superficial punctate (Thygeson's) keratitis
   - oedema
   - bullous keratopathy
   - filaments

– plaques
   exudative
   mucus
– iron
   Hudson–Stähli line
   Fleischer's ring (keratoconus)
   Ferry's line (filtration bleb)
   Stocker's line (pterygium)
– microcysts/map-dot-fingerprint
   dystrophy
– Meesman's dystrophy
– crystalline deposits
– verticillata

4. *sub-epithelial/Bowman's layer*:
   – pannus/fascicles
   – pterygium
   – band keratopathy
   – superficial vascularization
   – Reis-Bucklers' dystrophy

5. *stroma*:
   – keratitis
      infiltrates
      marginal
      nummular
      disciform
   – oedema
   – opacities/scars
   – dystrophy (lattice, macular, granular)
   – deposits/pigment
   – vascularization (active, ghost)
   – prominent nerves

6. *Descemet's membrane*:
   – guttata/Fuch's dystrophy
   – breaks/splits
   – folds
   – descemetocoele
   – posterior embryotoxon
   – posterior polymorphous dystrophy
   – copper (Kayser–Fleischer ring)

7. *endothelium*:
   – Krukenberg's spindle keratic precipitates
      mutton fat
      diffuse
      stellate
      pigmented

8. *sensation*:
   – neurotrophic keratopathy.

Episclera/sclera

● episcleritis (diffuse/nodular)
● scleritis

● blue sclera
● scleral discolouration/pigmentation.

NB: Always lift the upper lid during the examination so as to avoid missing superior corneal/scleral signs.

Anterior chamber

● depth (central and peripheral [van Herick test])
● activity: flare and/or inflammatory cells
● hyphaema
● fibrin
● hypopyon
● pigment
● anterior chamber intraocular lens
● foreign body.

Iris/pupil

● peripheral anterior synechiae
● posterior synechiae
● peripheral iridectomy/iridotomy
● atrophy/spiralling of fibres
● heterochromia (different iris colour)
● iris naevi/tumour(s)
● iris nodules
● pseudoexfoliation
● rubeosis (neovascularization)
● transillumination (degree and position)
● pupil size (possible iatrogenic miosis/dilation)
● pupil reaction (see also p. 19)
● pupil distortion
● polycoria
● iris clip intraocular lens
● iridodonesis.

Lens

● cataract (congenital or acquired; nuclear sclerotic, cortical, posterior subcapsular, anterior capsular [glass-blowers])
● aphakia
● pseudophakia (comment on clarity of posterior capsule)
● dislocation/subluxation
● pseudoexfoliation
● phakodonesis
● glaukomflecken.

Anterior vitreous

- cells
- veils
- pigment
- optical clarity
- haemorrhage
- asteroid hyalosis
- synchysis scintillans.

Lymphadenopathy

- enlargement of the preauricular lymph nodes may occur with viral or chlamydial conjunctivitis or eyelid/conjunctival tumours.

Depending on clinical findings the candidate should ask the examiner if he/she would like them to perform any additional examination (e.g. instilling stain, measuring IOP or performing gonioscopy). If pseudoexfoliation or pigment dispersion are diagnosed, glaucoma suspected, or if there is rubeosis the candidate should ask if he/she should extend the examination to the posterior segment.

Specific investigations

Stains

- fluorescein scanned using the cobalt blue filter (epithelial defects, Seidel positive leaks, tear film break-up-time, tonometry)
- rose bengal (devitalized cells, mucus threads, corneal filaments).

Tear film break-up time (BUT)

Fluorescein is instilled into the lower fornix and the patient is asked to blink once but then not to blink while the stained tear film is observed using the cobalt blue filter. The time taken for the tear film to break up due to drying is measured. The BUT is abnormal (i.e. less than 15 seconds) with mucin deficiency in the tear film (xerophthalmia).

Schirmer's tests

Commercially available Schirmer's test paper strips are folded and placed over the temporal third of the lower lid margin with 5 mm of the strip in the lower fornix. After 5 minutes the length of moist paper is measured:

- the total reflex and basic secretion is measured by asking the patient to gaze ahead with the eyes open, blinking as required (normal = 10–30 mm)
- the basic secretion is measured by the same test after instilling topical anaesthetic
- the reflex secretion is determined by determining the difference between the above two measurements
- reflex secretion is rarely abnormal
- basic or total secretion is reduced with aqueous deficiency in the tear film (e.g. keratoconjunctivitis sicca)
- basic or total secretion appears to be increased when there is failure of normal tear drainage.

Goldmann applanation tonometry

- Measurement of intraocular pressure (IOP).
- Fluorescein is instilled into the tear film of the patient and the tonometer head piece is placed against the cornea to flatten it. The diameter of the head piece is 3.06 mm which results in a capillary attraction force that is equal and opposite to the force provided by the rigidity of the cornea which resists flattening. Thus, the measured IOP is a more accurate reflection of the actual IOP. The head piece contains two prisms positioned in opposite directions such that when the head piece touches the central cornea two green semicircles are seen. The end-point, representing a uniformly flattened cornea is set by rotating the dial such that the inner two edges of the semicircles just touch. The dial and tonometer are calibrated such that the IOP is ten times the number read from the dial.

Gonioscopy

This is the assessment of the irido-corneal angle using an indirect goniolens (Goldmann or Zeiss-indentation) or direct goniolens (Koeppe). Normal angle structures include:

- Schwalbe's line
- trabecular meshwork (± pigmented part)
- scleral spur
- ciliary body
- angle recess
- iris processes
- normal angle vessels.

Schaffer angle width grading can be applied:

- Grade 0: (0°) closed
- Grade 1: (<10°) very narrow and close-able, only Schwalbe's line is visible
- Grade 2: (10–20°) open but narrow and closeable, Schwalbe's line and the trabecular meshwork are visible
- Grade 3: (20–35°) open and not closeable, scleral spur is visible
- Grade 4: (35–45°) wide open, ciliary body is visible.

Scheie grading is similar but uses a reversed numerical grading.

If there is difficulty in seeing the angle at gonioscopy it is worth asking the patient to move their eye a small amount in the direction of the goniolens mirror which usually provides a better view.

Pachymetry

Measurement of corneal thickness – the Goldmann pachymeter attachment of the slit-lamp provides a split image of the illuminated corneal section. The images are adjusted so that the anterior surface of one image is lined-up with the posterior surface of the other image. The thickness of the examined part of the cornea is read from the dial.

Microbiology/Virology/Mycology/Parasitology

- lid swabs
- conjunctival swabs/scrapings
- corneal scrapings
- aqueous and vitreous taps.

Other tests

- Serology/Antigen detection
- Histopathology/Cytology
- Immunology/Immunopathology.

Checklist for slit-lamp examination of the anterior segment

History

Symptoms of anterior segment disorders
- red eye
- swelling of the conjunctiva (oedema or chemosis)
- foreign body sensation
- discomfort or pain
- burning
- itchiness
- discharge
- dryness
- reduced visual acuity
- haloes
- photophobia
- lacrimation
- epiphora
- lymphadenopathy.

Clinical examination

1. General inspection
2. Eyelids
3. Precorneal tear film
4. Conjunctiva
5. Cornea
6. Episclera/sclera
7. Anterior chamber
8. Iris/pupil
9. Lens
10. Anterior vitreous
11. Lymphadenopathy.

Specific investigations

1. Stains
2. Tear film break-up-time
3. Schirmer's tests
4. Goldmann applanation tonometry
5. Gonioscopy
6. Pachymetry
7. Microbiology/Virology/Mycology/Parasitology
8. Serology/Antigen detection
9. Histopathology/Cytology
10. Immunology/Immunopathology.

10. Examination of the posterior segment and fundus

History

Symptoms relating to posterior segment pathology include:

- reduced visual acuity
- sudden loss of vision (usually vascular disease)
- obscurations (papilloedema)
- amaurosis fugax (vascular disease)
- impaired central vision (macular disease)
- reduced light brightness appreciation (optic nerve lesion)
- reduced colour vision (optic nerve lesion)
- reduced night vision (retinal disease)
- positive scotoma an obstruction to vision (macular disease)
- negative scotoma a hole in the visual field (optic nerve lesion)
- visual distortion (macular disease)
  - generalized
  - metamorphopsia (altered image shape)
  - micropsia (reduced image size)
  - macropsia (increased image size)
- photopsia (flashing lights) (vitreo-retinal disorders)
- floaters (vitreo-retinal disorders).

A carefully taken history can help the candidate distinguish optic nerve, macular/foveal, retinal, vascular or vitreous disorders.

Clinical examination

A candidate may be instructed to:

- 'Examine the posterior segment of this patient'
- 'Examine this patient's fundus'
- 'Comment on this patient's optic discs'
- 'Examine this patient's eye with a direct (or an indirect [not MRCP]) ophthalmoscope'.

Again it is often useful to look at the patient in general before examining the eye in isolation. An attempt to be systematic is advised. If you are not specifically asked to examine only one eye be sure to examine both fundi.

Optic disc

Various aspects of the disc have to be assessed:

- size
- colour
- cupping (physiological/pathological)
- vertical cup:disc ratio (VCDR)
- margin/neuroretinal rim
- disc cup rim notches
- baring of a circumlinear vessel
- disc rim haemorrhages
- peripapillary atrophy
- peripapillary pigmentation
- peripapillary retinal nerve fibre layer (RNFL) defects
- swelling
- drusen
- abnormal vessels
- congenital anomalies
- tumour.

In all aspects the degree of symmetry or asymmetry of the disc appearance should be noted.

Disc size

An important point to remember is that large 'physiological' discs tend to have large cups and small 'physiological' discs tend to have small cups – it is the area or volume of the neuro-retinal rim which is more constant. Disc size can be estimated fairly accurately using a 78D diagnostic lens and an adjustable slit beam height (correction factor = ×1.05, i.e. about unity).

Disc colour

A normal disc has a pink coloured neuroretinal rim. Pallor should not be confused with cupping, although, of course, both may co-exist. Confusion is best avoided by stereoscopic examination (slit-lamp biomicroscopy) rather than direct ophthalmoscopy. Generalized pallor with a flat or slightly concave appearance of the disc is a feature of optic atrophy. Bow-tie atrophy (pallor of the temporal and nasal portions of the disc) is a feature of chiasmal and retrochiasmal/pregeniculate lesions. Localized or generalized pallor of the neuroretinal rim, particularly if associated with cupping is a feature of glaucoma. The candidate should remember that a disc in an aphakic or pseudophakic eye appears more pale than in a phakic eye, particularly if there is any nuclear sclerosis.

Disc cupping and the VCDR

Most normal eyes have a VCDR of <0.3, although a VDCR of <0.3 may be pathological in small discs. A VDCR >0.4 should be regarded as suspicious of glaucoma or glaucomatous, the suspicion being less if the disc is large. Most discs with a VCDR of >0.6 are pathological. Asymmetry of VCDRs of >0.2 is highly suspicious of asymmetrical glaucoma.

Other signs of pathological glaucomatous cupping include:

- baring of circumlinear vessels
- sharply sloping or vertical cup walls
- apparent nasal shift of the central retinal artery/vein
- laminar dot sign (visible pores of the laminar cribrosa)
- bayonet sign (double angulation or kinking of blood vessels at the cup margin).

Although relatively uncommon, pathological cupping can occur in patients without glaucoma. Other rare aetiologies of pathological cupping include ischaemia, compression and inflammation.

The neuroretinal rim

In a normal disc the width of the neuroretinal rim follows the 'ISNT rule' where the rim is widest inferiorly, next widest superiorly, then nasally and least wide temporally. With glaucomatous damage, loss of the inferior (especially inferotemporal) and superior rims usually occurs before that of the nasal and temporal rims. In addition to loss of rim width there is also loss of rim thickness and the rim may take on a sloping appearance. Localized notches may be seen and are evidence of more focal damage. A rim notch may be associated with an arcuate shaped retinal NFL defect which are best identified using red-free light. The candidate should remember that nerve fibre layer defects are not specific to glaucoma but may occur in association with optic atrophy. Vessels in the region of a nerve fibre layer defect may appear slightly darker with slightly sharper margins due to loss of their neural covering. Disc rim haemorrhages may precede the development of rim notches and may be seen in early glaucoma. Signs of definite glaucomatous damage include:

- a rim notch
- a thinning of the rim to <10% of the vertical disc diameter
- a rim that is thinner inferiorly than superiorly.

Peripapillary atrophy and hyperpigmentation

These are features of a disc more commonly seen in a myopic eye or an eye of a glaucoma suspect.

Disc swelling

A swollen disc may be due to:

- papilloedema (including benign intracranial hypertension)
- pseudopapilloedema (includes buried drusen)
- malignant hypertension
- papillitis (many causes)
- hypotony
- acute angle closure glaucoma
- ischaemic optic neuropathy
- optic nerve compression
- diabetic papillopathy
- Leber's optic neuropathy
- spheno-orbital meningioma.

NB: Papilloedema is a specific term relating to swollen discs secondary to raised intracranial pressure.

Disc swelling is best identified by fundus stereoscopic biomicroscopy at the slit-lamp. However, various features can be identified by direct ophthalmoscopy, general ophthalmic or systemic examination:

1. *Papilloedema*
   - bilaterality
   - disc hyperaemia
   - peripapillary NFL opacification
   - absence of spontaneous venous pulsation
   - splinter haemorrhages, cotton-wool spots, exudates
   - peripapillary retinal folds
   - macular oedema
   - loss of disc cup
   - optic atrophy (end-stage).
2. *Papillitis*
   - may be unilateral
   - RAPD (if unilateral or asymmetrical)
   - intraocular inflammation (especially vitritis)
   - signs of associated systemic disease (e.g. multiple sclerosis, sarcoid, tuberculosis, syphilis, viral infection such as herpes zoster).

Congenital anomalies

These include:
- hypoplasia
- pit (± serous detachment of the sensory retina)
- coloboma
- tilt
- morning glory syndrome
- peripapillary nerve fibre layer myelination.

Patients with congenital disc anomalies should be examined for associated midfacial maldevelopment (hypertelorism, cleft lip and/or palate) or basal encephalocele and also for visual field defects.

Disc tumours
- melanocytoma
- rare neural tumours.

Macula

Remember that although common things are common, rarities appear in exams. Signs may be unrecognized by the candidate – but if this is the case the candidate should not panic, but methodically describe the lesion(s) in terms of position, distribution and depth within the retina and hope that further clues are forthcoming! Commonly seen signs include those of:

1. *diabetic maculopathy*
   - (microaneurysms, intra-retinal microvascular abnormalities [IRMA's], haemorrhages [dot, blot or flame], exudates [previously called hard exudates], oedema and cotton wool spots [previously misnamed soft exudates], neovascular complexes, traction retinal detachment or opaque membrane formation) and signs of previous laser therapy.
2. *age related macula degeneration*
   - (drusen, RPE pigmentary change, geographical RPE/(chorio-)retinal atrophy, subretinal neovascular membrane, RPE detachment, RPE rip, disciform scarring).

Signs which may be overlooked include:

- cystoid macula oedema
- central serous choroidoretinopathy
- angioid streaks
- lacquer cracks
- epiretinal membrane
- macular hole (full thickness, lamellar, pseudo-)
- myopic maculopathy (includes Fuchs' spot)
- chorioretinal folds
- retinal dystrophies (Best's dystrophy, adult pseudovitelliform macular degeneration, cone dystrophy, pattern dystrophies)
- bull's eye maculopathy
- 'flecked retina' syndromes (Stargardt's fundus flavimaculatus, autosomal dominant familial drusen, fundus albipunctatus, Kandori's syndrome, primary oxalosis)
- 'cherry-red spot' macular syndromes (sphingolipidoses)
- choroidopathies (including MIC and PIC).

Vessels

Follow the vascular arcades into each quadrant starting at the disc. Examine the arteries, veins and perivascular fundus. Look for:

- vessel attenuation, dilation, traction, tortuosity or sheathing
- emboli (describe the type of embolus if possible (dull grey = platelet/fibrin, sparkling yellow = cholesterol, dull white = calcium)
- neovascularization (peripheral or at the disc). There may be evidence for the

aetiology (e.g. diabetic retinopathy, retinal vein occlusion, sickle cell retinopathy)
- telangiectasis
- associated fundal signs.

Specific conditions include:

1. retinal vein occlusion (central, hemisphere, branch or arteriovenous crossing, macular branch, peripheral). Ocular features include dilated tortuous veins, flame haemorrhages, retinal oedema, cotton wool spots and late changes include vascular sheathing, collaterals and exudates. Central or hemisphere retinal vein occlusions may occur due to raised intraocular pressure and signs of glaucoma should be looked for.
2. retinal artery occlusion (central, branch, macular branch, cilio-retinal, pre-capillary). Ocular features include a RAPD, arteriolar narrowing, retinal oedema, 'cherry-red spot' (early sign only), segmentation of the blood column and cotton wool spots.
3. atherosclerotic changes (arterio-venous crossing abnormalities, copper-wire and silver-wire arterioles).
4. hypertensive retinopathy (mild generalized arteriolar attenuation = Grade 1, severe Grade 1 + focal arteriolar stenoses = Grade 2, Grade 2 + haemorrhages, exudates and cotton wool spots = Grade 3, Grade 3 + disc swelling = Grade 4). If hypertension is suspected all possible associated ocular signs should be looked for. These include:
   - atherosclerotic changes
   - retinal vein occlusion (central or branch)
   - a macroaneurysm
   - ischaemic optic neuropathy
   - ischaemic choroidal infarcts (Elschnig spots)
5. sickle cell retinopathy
   - (Proliferative: peripheral arteriolar occlusions, peripheral arteriovenous anastomoses, sea-fan neovascularization, vitreous haemorrhage, retinal detachment)
   - (Non-proliferative: tortuous veins, narrow arterioles, peripheral haemorrhages [salmon patches], peripheral chorioretinal scars [black sunbursts], retinoschisis, retinal holes, vascular occlusions, comma-shaped conjunctival vessels, iris atrophy).

6. retinopathy of prematurity (peripheral vasospasm, silver-grey line [mesenchymal ridge], dilated tortuous veins, retinal haemorrhages, neovascularization, vitreous haemorrhage, retinal detachment).
7. Eales' disease (retinal periphlebitis).
8. Coats' disease or Leber's miliary aneurysms.

Peripheral fundus

Examine each quadrant in turn, perhaps starting with the upper temporal quadrant where the common pathology is slightly more common. Look for:

Normal features of the fundus:
- ora serrata (junction between retina and pars plana)
- dentate processes (triangular extensions of retina at the ora serrata)
- normal neurovascular bundles (long posterior ciliary and short ciliary arteries and nerves, vortex veins)
- peripheral degeneration (microcystoid).

Retinal disorders:
- retinal detachment
  - (acute [rhegmatogenous – see also p. 177, tractional, serous]
  - long-standing [high water marks, retinal thinning, intraretinal cysts]
  - associated ocular signs)
- retinal breaks
  - type [U-tear, round-break, giant-tear]
  - position
  - size
  - number
- retinal dialysis
- subretinal fluid
- evidence of retinal reattachment (chorioretinal scarring, indentation)
- peripheral retinal degenerations (e.g. lattice, snail-track, paving-stone)
- white with or without pressure
- peripheral retinoschisis (look for breaks in both leaves)
- pigmentary retinopathy (retinitis pigmentosa or associated pigmentary retinopathy syndrome, old chorioretinitis, trauma, retinal reattachment)
- cotton wool spots (in the absence of other signs think of AIDS, hypertension, diabetes mellitus, autoimmune disease,

vascular occlusion, haematological abnormality)
- diabetic retinopathy
- retinal tumours (retinoblastoma, haemangioma, astrocytoma).

Chorioretinal, choroid and RPE disorders:
- chorioretinal laser photocoagulation scars (do not confuse with disease – e.g. toxoplasmosis)
- posterior uveitis
  - retinitis (cloudy white retina)
  - choroiditis (pale yellow/grey patches)
  - retinal vasculitis (sheathing)
  - retinal neovascularization
  - characteristic chorioretinal scarring (e.g. toxoplasmosis, toxocara)
  - associated ocular signs (vitritis and snow-banking, exudative retinal detachment, papillitis, optic nerve head granuloma, optic atrophy)
  - infective uveitis (toxoplasmosis, toxocariasis, CMV, tuberculosis, syphilis, herpes simplex, herpes zoster, BARN, candidiasis)
  - specific entities (Behçet's disease, sarcoidosis, intermediate uveitis, VKH syndrome, birdshot retinochoroidopathy, AMPPE, serpiginous choroidopathy, POHS, sympathetic ophthalmitis)
- choroidal dystrophies (choroideraemia, gyrate atrophy, central areolar choroidal atrophy)
- retinal pigment epithelialitis
- choroidal tumours (naevus, melanoma, haemangioma, osteoma, lymphoma [reticulum cell sarcoma], metastases).

Vitreous

- PVD (± Weis ring), syneresis, muscae volantes
- operculae
- haemorrhage (fresh, old or non-clearing)
- proliferative vitreoretinopathy (PVR) (see also p. 179)
- cells, snow-balls, snow-banks, precipitates, veils, pigment
- asteroid hyalosis (small spherical whitish particles, usually unilateral, relatively common)

- synchysis scintillans (highly refractile cholesterol crystals, associated with chronic vitreous haemorrhage or detachment)
- foreign body (size, type, site)
- persistent hyperplastic primary vitreous (anterior or posterior)
- hereditary vitreoretinal degenerations (e.g. Wagner's disease, Stickler's syndrome, familial exudative vitreoretinopathy, congenital retinoschisis, Goldmann–Favre disease)
- optical emptiness (feature of Wagner's hereditary vitreoretinal degeneration)
- amyloidosis.

If no obvious abnormality is found on initial survey double-check for the following since they commonly appear in exams:

- angioid streaks
- choroidal folds
- emboli
- pale disc or disc colour asymmetry
- peripheral retinoschisis
- albinism.

Specific investigations

Amsler grid testing

An Amsler grid or chart consists of a 10 cm square divided into 400 5 mm squares with a central spot. The patient fixates the central spot with one eye and with the chart held at 33 cm is asked to note whether any of the small squares are missing or distorted. The test is useful to screen for macular disorders or detect any change (e.g. the development of a sub-retinal neovascular membrane).

Macular photostress test

A simple test used to detect early macular dysfunction:

- a pre-test visual acuity is recorded
- a bright light is then held 3 cm in front of the patients eye for 10 seconds
- the time taken for recovery to a visual acuity to within a line of the pre-test visual acuity is determined (normal is <1 minute).

The Purkinje vascular entoptic test

A simple but relatively crude test of macular function used for eyes with opaque media:

- the eye is gently massaged, through closed lids, with the lighted end of a bright pen-torch
- if macular function is normal the patient will see a central red area and the super-imposed branching pattern of the retinal vasculature.

Watzke test

A simple slit-lamp test used to help determine the presence of a full thickness macular hole:

- using a 78/90D lens, a thin slit beam of light is projected to cross the suspected lesion and the patient is asked to report whether an unbroken line of light is seen or whether there is a central gap or region of dimness
- a Watzke positive test is relatively common with full thickness macular holes.

Fluorescein angiography

Angiography of the retinal and choroidal circulations is useful in the diagnosis and assessment of change for a multitude of disorders affecting the retinal vasculature, choriocapillaris, Bruch's membrane and/or the RPE. The present text cannot cover all issues and the interpretation of fluorescein angiography. However, a number of key points are listed below:

Fluorescein
- emits light of a longer wavelength when stimulated by light of a shorter wavelength (i.e. fluoresces)
- excitation peak: 490 nm (blue)
- emission peak: 530 nm (green)
- ~ 80% binds to serum proteins (especially albumin)
- ~ 20% is unbound
- under normal conditions fluorescein (bound or unbound) cannot cross the inner blood retinal barrier (retinal capillary endothelial cells and their tight junctions) or the outer blood retinal barrier (the RPE cells and their junctional complexes). Unbound fluorescein, however, is able to leak through the choriocapillaris and Bruch's membrane
- 5 ml of 10% fluorescein is injected intravenously
  - may cause nausea or vomiting
  - discolours urine and skin
  - rarely can cause syncope, bronchospasm and anaphylaxis.

The camera
- a fundus camera with filters (i) allowing red-free photography prior to angiography, (ii) allowing only blue light to enter the eye and a green light to reach the film during angiography
- used to take 15–20 fundus photographs from between 5 and 25 seconds and at 1, 2 and 5 minutes after rapid injection of the fluorescein. Late pictures (10–20 minutes) are taken when indicated.

The angiogram
Phases of the angiogram:
1. *Pre-arterial phase*
   - filling of the choroidal circulation occurs as a generalized flush or in segments
   - the unbound fluorescein rapidly leaks from the choriocapillaris except in areas of choroidal ischaemia
2. *Arterial phase*
   - reaches the retinal circulation about 1 second after the choroidal circulation
3. *Arterio-venous (capillary) phase*
   - complete filling of the arteries and early lamellar flow in the veins
4. *Venous phase*
   - early: complete laminar flow in the veins
   - late: complete venous filling
5. *Late phase*
   - usually shows the effect of recirculation and gradual dilution of the fluorescein but staining or pooling may be evident (see below).

Transit time:
- the normal arm to eye transit time is 15–20 seconds
- normal transit time through the retinal vasculature is within 5 seconds
- the transit time in the perifoveal area is the most rapid and characterized by the best resolution of the capillary bed due to the high level of RPE pigmentation which

blocks out the underlying choroidal fluorescence
- recirculation occurs in normal individuals at about 4 minutes
- transit times are slower in ischaemic conditions such as the ocular ischaemia syndrome.

Interpretation:
1. *Hypofluorescence*
   - reduced or apparently reduced fluorescence
2. *Hyperfluorescence*
   - increased fluorescence
3. *Pseudo-fluorescence*
   - due to leakage of fluorescein into the vitreous cavity
4. *Auto-fluorescence*
   - fluorescence from tissue rather than fluorescein (e.g. optic nerve head drusen)
5. *Pooling*
   - accumulation of dye in a tissue space (e.g. subretinal or between the RPE and Bruch's membrane following RPE detachment)
6. *Staining*
   - attachment of dye to the substance of a tissue (e.g. late staining of vitreo-retinal scars or of the optic nerve head, which is normal)
7. *Blocking*
   - obstruction of the underlying choroidal fluorescence by increased RPE thickness, increased choroidal pigmentation (e.g. naevus), retinal exudate or haemorrhage
8. *Filling defect*
   - area of decreased fluorescence due to occlusion of the choroidal or retinal circulation
9. *Window defect*
   - an area of RPE loss or depigmentation allowing the choroidal fluorescence to be seen more clearly.

Causes of hypofluorescence
- RPE hypertrophy
- cotton wool spots
- abnormal retinal deposits (haemorrhage, exudates, lipofuscin)
- choroidal/retinal vasculature obstruction (non-perfusion).

Causes of hyperfluorescence
- window defect (e.g. RPE atrophy overlying drusen, angioid streaks, associated with bull's eye maculopathy or macular hole)
- pooling (e.g. RPE detachment, central serous choroidoretinopathy)
- breakdown of the inner blood retinal barrier (e.g. macular oedema)
- leakage (e.g. retinal/choroidal neovascularization).

Electrodiagnostic tests

Based on the existence of a standing potential (6 mV) between the retina(−) and cornea(+) generated by the RPE and the photoreceptors.

Electro-oculogram (EOG)
- measured using electrodes placed at the medial and lateral canthi
- the pupils are dilated and the patient is placed in the dark for 15 minutes
- the patient fixates left and right target lights used to induce rhythmic 30° horizontal eye movements. Movements of the anterior-posterior potential induce a current detected by the electrodes which is amplified and recorded
- the dark adapted EOG is then compared to that after exposure to a bright light.

In normals the rise of the light EOG should be >180%. A reduced light rise indicates RPE disease (e.g. Best's disease, chloroquine toxic retinopathy).

Electro-retinogram (ERG)
- generated within the bipolar layer of the retina after photoreceptor stimulation
- measured using an active contact lens electrode placed on the cornea and a reference forehead skin electrode
- the standard ERG is a response to a flash of light
- flicker ERG responses can be recorded using a light flickering up to a frequency of 50Hz after which they are lost (critical flicker fusion frequency)
- pattern ERGs can be recorded but they are rarely used clinically
- ERGs are recorded in both dark-adapted (rod response) and light-adapted (cone response) states

The flash ERG is biphasic:

- a-wave: negative, arises from photoreceptors
- b-wave: positive, arises from the bipolar layer (including the Müller cells). The amplitude is measured from the trough of the a-wave to the peak of the b-wave.

The ERG is useful in the diagnosis and assessment of retinal disorders (e.g. retinal dystrophies, retinitis pigmentosa) but not those of the ganglion cells, optic nerve or retrobulbar pathways.

Visually evoked potentials (VEP)

- generated by retrobulbar neural pathways and the visual cortex (macula dominated)
- an adapted EEG of the retrobulbar neural pathways to the occipital cortex as a response to visual stimuli
- may be stimulated by a flash of light or an alternating chequerboard pattern
- recorded using active occipital scalp electrodes and reference apical scalp electrodes
- the stimulus is repeated as the patient fixates on a central spot
- the responses are averaged by computer averaging
- the amplitude of, and latency to the first peak are measured.

Used in combination with an EOG and ERG the VEP can be used to determine the site of a lesion in the visual system (e.g. a reduced VEP associated with a normal EOG and ERG indicates a lesion between the ganglion cells and the visual cortex). A delay in the VEP indicates possible optic nerve demyelination. Other uses of the VEP include detection of malingering, assessment of visual function in eyes with opaque media and determination of visual acuity in infants (see p. 6).

Ocular ultrasound

- uses high frequency (>18000 Hz) sound to produce reflective echoes from interfaces between acoustically differing structures
- A-scan ultrasonography (time-amplitude scanning) is used to measure the axial length of an eye prior to cataract surgery (biometry)
- B-scan ultrasonography (2-D scanning) is a useful, non-invasive investigation, particularly useful in examination of the eye with opaque media and of the orbit. Interpretation of scans is highly dependent on the skill of the examiner. Scans are useful in the diagnosis of posterior vitreous detachment, retinal detachment, proliferative vitreoretinopathy, choroidal detachments/haemorrhages, raised macular disciform lesions, intraocular foreign bodies, intraocular masses and their nature, posterior scleritis, optic disc cupping and various orbital conditions. Assessment of change (e.g. by measuring diameters and height of choroidal melanomas) can be monitored by B-scan.
- Doppler ultrasonography can be used to investigate vascular flow patterns within the eye and orbit.

Cardiovascular system investigations

- blood pressure
- auscultation (heart and carotids)
- angiography
- ultrasonography
- temporal artery biopsy.

Blood tests

- blood glucose
- ESR
- FBC + platelet count
- coagulation profile
- sickle cell test
- immunology profile.

Checklist for examination of the posterior segment and fundus

History

Symptoms of posterior segment disorders:

- reduced visual acuity
- sudden loss of vision
- obscurations
- amaurosis fugax
- impaired central vision
- reduced light brightness appreciation
- reduced colour vision
- reduced night vision
- positive scotoma
- negative scotoma
- visual distortion
- photopsia
- floaters.

Clinical examination

Optic disc
- size
- colour
- cupping (physiological/pathological)
- vertical cup:disc ratio (VCDR)
- margin/neuroretinal rim
- disc cup rim notches
- baring of the circumlinear vessel
- disc rim haemorrhages
- peripapillary atrophy
- peripapillary pigmentation
- peripapillary retinal nerve fibre layer defects
- swelling
- drusen
- abnormal vessels
- congenital anomalies
- tumour.

Macula
- diabetic retinopathy
- age related macula degeneration
- cystoid macula oedema
- central serous choroidoretinopathy
- angioid streaks
- lacquer cracks
- epiretinal membrane
- macular hole
- myopic maculopathy
- chorioretinal folds

- retinal dystrophies
- bull's eye maculopathy
- 'flecked retina' syndromes
- 'cherry-red spot' syndromes
- choroidopathies.

Vessels
- attenuation
- dilation
- traction
- tortuosity
- sheathing
- emboli
- neovascularization
- telangiectasis
- associated fundal signs
- specific conditions including:
  - retinal vein occlusion
  - retinal artery occlusion
  - atherosclerotic changes
  - hypertensive retinopathy
  - sickle cell retinopathy
  - retinopathy of prematurity
  - Eales' disease (retinal periphlebitis)
  - Coats' disease or Leber's miliary aneurysms.

Peripheral fundus
- normal features
- retinal detachment
- retinal breaks
- retinal dialysis
- subretinal fluid
- retinal reattachment
- peripheral retinal degenerations
- white with or without pressure
- pigmentary retinopathy
- diabetic retinopathy
- retinal tumours
- laser scars
- posterior uveitis
- choroidal dystrophies
- retinal pigment epithelialitis
- choroidal tumours.

Vitreous
- posterior vitreous detachment (PVD)
- operculae
- haemorrhage

▶

◀

- proliferative vitreoretinopathy (PVR)
- cells
- asteroid hyalosis
- synchysis scintillans
- foreign body
- persistent hyperplastic primary vitreous
- hereditary vitreoretinal degenerations
- optical emptiness
- amyloidosis.

Specific investigations

- Amsler grid testing
- Macular photostress test
- The Purkinje vascular entoptic test
- Watzke test
- Fluorescein angiography
- Electrodiagnostic tests
- Ocular ultrasound
- Cardiovascular system investigations
- Blood tests.

11. Refraction

(By Michael Wearne BSc FRCOphth)

History

Age

- infants up to the age of five years may require a cycloplegic refraction with either cyclopentolate or atropine, particularly if there is an esotropia (Oc atropine 1% bd for three days prior to refraction). Beware systemic toxicity: initially restlessness/excitement, dry mouth, flushed appearance, tachycardia, confusion
- over the age of five years, cyclopentolate is often adequate (G cyclopentolate 1% two drops separated by five minutes), waiting a period of 30–40 minutes before retinoscopy
- presbyopia is usually apparent in Caucasians by their mid-forties, but can be 5–10 years earlier in the Afro-Caribbean population
- accommodation is usually 1.0D or less by the age of 60 years in all racial groups.

Current spectacles

- single vision (distance/near)
- bifocals
- multifocals
- tint
- safety/sports goggles.

This information may give a clue about the patient's refractive status (e.g. a 55 year old lady who reads unaided but wears glasses for distance is likely to be a low myope). In addition, such information must be taken into account when prescribing new glasses.

Visual symptoms

- blurred vision (distance, intermediate, near)
- asthenopia ('eye-strain'), often after visually demanding tasks
- diplopia
- scotoma

- glare
- headache (rarely caused by refractive problems).

It is essential to enquire about any visual difficulties, since some refractive errors do not need correcting. Furthermore, some symptoms suggest a particular problem that can be given careful attention (e.g. asthenopia after long periods using a Visual Display Unit may be due to an extra-ocular muscle imbalance).

Occupation/hobbies

Visual demands vary widely, and some occupations require a minimum level of visual acuity:

1. British Army – minimum corrected visual acuity of 6/6 in one eye and not less than 6/36 in the other.
2. Royal Air Force (pilot entry) – 6/12 in each eye separately correctable to 6/6 within the refraction range of −1.25D to +3.00D in any meridian, with an astigmatic element < +1.25D.
3. British Rail (train driver) – 6/9 in one eye and 6/12 or better in the other with glasses if worn; if corrected, the unaided vision must not be worse than 6/12, 6/18.
4. Motor vehicle driver – current requirement is the ability to read a number plate at 20.5 m (67 feet) – approximately 6/10 Snellen equivalent.

Past medical and ophthalmic history

It is important to enquire about:

- general health (e.g. diabetes mellitus)
- medications (e.g. topical miotics, systemic steroids)
- past and present ocular history (e.g. strabismus, amblyopia, aphakia/pseudophakia, family ocular history – glaucoma, retinitis pigmentosa).

Objective/subjective refraction

It is essential to spend a few minutes becoming familiar with the equipment and room layout before starting. Ideally, candidates should take their own equipment to the exam:

- trial frame
- retinoscope
- ophthalmoscope
- occluder/pin-hole
- ruler
- pen-torch
- cross-cylinders (0.50D and 1.00D)
- near fixation target.

In order to refract any patient using a streak retinoscope and negative cylinders, the following routine is suggested:

1. Record monocular visions (see 'Assessment of visual acuity'); glasses belonging to the patient may not be available.
2. Perform a cover test for distance using a suitable fixation target, depending on the vision in the worst eye; it is valuable to know the presence or absence of a strabismus at this stage (see 'Assessment of strabismus').
3. Measure the interpupillary distance (IPD) from limbus to limbus; this is necessary in order to centre the trial frame correctly, and also needs to be documented when prescribing glasses. Remember that in patients with strabismus it is important to occlude one eye at a time when measuring the IPD, and that in infants the best estimate is often the distance from the outer canthus of one eye to the inner canthus of the other eye.
4. Fit the trial frame on the patient and adjust it so that it is comfortable and correctly centred. Place the retinoscopy working distance correction (+1.50D for 0.66 m, +2.00D for 0.50 m) in the back cells of the trial frame, warning the patient that the distance vision is likely to be temporarily blurred.

Objective refraction
- Instruct the patient to fixate on a non-accommodative target (either the green on the duochrome or a white spot light).
- If starting with retinoscopy on the right eye it is necessary to quickly obtain an 'against' movement of the reflex in the left eye, thus ensuring that the eye is slightly 'fogged', which encourages relaxation of accommodation (this is particularly important in children and young hyperopes with active accommodation).
- Neutralize the reflex in the right eye by placing spherical lenses in the front cell of the trial frame (a 'with' movement requires the addition of plus spheres, and an 'against' movement, minus spheres).
- If there is astigmatism present, then neutralize one meridian with spheres to leave an 'against' movement in the other meridian; place a minus cylinder in the trial frame with the axis in the same direction as the long axis of the streak light (remember that the long axis of the streak is at right angles to the power meridian being measured). Modify the power and axis of the cylinder to achieve neutrality.
- The right eye will obviously be 'fogged' by having the working distance in the back cell of the trial frame, and so one can simply move over to perform retinoscopy of the left eye in a similar manner.

Recording retinoscopy findings ('power-cross'): a cross is drawn in the orientation of the principal meridians and the angle of one meridian is marked; the dioptric value of the point of reflex reversal is marked on each meridian and the working distance is recorded.

When transposing into a lens prescription corrected for the working distance, remember that the axis of any cylinder lies at 90° to the angle of the power line. As an example:

$$+1.00/-0.50 \times 140 \text{ (or } +0.50/+0.50 \times 50)$$

NB_1 – if spherical aberrations are present during retinoscopy (e.g. with a widely dilated pupil), concentrate on the central 3–4 mm reflex)

NB_2 – in infants, where speed is essential, it is often helpful to vary the retinoscopy working distance to find the neutral reflex rather than changing lenses

NB_3 – a very dull retinoscopy reflex may be due to high refractive error, and it is worth trying with ±10.0D lenses before stating that there is no useful reflex

NB₄ – consider keratoconus if there is a 'swirly' reflex with a non-definable end-point.

Subjective refraction
- Remove the working distance correction lenses from the back cells of the trial frame and occlude the left eye; check the visual acuity in the right eye and make sure that the spherical component present is the 'best sphere' by adding plus spheres unless there is a reduction in visual acuity. Only modify with minus spheres for a definite improvement in visual acuity (it is essential to relax the patient's accommodation).
- Even if no cylinder was detected on retinoscopy, check for astigmatism (unless the visual acuity is 6/5 or better in both eyes with the spherical correction); the most commonly used method is the cross-cylinder technique. The basis of this technique is that the circle of least confusion is placed on the retina whilst the patient determines which of two lenses, presented in a forced-choice manner, is clearer; the patient will automatically keep the circle of least confusion on the retina if allowed to accommodate. It is therefore beneficial to add −0.50D or −0.75D to the spherical component in the trial frame prior to commencing the cross-cylinder tests in phakic patients (although this does not apply to patients >60 years of age with little or no accommodation).
- Using a suitable target (usually a letter 'O' on the 6/9 line) first verify the cylinder axis. Hold the handle of the cross-cylinder parallel to the axis of the cylinder in the trial frame, and move the angle of the cylinder in the direction of the minus power on the cross-cylinder until no difference is detected between the two choices. Ideally, the patient should appreciate that the two lenses shown make the 'O' appear equally blurred when the correct angle has been found. Now hold first one and then the other axis of the cross-cylinder parallel to the trial frame cylinder (handle of the cross-cylinder at 45°) in

order to check the power component (NB: for every 0.50D added to the cylinder it is necessary to modify the sphere by 0.25D in the opposite direction, in order to help keep the circle of least confusion on the retina). If a large adjustment is required in the cylinder power then it is necessary to go back and recheck the best sphere. Having completed the cross-cylinder testing, add the +0.50D or +0.75D back to the sphere and test the visual acuity. Once again, make sure that no more plus can be added to the sphere without a loss of clarity (if the patient is 6/5 a +0.50D lens should reduce the visual acuity to 6/9 and a +1.00D lens to 6/18). If a final visual acuity of 6/6 or better has not been achieved, then place a pin-hole in front of the eye: any improvement with the pin-hole requires that the refraction be rechecked (especially in the absence of ocular pathology). If no improvement can be achieved with the pin-hole, then occlude the eye and carry out a similar monocular refraction on the other eye.

5. With the monocular refraction completed, record the binocular visual acuity. If the patient has similar visual acuity in both eyes (not more than one line difference between the two eyes and no less than 6/9 in the worst eye), one can check that the accommodation has been relaxed equally in both eyes by performing binocular balancing. The most commonly used method is the Humphriss technique:
   - add +0.75D to the left eye and ask the patient to concentrate on the lowest line that can be read (it is often unchanged from the binocular visual acuity, but not as sharp)
   - offer plus and minus 0.25D spheres to the right eye, but only modify the trial frame spherical correction for a definite improvement in clarity or comfort
   - move the +0.75D to the right eye and repeat the process. If the patient accepts >0.50D in either direction, then recheck the monocular refraction on that side.

6. *Duochrome test*
   - chromatic aberration in the eye means that there is a difference in the refraction of red wavelengths compared to green

wavelengths in the order of 0.50D; this cannot usually be appreciated if the visual acuity is worse than 6/9
- colour blindness is not a contraindication to the test
- the test can be performed either monocularly or binocularly to help determine the end-point of the refraction
- in practice, it is useful to check binocularly that young hyperopes are not overcorrected or that young myopes are not under-corrected (red clearer than green in both cases). However, be aware that the latter statement is controversial, as many texts recommend leaving myopes on the red and therefore under-corrected. In practice most myopes actually dislike being left under-corrected (probably due to the fact that the refraction is carried out at six metres and not infinity, and that the Purkinje shift causes a myopic shift in twilight), and this is a significant cause of non-tolerance to new spectacles.

7. *Maddox rod/wing testing*
- dissociates the eyes to enable testing for extraocular muscle imbalance, which may be difficult to appreciate on a cover test
- place the Maddox rod in front of the right eye (by convention) with the axis of the convex cylindrical lenses horizontal, and direct the patient to fixate on a white spot of light in the distance
- demonstrate that a vertical red line is seen by the right eye, and a white spot of light by the left eye
- horizontal muscle imbalance can be determined by asking the patient to state whether the line is to the right, left or through the centre of the spot
- any deviation is measured by placing prisms in front of the left eye until orthophoria is achieved (remember that if the line is seen to the left of the spot then this is 'X'ed diplopia and signifies an eXo deviation requiring base-in prism)
- now rotate the Maddox rod in order to obtain a horizontal red line in front of the right eye and allow detection of any vertical imbalance (when correcting to orthophoria, remember that the prism in front of the left eye is placed with the base in the opposite direction to the

displacement of the line in front of the right eye)
- the Maddox wing test can be used to assess imbalance for near but needs to be done after the reading addition has been determined in presbyopes
- the findings of both of these techniques must be considered in conjunction with any visual symptoms apparent from the history
- prisms would usually be prescribed on demonstrating increased subjective visual comfort, but the full value of prism found is rarely required, although any vertical deviation is more likely to be significant.

8. *Near addition*
- Either measure the patient's accommodation and then apply the equation:

$$\text{Near addition (D)} = \text{reading distance (D)} \\ - 2/3\text{rds available} \\ \text{accommodation (D)}$$

e.g.   reading distance 33 cm = 3.00D patients accommodation = 3.00D, i.e. 2.00D available accommodation near addition = 3.00 − 2.00 = 1.00D
- Or, more commonly, estimate the near addition from the patients age:

$$\begin{array}{ll} 45\text{–}50 \text{ yrs} = 1.00\text{D} \\ 50\text{–}55 \text{ yrs} = 1.50\text{D} \\ 55\text{–}60 \text{ yrs} = 2.00\text{D} \\ >60 \text{ yrs } = 2.50\text{D} \end{array}$$

- Whichever method is used, it is necessary to incorporate the near addition into the trial frame and check the patient's reading distance and range of clear near vision; any occupational considerations and/or hobbies may also need to be taken into consideration before reaching a final decision.

NB: Be careful not to 'over-plus' the patient for near and make the working distance too short since this is the commonest reason for non-tolerance to new spectacles. Occasionally a higher addition may be required in aphakic/pseudophakic patients, or if there is any ocular pathology.

9. *Final refraction result*
- decide on the final refraction result and write it down for distance and near in a conventional manner

- the glasses prescribed may not always be the exact findings, as there are often other factors to take into account
- astigmatism of >1.00D in children should be fully corrected
- correct any anisometropic hyperopia of >1.00D in children. Modification may be necessary depending on the presence of a latent or manifest deviation
- only change a cylinder axis/power for a definite improvement in visual acuity in adults
- add a prismatic component only if convinced of benefit to vision or comfort
- aphakes and pseudophakes tolerate the full astigmatic correction well
- specify the lens material and type (e.g. glass vs. plastic, single vision, bifocals, multifocals and tint)
- document the IPD and the back vertex distance (BVD) if the lens power is >±5.00D in any meridian
- advise on timing for next refraction (e.g. 6 months for 12 year old myope).

Checklist for refraction

History

- age
- visual symptoms
- occupation/hobbies/driver
- general health/medications
- past ocular history/family ocular history.

Refraction

1. Monocular visions
2. Cover test/IPD
3. Retinoscopy (expressed as power cross)
4. Cross-cylinder
5. ± Binocular balancing
6. ± Duochrome test
7. ± Maddox rod/wing
8. ± Reading addition
9. Conventional documentation of final prescription with IPD (± BVD)
10. Retest date.

Section B
Medical and surgical cases

12. Cataract

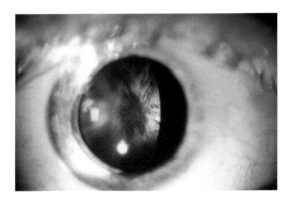

Figure 1 A posterior subcapsular cataract (courtesy of Jane Gardiner MD).

Definition

Any lens opacity.

Classification

May be classified by:

- age (congenital to senile)
- stage (early to hypermature)
- morphological type
- aetiology.

Clinical features

Morphological types of cataract

Capsular
1. *Congenital*:
   - Anterior polar
2. *Acquired*:
   - glassblowers infra-red radiation
   - chlorpromazine toxicity (white-star)
   - alkali burn
   - mercury toxicity (grey).

Subcapsular
1. *Anterior*:
   - Wilson's disease (green sunflower)
   - glaucomflecken
   - topical miotic therapy
2. *Posterior*:
   - senile (cupuliform)
   - secondary: steroid-induced; associated with systemic disease.

Cortical
1. *Congenital*:
   - blue dot
   - coronary
2. *Acquired*:
   - senile (cuneiform).

Nuclear
1. *Congenital*:
   - embryonal
   - lamellar (± riders)
2. *Acquired*:
   - senile nuclear sclerosis.

Exam questions

Question: *What systemic conditions are associated with cataract formation?*

Answer: Development of cataract can be associated with a number of metabolic disorders, certain syndromes, drug toxicity and maternal infections.

Metabolic disorders include:

- diabetes mellitus
- galactosaemia (galactose-1-phosphate uridyltransferase [GPUT] or galactokinase [GK] deficiency)
- hypocalcaemia (hypoparathyroidism or pseudohypoparathyroidism)
- hypoglycaemia
- hypothyroidism

- Wilson's disease (α-2-globulin ceruloplasmin deficiency)
- Lowe's (oculocerebrorenal) syndrome (an inborn error of amino acid metabolism)
- Fabry's disease (α-galactosidase A deficiency)
- Mannosidosis (α-mannosidase deficiency)
- Homocystinuria.

Syndromes include:

- Down's (trisomy 21, mongolism)
- Edwards' (trisomy 18)
- Patau's (trisomy 13)
- Turner's (XO syndrome)
- Cri-du-chat (−5p syndrome)
- Conradi's (autosomal recessive disorder)
- Crouzon's (craniofacial syndrome)
- Marfan's (arachnodactyly)
- Alport's (autosomal dominant renal disorder)
- Werner's (scleropoikiloderma)
- Rothmund's (infantile poikiloderma)
- Schaefer's (congenital dyskeratoses).

Drug toxicity due to the following:

- corticosteroids
- antimitotics
- chlorpromazine
- haloperidol
- topical miotics
- radiation.

Maternal infections include:

- rubella
- cytomegalovirus (CMV) inclusion disease
- toxoplasmosis
- syphilis
- herpes simplex.

Other conditions associated with cataract include:

- atopic dermatitis
- congenital ichthyosis
- pemphigus
- dystrophia myotonica
- syphilis.

Question: *Can the presence of a cataract improve vision?*

Answer: Yes.
The development of a nuclear sclerotic cataract may be associated with the return of clearer near vision in presbyopic individuals. This so-called 'second sight' is thought to be due to the increased refractive power of the nuclear part of the lens as it yellows. The improvement is only temporary, since maturation of the cataract results in increasing opacification. Development of a significant unilateral cataract may also be associated with apparent improvement in vision, or at least reduced visual symptoms, in patients with diplopia, anisometropia or ipsilateral visual symptoms such as glare from corneal disease, vitreous floaters or distortion from macular disease.

Question: *What exactly is phakoemulsification?*

Answer: Phakoemulsification is the currently fashionable method used to perform extracapsular cataract extraction through a small (usually sutureless) incision. A titanium probe vibrating at ultrasonic frequencies (about 40000 cps) is used to disrupt the lens nucleus, which is aspirated through the same probe.

Question: *What is the Irvine–Gass syndrome?*

Answer: This is cystoid macular oedema which develops after cataract surgery, particularly following intracapsular extraction with rupture of the anterior vitreous face or extracapsular surgery with vitreous loss. In the original description, the macular oedema was accompanied by optic nerve head oedema. There is some evidence that the peri-operative use of topical inhibitors of prostaglandin synthesis (e.g. diclofenac) reduces the incidence of this complication. Most cases resolve spontaneously within six months following surgery. Treatment with a low dose of acetazolamide has proved useful in many cases.

Question: *What is Wolter's membrane?*

Answer: This is the ultra-thin proteinaceous membrane that is deposited on intraocular lenses (IOLs) following cataract surgery with IOL implantation. Such membranes which vary in thickness from about 0.01 mm to 0.1 mm, have been demonstrated on polymethyl methacrylate (PMMA), silicone and surface-modified IOLs.

Question: *What are the potential complications of Nd:YAG (neodymium:yttrium–aluminium–garnet) laser capsulotomy?*

Answer: Complications are rare, but include:

- posterior vitreous detachment (PVD)

- retinal breaks
- retinal detachment
- cystoid macular oedema
- macular hole

- transiently raised intraocular pressure (IOP): common
- permanently raised IOP: rare
- laser damage (pitting/cracking) of IOL.

13. Anisocoria

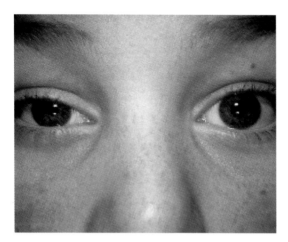

Figure 2 Anisocoria: a right-sided congenital Horner's pupil (courtesy of Duncan Anderson MD).

Definition

Asymmetry of pupil size.

Clinical features

In addition to the asymmetry of the pupils the candidate should ask about symptoms and look for other signs that may aid in making a diagnosis (see 'Examination of the pupils', and below).

Exam questions

Question: *What is the most common cause of anisocoria?*

Answer: Simple or essential anisocoria. This is present in about 20% of individuals in a normal population, is associated with normal pupil reactions and is of no pathological importance.

Question: *What are the features of Adie's tonic pupil?*

Answer: This is a form of benign internal ophthalmoplegia, characterized by:

- pupil dilation
- absent or poor reaction to light
- reduced and slow reaction with accommodation followed by a tonic response (slow dilation) after near vision effort
- sectoral vermiform movements due to segmental iris palsy (with either light or accommodation)
- there is often a temporary accommodative paresis
- there is often supersensitivity to 0.125% (weak) pilocarpine or 2.5% methacholine. If pupil dilation is a problem, treatment with 0.125% pilocarpine can be useful.

The condition, which is usually idiopathic, affects young adults and is more common in women. In 80% of cases the abnormality appears to be unilateral at presentation, but it tends to become bilateral at a rate of about 5% each year. The lesion is located in the ciliary ganglion and is thought to be due in at least some cases to post-viral infection degeneration. The Holmes–Adie syndrome is the association between Adie's tonic pupil and deep tendon hyporeflexia.

Question: *What are the features of Horner's syndrome?*

Answer: The complete picture is rarely clinically apparent, but features include:

- miosis (the anisocoria being greater in dim illumination–dilation lag)
- partial (upper eyelid) ptosis (usually 2–3 mm)
- lower lid elevation (inferior tarsal muscle paresis)
- apparent enophthalmos (actually due to a narrowing of the palpebral aperture)

- ipsilateral hemifacial anhydrosis (if lesion is above bifurcation of the common carotid artery)
- iris heterochromia (affected iris is lighter) in congenital or long-standing cases
- transient fall in IOP, conjunctival vessel dilation, facial flushing and increased accommodative power.

In addition to the ocular and facial features, there may be clinical features associated with the causative lesion.

Question: *How is a suspected case of Horner's syndrome confirmed pharmacologically?*

Answer: The topical cocaine test. Cocaine 4% drops cause dilation of a normal pupil, but no reaction in a Horner's pupil. Thus, instilling cocaine into both eyes increases the anisocoria when there is a Horner's syndrome. The test is based on the fact that cocaine exerts its sympathomimetic effect by blocking noradrenaline receptors at the iris dilator myoneural junction, thus prolonging the dilating effect of noradrenaline. This requires the normal release of noradrenaline at the myoneural junction and therefore only occurs when the normal three neurone oculosympathetic pathway is functioning normally and not when there is a Horner's syndrome.

Question: *How are pre- and postganglionic lesion causes of Horner's syndrome differentiated pharmacologically?*

Answer: Topical hydroxyamphetamine 1% dilates the normal pupil, but only dilates a Horner's pupil normally if the causative lesion is preganglionic (i.e. of the first or second order neurones). The test is therefore ideal for identifying a postganglionic (third order neurone) lesion, when the dilation is subnormal. The test is based on the fact that hydroxyamphetamine exerts its sympathomimetic effect by stimulating release of noradrenaline at the iris dilator myoneural junction. This action is dependent on an intact postganglionic (third order neurone) with normal formation and transfer of noradrenaline at the nerve ending.

An alternative test utilizes topical phenylephrine 1%, which only dilates a Horner's pupil if the causative lesion is postganglionic (i.e. of the third order neurones), on the basis of denervation hypersensitivity.

There is no pharmacological test that can differentiate a Horner's syndrome secondary to a lesion of a first order from a second order neurone.

Question: *What are the causes of anisocoria?*

Answer: The main causes of anisocoria are:

- simple anisocoria
- trauma/iris damage
- posterior synechiae
- Horner's syndrome
- Adie's pupil
- third cranial nerve palsy
- topical drug induced (unilateral administration of a miotic or mydriatic).

14. Manifest concomitant squint (non-paralytic strabismus)

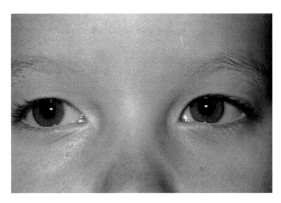

Figure 3 Non-paralytic strabismus: A left esotropia (courtesy of Duncan Anderson MD).

Definition

A manifest squint of consistent size not due to an extraocular muscle paresis or mechanical restriction. This may be a convergent squint (esotropia) or divergent squint (exotropia).

Some terminology

- a 'primary' squint is a squint unrelated to other pathology, in which the deviation is the only known defect
- a 'secondary' squint is a squint related to additional ocular pathology
- a 'consecutive' squint refers to a deviation which replaces a previous squint of opposite direction (e.g. following surgery, or after a long period of time)
- a 'constant' squint occurs at all times
- an 'intermittent' squint only occurs at certain times, or is only manifest for either near or distance fixation
- a 'unilateral' squint affects one eye. The squinting eye fixates when the other eye is covered, but deviates as soon as the cover is removed (i.e. the patient prefers to fixate with the same eye)

- an 'alternating' squint affects both eyes. The squinting eye fixates when the other eye is covered and retains this fixation when the cover is removed whilst the other eye takes up the deviated position (i.e. fixation is possible with either eye)
- a 'concomitant' squint exists when the deviation is of the same size/angle irrespective of which eye is fixating or the position of gaze – it is non-paralytic
- an 'incomitant' squint exists when the size of deviation varies with the position of gaze or depends on which eye is used for fixation – it is usually paralytic or due to mechanical defects, but can be due to unequal accommodative effort in uncorrected anisometropia
- an 'accommodative' squint is influenced by the degree of accommodation being exerted (and can be altered by the correction of a refractive error)
- a 'microtropia' is a manifest squint of <5° or <10D
- 'binocular single vision – BSV' is the normal, simultaneous use of the two eyes in order to produce a single perceived image.

Classification

Esotropia
Primary esotropia (commonest type)

1. *Non-accommodative*
   a) Constant
      - early-onset (infantile) esotropia
      - nystagmus blocking syndrome
      - later-onset esotropia
      - myopia associated esotropia
   b) Intermittent
      - near esotropia
      - divergence insufficiency (distance esotropia)
      - cyclic esotropia

2. *Accommodative*
   - partially accommodative
   - fully accommodative (refractive)
   - convergence excess (non-refractive).

Secondary esotropia (usually associated with visual loss).

Consecutive esotropia (i.e. previously divergent).

Exotropia

Primary exotropia
1. *Constant*
   - early-onset exotropia
   - later-onset/decompensated intermittent exotropia
2. *Intermittent*
   - near exotropia
   - distance exotropia (divergence excess)
   - non-specific.

Secondary exotropia (usually associated with visual loss).

Consecutive exotropia (spontaneous or post-operative).

Clinical features

(See 'Examination of eye movements', p. 14, and 'The cover tests', p. 33.)

Primary esotropia

Early-onset (infantile) esotropia
Onset is before six months of age, and there may be a positive family history. The child is usually systemically normal, but overall there is an increased incidence of associated developmental abnormalities. Refractive error is rare, although there may be low hypermetropia. The squint is constant with a large angle of deviation ($\geq$30D) and is usually alternating, frequently with preference to one eye. Associated features may include:

- crossed fixation
- an abnormal head posture (debatable)
- dissociated vertical deviation (DVD)
- latent (or occasionally manifest) nystagmus
- asymmetrical optokinetic nystagmus (OKN)
- extorsion
- inferior oblique overaction.

Management is surgical, and of any associated amblyopia. Ideally, surgical correction should be performed before two years of age. The patients never achieve normal BSV; the best one can expect is a microtropia. Some patients have no sign of binocularity, with alternating suppression and a lack of retinal correspondence. Surgery can be either bimedial recessions or a recession/resection procedure. Both types of surgery can work, but the disadvantage of bimedial recessions is that further surgery to the medial rectus is less satisfactory in the cases when, postoperatively, there is a significant esotropia for near. However, it seems to be a good procedure for the smaller alternating squint. Postoperatively, the patients need to be carefully monitored for amblyopia. Some children stop alternating, so the parents think that they are cured and fail to bring them back for follow-up and amblyopia ensues.

Nystagmus blocking syndrome
(See p. 82.)

Late-onset esotropia
Presentation is usually at two to four years of age. The squint is constant with a large angle of deviation, and associated features include:

- emmetropia or low hypermetropia
- non-accommodative
- normal retinal correspondence and fusion.

Management is surgical, and of any associated amblyopia.

Myopia associated esotropia
This is uncommon, usually presents in adulthood (although occasionally in childhood) and is associated with moderately high or high myopia. The squint is constant, and the degree of deviation tends to increase with time. Additional features may include:

- other features of myopia
- limitation of abduction
- normal retinal correspondence and fusion.

Management is essentially conservative, surgery being risky and results poor due to scleral thinness.

Near esotropia
Presentation is usually in childhood or early adulthood. The squint is intermittent, being

manifest for near and controlled for distance (i.e. there is BSV for distance). The condition looks like convergence excess but is not accommodative. Other features may include:

- emmetropia or low hypermetropia
- a normal (or even low) AC/A ratio
- no influence of refractive correction
- rare, early presentation (at less than one year) often associated with some esotropia for distance, amblyopia, and nystagmus
- superior oblique underaction.

Management involves correction of any ametropia and surgery (bilateral medial rectus recessions).

Divergence insufficiency (distance esotropia) (less common)

Onset may be at any age, the most common initial symptom being homonymous diplopia with distance fixation. The patient is usually emmetropic and the squint is intermittent, being manifest for distance but controlled for near. Abduction is normal for both eyes. Amblyopia is not a feature. Management involves exclusion of intracranial pathology (i.e. a mild sixth cranial nerve palsy or divergence paralysis – rare), and treatment with base-out prisms if the angle of deviation is small or surgery (bilateral lateral rectus resections) for stable larger deviations.

Cyclic esotropia (alternate day squint)

Presentation of this time-dependent, intermittent squint is usually at about four to five years of age. The squint is intermittent with respect to time, rather than distance. The unilateral squint occurs at regular intervals of time, with normal BSV present at other times. A 48-hour cycle is common, although phases of strabismus and normality are not always equal. Diplopia is not usually a feature. Other features include:

- emmetropia
- no amblyopia
- no latent deviation during normal phases
- development of a constant esotropia with time (usually within a year).

Management is surgical, once the deviation has become constant.

Partially accommodative esotropia

Onset is at one to three years of age in a hypermetropic child. The squint is usually unilateral, the deviation being maximum with near fixation and reduced with distance fixation or the hypermetropic correction. It is a constant type of squint with an accommodative element. Other features include:

- astigmatism and/or anisometropia
- amblyopia
- inferior oblique overaction (uni- or bilateral).

Management involves cycloplegic refraction, correction of hypermetropia, assessment of BV to determine whether the outcome will improve function as well as cosmesis, treatment of amblyopia and surgery. If there is fusion, the visual axes should be placed parallel and regular orthoptic follow-up organized so as to maintain it. If there is no BV the deviation should be slightly under-corrected, since the risk of consecutive exotropia is relatively high.

Fully accomodative esotropia (refractive esotropia)

Onset is usually at two to five years of age, and occurs due to uncorrected moderate hypermetropia. There is frequently a positive family history. Presentation of the intermittent squint occurs when the child is tired or suffering a febrile illness. The child attempts to clear the blurred image induced by the hypermetropia by accommodating, and this results in the esotropia (i.e. there is a manifest squint without glasses when accommodating). The deviation is usually similar in degree for both near and distance fixation. Other features include:

- normal BSV with glasses
- occasionally a microtropia (with anomalous BSV)
- a normal AC/A ratio
- usually no amblyopia.

Management is usually successful with correction of the hypermetropia alone. The child should be given glasses with the full plus correction. When older, orthoptic exercises are useful to teach the child to control the squint without glasses. The exercises include the teaching of diplopia appreciation (without glasses), the joining of diplopia images by relaxing accommodation, and improving negative relative convergence so as to see clearly (i.e. obtain good BSV without squinting). Eventually most patients are able to leave their glasses of less than +3.00DS off; others keep glasses for close work.

Accommodative esotropia with convergence excess (non-refractive esotropia)

This type of squint has many similarities to a fully accommodative (refractive) esotropia, but is due to a high AC/A ratio rather than hypermetropia. The refraction is often of mild hypermetropia (i.e. normal for age). Similarities include:

- onset between two to five years of age
- intermittent
- normal BSV for distance
- occasionally a microtropia (with anomalous BSV)
- usually no amblyopia.

Differences include:

- a high AC/A ratio (e.g. >6:1)
- mild hypermetropia, emmetropia or mild myopia rather than moderate hypermetropia
- deviation greater for near fixation relative to distance fixation.

Management requires:

- correction of refractive error (slight under-correction if myopic)
- treatment of amblyopia if required
- conservative therapy (miotics, executive bifocals, contact lenses, orthoptic exercises) if appropriate, but,
- surgery (bimedial recessions or Faden) if the deviation is large, the AC/A ratio is very high or conservative therapy fails.

Primary exotropia

Early-onset exotropia

Onset of this rare form of squint is before six months of age, and is often associated with neurological abnormalities. Refractive error is rare. The squint is usually constant with a large angle of deviation (≤30D). Associated features include:

- homonymous (uncrossed) fixation in some alternating cases
- DVD
- nystagmus
- closure of one eye in bright light.

Management involves careful fundal examination to exclude pathology (secondary exotropia), followed by surgery when the deviation is stable.

Later-onset exotropia

This constant squint is usually due to decompensation of an intermittent exotropia.

Near exotropia

Onset is usually in late childhood or adulthood, with diplopia on near fixation, jumbling of print, blurred vision or asthenopia and headaches induced by attempts to control the intermittent squint. Additional features include:

- poor binocular convergence (i.e. convergence weakness)
- normal retinal correspondence and fusion
- myopia (in some cases)
- no amblyopia
- no closure of one eye in bright light.

Management involves correction of refractive error and orthoptic exercises if the patient has symptoms. It is important that the patient is taught to perform relaxation exercises after convergence exercises to avoid precipitating accommodative spasm. Base-in prisms for near vision or surgery (bimedial resections) may be required if conservative therapy fails. If the patient is hypermetropic, the refractive error should be under-corrected. If the patient is myopic, a full correction should be provided – this alone may abolish the exotropia.

Distance exotropia (intermittent divergence excess)

Onset is at two to five years of age, and the squint tends to occur when the child is tired or ill. The squint is greater for distance fixation than for near fixation. Associated features include:

- suppression or abnormal retinal correspondence when the deviation is manifest
- closure of one eye in bright light
- may decompensate to cause a constant later-onset exotropia.

Simulated (cf. true) exotropia differs in that the angle measures the same for distance and near if tested with a +3.00DS or prolonged occlusion. Management of a true distance exotropia includes full-correction of any myopia, under-correction of any hypermetropia, and in most cases surgery (bilateral lateral rectus recessions), although the ideal age for this is unknown. Late surgery (e.g. at about six years of age) has the advantage that more accurate preoperative measurements can be made. An additional problem with surgery in the younger patient is that if there is any post-operative over-correction, there will be rapid development of suppression, amblyopia and loss of binocularity. Some clinicians favour early surgery on the grounds that normality may be achieved as early in life as possible. However, if the control for near deteriorates, surgery should be considered whatever the age. Management of a simulated distance exotropia is similar, although for surgery, a unilateral recession/resection procedure is favoured.

The results are not always as good as they should be in theory with a patient who has fusion and good visual acuity. Redivergence is relatively common, and the best results tend to occur when there has been a small over-correction with diplopia in the early post-operative period.

Non-specific intermittent exotropia
This type of exotropia is characterized by being intermittent at any distance.

Exam questions

Question: *What are the features of a consecutive exotropia?*

Answer: By definition, a consecutive exotropia follows a primary esotropia. Onset may be either spontaneous or occur following surgical correction of the primary squint. The patient may complain of diplopia, but the usual symptom is of poor cosmesis. When spontaneous, the exotropia develops in late childhood or adulthood and is most common in patients with hypermetropia and no fusion. The post-operative type may be immediate or may develop after a long period of time. The latter is more common in patients whose esotropia developed

at an early age, those with amblyopia and/or marked hypermetropia and when there has been failure to slightly over-correct the primary deviation. There is usually poor or no fusion. Management includes a reduction of the hypermetropic correction. Surgery may be required to improve the cosmetic appearance.

Question: *What are the features of secondary strabismus (exotropia and esotropia), and what are the principles behind their management?*

Answer: Secondary strabismus occurs when there is severe visual loss in one eye, or asymmetrical visual disturbance. With long-standing severe visual loss in one eye, adults with secondary strabismus usually develop an exotropia. Rarely, secondary exotropia occurs in childhood, although it is much more common for a child's eye with poor vision to converge due to powerful convergence and accommodative reflexes. Congenital or infantile loss of function may result in either a secondary esotropia or an exotropia. Management of secondary squints involves correction of any visual loss where possible. Surgery should be avoided until the deviation is known to be stable, and in cases where intractable diplopia will occur post-operatively. If there is no risk of diplopia, cosmetic surgery performed on the eye with poor vision may be indicated. For a longer lasting result, the surgery should aim for a slight eso-deviation post-operatively. Surgery on severely abnormal eyes may carry additional risks, such as anterior ischaemia or prolonged painful post-operative inflammation. In the latter cases, the use of botulinum toxin or the fitting of a cosmetic contact lens may be the most appropriate forms of management.

Question: *What is the nystagmus blocking syndrome?*

Answer: Also known as the nystagmus compensation syndrome, this occurs in some patients with manifest congenital nystagmus that is characterized by horizontal increased oscillations on abduction and decreased oscillations on adduction. It is a 'physiological-like' process, the aim of which is to minimize the amount of nystagmus. Features include:

- onset within the first six months of life
- adduction of the fixing eye
- a head turn towards the side of the fixing eye

- esotropia of the non-fixing eye
- bilateral pseudo-palsy of abduction
- occurs for near and distance vision
- amblyopia is common
- a high incidence of neurological abnormalities.

The condition may be confused with infantile esotropia (large angle, early onset esotropia), but the angle may be variable and it may have been noticed that the squint was preceded by nystagmus.

Surgery, with a medial rectus recession and a lateral rectus resection, may be successful, but there is some controversy as to which eye should undergo surgery and the results in general are unpredictable. In view of this, some advocate that the surgery should be in the form of bimedial recessions and Faden procedures.

Question: *What is amblyopia and how is it classified?*

Answer: The term amblyopia (Greek – amblus: dull, dim) refers to reduced visual acuity that is unrelated to a pathological obstruction to vision, and that persists following correction of refractive error. The types of amblyopia include:

- strabismic (squint related)
- stimulus deprivation (e.g. related to congenital cataracts – may be uni- or bilateral)
- anisometropic (differing refractive errors in the two eyes)
- ametropic (high bilateral refractive error, includes meridional when there is high astigmatism).

Question: *Is amblyopia a frequent finding in patients with an infantile esotropia?*

Answer: No, this is relatively rare because most infants with an infantile esotropia have alternate fixation in the primary position of gaze and crossed fixation on lateral gaze. Crossed fixation is such that the child uses the right eye to fixate in the left visual field and the left eye to fixate in the right visual field. However, there is a risk of amblyopia in the rare cases with non-alternating strabismus. If untreated, the amblyopia develops in the non-preferred eye, which may have eccentric fixation.

Question: *What is a pseudo-squint?*

Answer: A pseudo-squint is the deceptive appearance of a squint when a 'true' squint is not present and BSV is maintained constantly.

Pseudo-esotropia is most commonly diagnosed in patients with prominent epicanthal folds, which result in the apparent shift of the globe nasally. Other causes of pseudo-esotropia include facial asymmetry, a wide flat nasal bridge, a narrow IPD (interpupillary distance), enophthalmos and a negative angle kappa (nasal shift of the fovea).

Pseudo-exotropia is less common, but may occur with facial asymmetry, exophthalmos, a wide IPD (hypertelorism), an increased positive angle kappa (temporal shift of the fovea) or iris heterochromia, when the eye with the lighter iris appears to diverge.

Pseudo-hypertropia may be seen in patients with an ipsilateral unilateral ptosis or asymmetrical bilateral ptosis.

Pseudo-hypotropia may be present in an eye with a coloboma, although there may well be a true squint in addition.

It is particularly important to exclude retinopathy of prematurity or other posterior segment pathology with displacement of the fovea before making the diagnosis of a pseudo-squint in isolation.

Question: *What are 'A-' and 'V-' patterns?*

Answer: These terms are used to describe deviations which vary in horizontal degree as patients alter their vertical fixation. An A-pattern is associated with increased convergence/decreased divergence on elevation and increased divergence/decreased convergence on depression. A V-pattern is the opposite. It is thought that A-patterns are often due to bilateral superior oblique overactions, and that V-patterns are often due to bilateral inferior oblique overactions. However, there are other theories.

Question: *What is asthenopia?*

Answer: This term is more commonly called 'eye-strain', the symptoms of which may occur due to the attempted maintenance of binocular single vision. The symptoms include 'eye-ache', headache, nausea, dizziness, blurred vision, photophobia, difficulty in changing focus and poor judgement of distance.

Question: *What is a heterophoria, how are the different types classified, and how are patients affected managed?*

Answer: A heterophoria is a latent deviation/squint, which is held in check by fusion. It is classified by direction and according to the distance at which the angle is the greatest:

1. *Esophoria*
   - convergence excess (>N)
   - divergence weakness (>D)

2. *Exophoria*
   - divergence excess
   - convergence weakness

3. *Hyperphoria*
   - usually incomitant.

Small degrees of heterophoria are normal and require no treatment. Management of significant heterophoria should be conservative in the first instance. As in tropias, +ve lenses improve esophorias and −ve lenses improve exophorias. Orthoptic exercises should be tried if the fusion range is reduced. If symptoms persist, or if the phoria is vertical, prisms should be tried. Surgery should be considered if the angle is large, especially if the patient is young and does not wear glasses. If the deviation is greater for near, a greater amount of surgery should be performed on the medial recti. If the deviation is greater for distance, a greater amount of surgery should be performed on the lateral recti. The use of botulinum toxin can be useful to reduce the angle in these cases. Control can be improved as the effect of the toxin wears off.

Question: *What is orthophoria?*

Answer: This term indicates perfect alignment of the eyes, with neither eye having a tendency to deviate when fusion is artificially interrupted (e.g. on cover testing). Orthophoria is rare, and most 'normal' individuals have a small degree of heterophoria.

Question: *What is a binocular visual acuity (BVA), and why is it of value in the assessment of strabismus?*

Answer: Binocular visual acuity, as the name implies, is a visual acuity obtained using both eyes. This measurement is useful in all patients since it is the visual acuity that is actually used outside the clinic setting and is used in the assessment of intermittent squints to record the lowest Snellen visual acuity line that can be seen while maintaining BSV. If a near BVA is not obtained it is easy to mistake a convergence excess type of squint for a fully accommodative type of squint.

Question: *What is a microtropia?*

Answer: A microtropia is a small angle manifest squint of <5° or <10D. The patient with microtropia has subnormal binocular vision and gross stereopsis, and may have an associated condition (e.g. a fully accommodative squint or convergence deficiency). There is some form of binocular function, usually ARC but sometimes NRC with central suppression and peripheral fusion. Patients may have central or eccentric fixation. If the eccentric point coincides with the point used for ARC, then the condition is known as a microtropia with identity. In this condition at cover testing, no manifest squint is observed, but a small central suppression scotoma can be detected using the four dioptre prism test – this is common with anisometropic amblyopia.

15. Optic atrophy

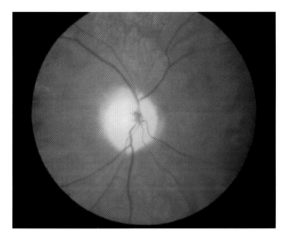

Figure 4 Optic atrophy: disc pallor associated with optic atrophy secondary to demyelination (courtesy of Peng Khaw PhD MRCP FRCS FRCOphth).

Definition

Atrophy of the optic nerve due to degeneration of axons between the retina and the lateral geniculate nuclei.

Classification

Congenital/hereditary/familial
- *Autosomal dominant*
  - Kjer's/infantile/juvenile
- *Autosomal recessive*
  - congenital/simple
  - Behr's/complicated
  - diabetic (± deafness)
- *Mitochondrial disease*
  - Leber's disease.

Consecutive (following retinal ganglion cell axon injury/death)
- traumatic (e.g. physical, radiation)
- compressive (e.g. tumours, aneurysm, dysthyroid eye disease, Paget's disease)

- vascular (e.g. ischaemic optic neuropathy, central retinal artery occlusion [CRAO])
- inflammatory (e.g. syphilis, Behçet's disease)
- infiltrative (e.g. sarcoidosis, lymphoma, leukaemia)
- toxic (e.g. drug-induced, nutritional deficiency)
- degenerative (e.g. retinitis pigmentosa)
- metabolic (e.g. mucopolysaccharidoses)
- demyelination
- paraneoplastic
- glaucoma.

Secondary
- following papillitis
- following chronic papilloedema.

Clinical features

Ophthalmoscopic appearance

- pallor of the disc
- flattening of the neuroretinal rim
- exposure of the lamina cribrosa
- attenuation of the retinal arteries
- nerve fibre layer defects.
- disc cupping (in the absence of glaucoma)

Exam questions

Question: *What is Wallerian degeneration?*

Answer: When an axon is cut, the segment that ascends towards the brain atrophies, disintegrates and eventually disappears. This is called Wallerian degeneration. If an optic nerve axon is cut, Wallerian degeneration takes approximately one week. The segment of the axon connected to the ganglion cell body also undergoes degeneration, but this only occurs after a delay of about a month (descending degeneration).

Question: *What is bow-tie optic atrophy?*

Answer: This refers to a specific pattern of nerve fibre layer and optic nerve atrophy, characterized by a bow-tie shaped or horizontal band of disc pallor, which is occasionally seen in an eye contralateral to an optic tract lesion. There is atrophy of nasal and temporal parts of the disc with relative sparing of superior and inferior arcuate bundles, since these arise from ganglion cells both temporal and nasal to the disc. The optic tract lesion will also give rise to an incongruous homonymous hemianopia.

Question: *What are the features and causes of toxic optic neuropathy?*

Answer: Toxic optic neuropathy is a bilateral retrobulbar optic neuropathy characterized by central or centrocaecal visual field defects, occasional peripheral visual field constriction, reduced colour perception and eventual severe visual loss. In its early stages, the disc may appear normal or even hyperaemic, but it can become pale eventually. If recognized early enough and administration of the toxin is stopped, recovery can occur. In some cases there appears to be a response to therapy with hydroxocobalamin.

Causes include toxicity from drugs such as:

- ethambutol
- isoniazid
- streptomycin
- chloramphenicol
- chloroquine
- chlorpropamide
- digitalis

or from heavy metals and other toxins such as:

- lead
- arsenic
- hexachlorophene.

Question: *What is tobacco–alcohol amblyopia?*

Answer: This has similar clinical features to toxic optic neuropathy, classically with characteristic bilateral centrocaecal visual field defects and associated atrophy of the papillomacular bundle. As the name implies, it occurs in individuals who smoke tobacco and drink alcohol to excess. It is unknown whether the condition is due to a deficiency of Vitamin B (cobalamin [B_{12}], pyridoxine [B_6], thiamine [B_1], riboflavin [B_2], niacin) and/or folic acid, a toxic effect of cyanide, or a combination of deficiency and toxicity.

Question: *What is Leber's optic atrophy?*

Answer: This is a hereditary optic neuropathy, frequently due to a point mutation of mitochondrial DNA at position 11778 (60%), 3460 (25%), 14484 or 4160. It thus affects males, whereas females can only be carriers of the condition. It usually presents between 10 and 30 years of age with sudden loss of vision (to 6/60 or less) and a centrocaecal visual field defect in one eye, followed by a similar event in the fellow eye a few weeks or months later. The classic clinical signs are of peripapillary telangiectasia (with no leakage from the telangiectatic vessels at fluorescein angiography), pseudo-oedema of the disc and vessel tortuosity, although a normal fundal appearance does not exclude the diagnosis. There is no effective treatment, vision usually remains severely impaired, and these patients eventually develop optic atrophy. The different mitochondrial genotypes are associated with some variation in phenotype. Patients with a 14484 mutation, for example, have associated neurological manifestations and recovery of vision. It is an important diagnosis to recognize, so as to avoid unnecessary investigations.

16. Internuclear ophthalmoplegia (INO)

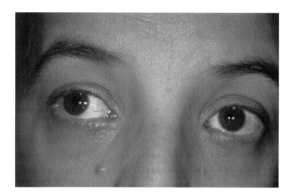

Figure 5 Internuclear ophthalmoplegia: reduced adduction of the left eye on attempted right gaze in a woman with multiple sclerosis (courtesy of Duncan Anderson MD).

Definition

An ophthalmoplegia due to a lesion in the medial longitudinal fasciculus, which disrupts the connection between the contralateral para-median pontine reticular formation (PPRF) and the ipsilateral third cranial nerve nucleus.
NB: The PPRF is also known as the 'horizontal gaze centre'.

Clinical features

Symptoms

There may be diplopia, but this is not always a feature.

Eye movements

- reduced or absent adduction on attempted conjugate gaze away from the side of the lesion
- abduction/ataxic nystagmus of the 'normally' abducting eye on attempted conjugate gaze away from the side of the lesion
- apparent normal medial rectus function upon convergence (Cogan's posterior INO)
- thus the lesion is on the same side as the eye with the adduction weakness.

An INO can be unilateral or bilateral, and if bilateral, may be symmetrical or asymmetrical.

Exam questions

Question: *What is the most likely cause of an INO in a young patient?*

Answer: Demyelination.

Question: *What is the most likely cause of an INO in a patient over 50 years of age?*

Answer: Brainstem vascular disease, usually due to arteriosclerosis.

Question: *What is Cogan's anterior INO?*

Answer: This is usually a bilateral INO with an associated failure of convergence. It occurs secondary to a mesencephalic lesion.

Question: *What is WEBINO syndrome?*

Answer: This is the occurrence of exotropia in a patient with a bilateral INO – the so-called Wall Eyed Bilateral Inter-Nuclear Ophthalmoplegia. The most common causes are multiple sclerosis or brainstem vascular disease.

Question: *What is the 'one-and-a-half syndrome'?*

Answer: This syndrome is characterized by a pontine gaze palsy to the ipsilateral side together with an INO on gaze to the contralateral side. The condition is due to a unilateral pontine lesion, which affects the PPRF and the ipsilateral medial longitudinal fasciculus (MLF). Thus a right-sided lesion results in an inability to move the eyes horizontally except for left eye abduction, and this occurs with ataxic nystagmus.

17. Papilloedema

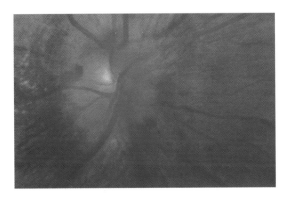

Figure 6 Papilloedema secondary to cerebral metastases (courtesy of Duncan Anderson MD).

Definition

Bilateral optic disc swelling secondary to raised intracranial pressure.

Do NOT use the term 'papilloedema' to describe a 'swollen disc' unless the cause is known to be (or is thought to be) due to raised intracranial pressure.

Clinical features

Stages

1. *Acute (non-decompensated)*
   - mild nerve fibre layer (NFL) swelling at disc margin
   - disc capillary dilation/hyperaemia
   - absence of spontaneous venous pulsation
   - peripapillary haemorrhages
   - peripapillary retinal folds (concentric striae)
2. *Acute (decompensated)*
   - gross NFL swelling with vessel masking, loss of any cup and disc tissue elevation
   - gross disc hyperaemia
   - peripapillary cotton wool spots
   - peripapillary and disc haemorrhages
   - peripapillary retinal folds
   - macular oedema
3. *Chronic/vintage*
   - champagne cork appearance
   - macular star
   - resolving peripapillary and disc haemorrhages
4. *End-stage*
   - peripapillary gliosis
   - optic atrophy (pale, flat disc)
   - arteriolar attenuation and sheathing.

Exam questions

Question: *Does raised intracranial pressure always cause papilloedema?*

Answer: No. The level of intracranial pressure has to be sufficiently raised for at least 24 hours and often up to five days (unless there has been an acute massive intracranial bleed) to produce it. Even if this is the case, papilloedema may not be clinically apparent in an eye with optic atrophy or high myopia.

Question: *What are the ocular symptoms of early papilloedema?*

Answer: Vision is usually good in the early stages, and transient visual obscurations are commonly the only symptoms reported. These occur in about 25% of cases, last less than one minute and are characterized by sudden blurring of vision and reduced colour vision. There may be associated diplopia secondary to a sixth cranial nerve palsy.

Question: *What is the pathogenesis of early papilloedema?*

Answer: It is thought that early papilloedema occurs when the raised intracranial CSF pressure around the optic nerve results in transudation of fluid into the nerve with subsequent obstruction of axoplasmic transport, particularly at the relatively inelastic lamina cribrosa. It is the intra-axonal swelling of optic disc axons with accumulation of mitochondria and not extracellular extravasation of fluid that is considered to be the main cause of the early disc swelling. Vascular changes and oedema are thought to be later, secondary changes.

Question: *How long does resolution of papilloedema take?*

Answer: Following normalization of intracranial pressure, resolution of fully established papilloedema takes six to eight weeks. If optic atrophy follows, it usually takes about six to eight months to develop.

Question: *What are Uhthoff's and Pulfrich's phenomena?*

Answer: These are phenomena usually associated with optic neuritis secondary to demyelination (and not papilloedema). Uhthoff's phenomenon refers to blurring of vision that occurs with physical exertion or during a hot bath. Pulfrich's phenomenon refers to impairment of depth perception, particularly with moving objects.

Question: *What are the causes of optic disc swelling?*

Answer: There are numerous causes of optic disc swelling, including:

- papilloedema
- optic neuritis/papillitis (demyelination, inflammatory eye disease, idiopathic)
- ischaemic optic neuropathy
- central retinal vein occlusion
- ocular hypotony
- diabetic papillitis
- malignant hypertension
- toxic optic neuropathy
- Leber's optic neuropathy
- optic nerve compression (e.g. glioma, meningioma)
- 'pseudo-swelling' of infiltrative optic neuropathy (e.g. lymphoma, leukaemia, metastasis), of congenital optic disc anomalies (e.g. tilted disc, coloboma, hypoplasia, morning-glory syndrome, peripapillary nerve fibre myelination, optic disc drusen), and of hypermetropia.

18. Nystagmus

Definition

An involuntary, rhythmic (to-and-fro) oscillation of the eyes.

Classification by aetiology

1. Physiological
2. Pathological
   - congenital;
   - acquired
   - localizing or specific;
   - non-localizing or non-specific
3. Idiopathic (drug-induced)
4. Hysterical ('voluntary').

Clinical features

Although it is not always available in short case examinations, the clinical history can aid in making a diagnosis. Key points to ascertain are:

- whether the nystagmus is congenital or acquired
- whether there is associated ocular, neurological or vestibular disease
- any drug history
- any family history (congenital nystagmus can be X-linked or autosomal dominant).

The eye movements should be carefully examined, and the nystagmus defined in terms of its type, plane, rate, amplitude and symmetry.

Classification by examination

1. *Type*:
   - jerk
   - pendular
2. *Plane*:
   - horizontal
   - vertical
   - rotary
   - circular
   - mixed
3. *Rate*:
   - rapid/fast
   - slow
4. *Amplitude*:
   - coarse
   - fine
5. *Symmetry*:
   - conjugate
   - dissociated
6. *Constancy*:
   - constant
   - periodic/cyclical.

In addition to examination of the nystagmus, it is important to examine:

1. The patient in general (signs of potentially causative neurological and vestibular disease: stroke, demyelination, head trauma/surgery, deafness, vertigo)
2. Visual acuity
3. Eye movements and cover tests
4. Anterior segment (e.g. congenital cataracts, buphthalmos, aniridia, ocular albinism)
5. Posterior segment (e.g. optic nerve or macular hypoplasia, retinopathy of prematurity)
6. Head posture and movements (spasmus nutans).

Specific, localizing, pathological nystagmus

Latent
- congenital
- a jerk nystagmus occurring when one eye is covered, in a direction away from the covered eye
- onset associated with a fall in visual acuity
- often associated with a DVD and strabismus.

Spasmus nutans

- congenital, with onset before two years of age
- characterized by head nodding, head turn and nystagmus, which is often asymmetrical
- a pendular horizontal or vertical nystagmus of low amplitude but high frequency
- resolves by three years of age (but need to exclude glioma).

Downbeat

- a vertical jerk nystagmus with a downwardly directed fast phase
- often increases with lateral gaze
- due to a lesion at the cervicomedullary junction near the foramen magnum (e.g. Arnold–Chiari malformation, demyelination, brainstem cerebrovascular accident.

Upbeat

- a vertical jerk nystagmus with an upwardly directed fast phase
- can be congenital, drug-induced or due to brainstem disease.

See-saw (see p. 92)

Convergence-retraction

- jerk retraction movements due to co-contraction of extra-ocular muscles on attempted convergence or up gaze.

Periodic alternating

- a cyclical, horizontal, jerk nystagmus
- the fast component occurs in one direction for one to two minutes, and then (after a short rest period of about five seconds) the nystagmus returns with the fast component in the opposite direction for one to two minutes. After another rest period the cycle repeats
- can be congenital, due to vestibulo-cerebellar disease (vascular, demyelinating or degeneration) or associated with severe bilateral visual loss.

Vestibular

- a horizontal or rotary jerk nystagmus which usually lessens with fixation
- due to a disorder of the vestibular apparatus, the eighth cranial nerve or nucleus (i.e. can be peripheral or central)
- often associated with deafness, tinnitus and/or vertigo (particularly with peripheral lesions).

Dissociated

- asymmetrical nystagmus with the nature (e.g. plane or amplitude) of the nystagmus differing between left and right eye
- usually indicates posterior fossa disease
- occurs with the ataxic nystagmus of an INO.

Sensory deprivation (see p. 92)

- always occurs when visual loss occurs before two years of age
- does not occur when visual loss occurs after six years of age.

Non-specific, non-localizing, gaze-evoked, pathological nystagmus

Differs from specific, localizing nystagmus:

- non-localizing nystagmus is not present with the eyes in the primary position of gaze
- occurs with eccentric gaze, with the direction of the fast phase in the direction of the gaze.

The nystagmus is usually due to either drug toxicity or posterior fossa disease (bilateral brainstem and/or cerebellar disorders), but does not aid specific lesion localization.

Exam questions

Question: *What is a jerk(!)?*

Answer: A 'jerk' refers to the movement of an eye with jerk nystagmus. Jerk nystagmus is characterized by phases of unequal velocity, one fast and one slow, and the direction of the nystagmus is defined as the direction of the fast component. The amplitude of 'jerk' nystagmus often increases when gaze is in the direction of the fast phase (Alexander's rule), and may have a null zone (that is, a field of gaze in which the amplitude of nystagmus is minimal and the visual acuity maximum). The null zone may coincide with the neutral zone, which is the field of gaze in which bilateral jerk nystagmus reverses direction. The other type of nystagmus is 'pendular', which is characterized by phases of equal velocity. Jerk nystagmus tends to indicate CNS disease, whereas pendular nystagmus is more common with sensory deprivation or certain types of congenital nystagmus (e.g. spasmus nutans).

(NB: Do not be tempted to say 'An examiner'!)

Question: *What is physiological nystagmus?*

Answer: Physiological nystagmus is normal, and there are various types.

1. End-gaze nystagmus is a symmetrical/conjugate, fine, horizontal jerk nystagmus which usually lasts only about ten seconds following extreme left or right gaze.
2. Physiological optokinetic nystagmus occurs when individuals observe an object (or series of objects) moving relative to themselves (e.g. whilst looking from the window of a moving train, or observing a rotating optokinetic drum). The nystagmus occurs due to a repetitive, alternating combination of a slow pursuit movement followed by a fast saccade movement aimed at picking up fixation on the next target object or drum stripe. The jerk nystagmus is symmetrical and of a variable rate. Physiological optokinetic nystagmus can be used to indicate the presence of sight in a patient with hysterical blindness.
3. Caloric nystagmus is induced by unilateral irrigation of the external auditory meatus with either cool or warm water. The stimulus induces movement of endolymph within the semicircular canals, producing a vestibular induced slow phase eye movement, which is followed by a compensatory fast saccade producing a jerk nystagmus. The nystagmus can be horizontal, oblique or rotary, depending on the position of the head (and hence semicircular canals). With the head inclined back 60° for maximum effect, cool water irrigation induces horizontal jerk nystagmus in the direction away from the side of the stimulus (COWS – cool : opposite; warm : same).

4. Rotational nystagmus is associated with rotating head movements, and also occurs due to movement of endolymph within the semicircular canals. The jerk nystagmus occurs in the direction of rotation and reverses upon cessation of rotation (post-rotary nystagmus). Rotational nystagmus can be used to examine eye movements in infants.

(NB: Never say 'There are four types of ...', since you may not remember all of them in the heat of an exam. This general rule applies to many types of question that you may be asked!)

Question: *What are the features of congenital nystagmus associated with visual loss before the age of two years?*

Answer: Early-onset sensory deprivation is usually a symmetrical/conjugate, bilateral, horizontal, pendular nystagmus with an identifiable null zone; although it can be vertical, circular or mixed and/or of the jerk type. Other classic and potential features include:

- lack of oscillopsia
- cessation with sleep
- a constant plane of nystagmus in all positions of gaze
- reduction with convergence
- increasing on attempted fixation
- direction reversal of physiological optokinetic nystagmus
- an abnormal head posture (keeping the eyes in the null zone)
- associated head oscillation (spasmus nutans)
- superimposed latent nystagmus (increased when one eye is covered).

In addition, there may be evidence of the cause of visual loss.

Question: *What is see-saw nystagmus?*

Answer: The see-saw nystagmus of Maddox is characterized by one eye intorting and rising while the other extorts and falls, giving the two eyes movements reminiscent of a see-saw. The nystagmus is pendular in nature and although it may be congenital it is often associated with a bitemporal hemianopia due to a suprasellar and chiasmal lesion.

Question: *What is Parinaud's syndrome?*

Answer: Also known as Sylvian aqueduct or dorsal midbrain syndrome, this condition is characterized by convergence-retraction nystagmus, poor convergence, light-near dissociation of the pupils and defective vertical gaze. The nystagmus is best identified using a down-rotating optokinetic drum. Other features can include lid retraction and accommodative spasm. The syndrome can be congenital, secondary to Sylvian aqueduct stenosis. In the young, causes include pinealoma, vascular malformations of the brainstem and trauma. In the older patient, causes include basilar artery cerebrovascular accident (CVA), metastasis and chronic demyelination. A tumour of the pineal gland is the most common cause.

Question: *Can drugs induce nystagmus?*

Answer: Yes. Various anticonvulsants such as phenobarbitone, carbamazepine and phenytoin can cause non-localizing, gaze-evoked nystagmus. The same can occur with virtually all kinds of tranquillizer and sedative, such as diazepam. In addition, streptomycin, neostigmine, salicylate and gold toxicity have been reported to cause nystagmus.

Question: *What type of nystagmus occurs following labyrinth destruction in Ménière's disease?*

Answer: None; there is central compensation for the lack of any input from the vestibular pathway and so nystagmus does not occur.

19. Entropion

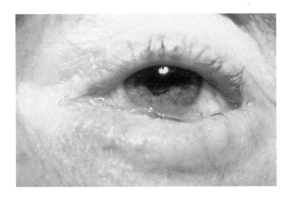 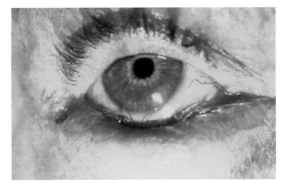

Figures 7 and 8 Examples of lower lid entropion (courtesy of Peng Khaw PhD MRCP FRCS FRCOphth).

Definition

Inversion of the eyelid(s).

Classification

1. Involutional
2. Congenital
3. Cicatricial
4. Acute spastic.

NB: Trichiasis is an acquired disorder in which the lashes are directed posteriorly towards the globe. Although trichiasis may occur in association with entropion, they are not the same abnormalities and trichiasis can occur in isolation from entropion.

Examination

1. Establish whether unilateral/bilateral, upper lid/lower lid involved.
2. Remember a dynamic examination (i.e. asking the patient to blink) may reveal the abnormality.

3. Determine cause by further examination:
   - age of patient:
     - old – more likely to be involutional;
     - young – more likely to be congenital or cicatricial (e.g. Stevens–Johnson syndrome)
   - note presence/absence of facial spasm or blepharospasm
   - remember to evert eyelids to check for cicatricial changes
   - examine the cornea for complications of the entropion (or for trachomatous pannus)
   - note presence/absence of previous surgical scarring.

4. Determine factors relating to choice of treatment
   - cicatrization
   - degree of horizontal lid laxity (can be assessed by either pinching the eyelid or by retracting the lower lid down and away from the globe, releasing, and determining the speed of return)
   - degree of canthal tendon laxity.

Clinical features

Involutional

- the most common in the United Kingdom (UK)/United States of America (USA)
- patient is usually elderly
- affects lower lid(s).

Occurs due to:

- preseptal over-riding of pretarsal orbicularis
- horizontal lid laxity
- dehiscence and weakening of the lower lid retractors with subsequent vertical instability
- weakening of the tarsal plate.

Congenital

- rare
- affects both lower lids (especially in oriental races)
- usually mild and self-limiting over the age of two years
- associated with hypertrophy of orbicularis and skin
- rarely associated with tarsal hypoplasia or microphthalmia.

Cicatricial

- may affect upper and/or lower lids
- caused by scarring and shortening of the posterior lamella
- often associated with trichiasis, dry eye and punctal occlusion
- common in the developing world, due to trachoma.

Acute spastic

- associated with ocular irritation and orbicularis spasm or essential blepharospasm
- may be intermittent
- often associated with involutional entropion.

Exam questions

Question: *How is simple congenital entropion managed?*

Answer: Congenital entropion is best managed conservatively since it is usually mild and self-limiting by the age of two years. In the rare, severe or persistent cases, a blepharoplasty involving excision of the hypertrophic orbicularis muscle and overlying skin should be performed. The skin edges should be sutured to the lower border of the tarsus to prevent over-riding of the pretarsal by the preseptal orbicularis.

Question: *What is epiblepharon?*

Answer: This congenital anomaly refers to the presence of an extra fold of skin just below each of the lower lid margins, particularly medially. The excessive amount of skin is not associated with hypertrophy of the underlying orbicularis (in contrast to congenital entropion). It is rare, usually mild, and self-limiting by two years of age, requiring no treatment. If surgery is required for persistent inturning of the lashes, excision of the excess skin alone is curative.

Question: *What mechanical factors give rise to the increased horizontal lid laxity of the older patient?*

Answer: Lid laxity is increased due to both degeneration with stretching of the canthal tendons and atrophy of orbital fat which gives rise to a relative enophthalmos. The laxity is considered excessive if the central part of the lower lid can be pulled more than 1 cm away from the globe, and if it fails to spring back briskly following release.

Question: *What are the surgical principles behind the treatment of involutional lower lid entropion?*

Answer: If a temporary cure (for up to a year) is all that is required, either transverse sutures are placed through the lid to prevent upward movement of the preseptal orbicularis, or oblique everting sutures are placed through the lid so as to incorporate and shorten the lower lid retractors, thus transferring their pull to the upper border of the tarsus to evert the lid.
If a more permanent cure is required, the choice of procedure depends on the degree of any associated horizontal lid laxity. If there is little

laxity, a transverse lid split together with everting sutures (Wies procedure) is sufficient. If laxity is the sole problem or entropion recurs following a Wies procedure, simple horizontal lid shortening or a lateral canthal sling procedure is indicated. If there is excessive laxity together with orbicularis over-riding, a transverse lid split, everting sutures and simple horizontal lid shortening is indicated (Quickert procedure). Should recurrence of the entropion occur following a Quickert procedure, a plication of the lower lid retractors (Jones procedure) should be performed.

Question: *What are the causes of cicatricial entropion?*

Answer: Cicatricial entropion, which can affect both upper and lower lids, can occur with any condition associated with scarring of the palpebral conjunctiva sufficient to pull the lid margin towards the globe. Causes include:

- ocular cicatricial pemphigoid
- Stevens–Johnson syndrome
- trachoma
- trauma (including chemical burns).

20. Ectropion

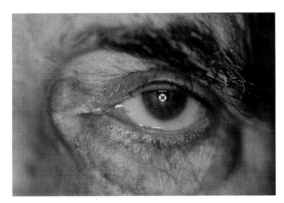

Figure 9 Left medial ectropion of the lower eyelid (courtesy of Jane Gardiner MD).

Definition

Eversion of the eyelid(s).

Classification

1. Involutional
2. Mechanical
3. Paralytic
4. Cicatricial
5. Congenital.

Clinical features

The approach to examination of the lids should be methodical and similar to that for diagnosing entropion so as to determine both the cause and ideal course of management. The types of ectropion are as follows.

Involutional

- the most common in the UK/USA
- patient is usually elderly
- affects lower lid(s)
- as with involutional entropion, there is increased lid tissue laxity, but this occurs in the absence of preseptal over-riding of pretarsal orbicularis
- lid eversion is accompanied by conjunctival exposure, secondary inflammation, keratinization and hypertrophy with a resultant element of mechanical ectropion.

Mechanical

- affects lower lid(s)
- classically due to tumours or cysts near the eyelid margin.

Paralytic

- affects lower lid(s)
- due to a 7th cranial (facial) nerve palsy
- may be temporary (Bell's palsy).

Cicatricial

- may affect upper and/or lower lids
- caused by cicatricial skin changes (shortage of skin), which pull the lid away from the globe.

Congenital

- rare
- may affect upper and/or lower lids
- usually due to a shortage of skin (i.e. cicatricial-like)
- may be associated with blepharophimosis.

Associated features

- epiphora
- chronic conjunctivitis
- exposed conjunctival keratinization
- exposure keratopathy.

Exam questions

Question: *How are cases of congenital ectropion managed?*

Answer: Congenital ectropion is usually mild, and rarely requires active treatment. In severe cases, which are invariably due to a shortage of skin, replacement of a vertical skin defect with a full-thickness skin graft is required.

Question: *What are the causes of cicatricial ectropion?*

Answer: Any periorbital scarring or contracture of skin may induce an ectropion due to a combination of skin traction and tissue loss. Causes include trauma, burns, cicatrizing skin tumours and dermatitis.

Question: *What is a lazy-T operation, and for what type of ectropion is it the surgical procedure of choice?*

Answer: A lazy-T procedure involves excision of a full-thickness pentagon of lid to shorten the medial aspect of the lower lid, together with excision of a diamond-shaped piece of tarso-conjunctiva to invert the lower lacrimal punctum. It is thus of most benefit in the treatment of an involutional ectropion, which is mainly medial and associated with horizontal lid laxity but where there is no significant medial canthal tendon laxity.

Question: *Are surgical procedures indicated in a patient with an ectropion associated with a facial nerve palsy?*

Answer: Not always. In temporary cases, such as those due to a Bell's palsy, surgery should not be carried out and treatment should be aimed at preventing exposure keratopathy with regular topical lubricants and nocturnal lid taping. If resolution is not going to occur it is appropriate to perform a tarsorrhaphy, a medial canthoplasty together with a lateral canthal sling (which is more cosmetically acceptable than a tarsorrhaphy), a medial canthoplasty alone if the ectropion is only medial, or a medial canthal resection if there is medial canthal tendon laxity.

Question: *What surgical procedure is indicated for involutional ectropion?*

Answer: The procedure of choice depends on the exact nature of the ectropion. If the ectropion is mainly medial and there is no horizontal lid laxity, excision of a diamond-shaped piece of tarsoconjunctiva below the lower punctum is sufficient. If there is significant horizontal lid laxity, a lazy-T procedure should be performed unless there is medial canthal tendon laxity, in which case a medial canthal tendon plication or resection is indicated. If the ectropion affects the whole lid length, a horizontal lid shortening, with or without a blepharoplasty if there is an excess of skin, or a lateral canthal sling procedure is indicated.

21. Blepharitis

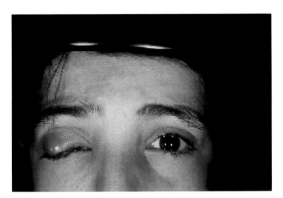

Figure 10 Blepharitis: a right upper eyelid chalazion (courtesy of Gordon Douglas MD).

Definition

A common, chronic, inflammatory condition of the eyelid margins.

Classification

1. Staphylococcal
2. Seborrhoeic
3. Mixed.

Clinical features

Staphylococcal blepharitis

- scarred, notched, thickened, inflamed lid margins
- dilated lid margin blood vessels (rosettes)
- adherent, brittle scales at the lash bases
- trichiasis (inward misdirection of eyelashes)
- madarosis
- poliosis
- ectropion or entropion
- external hordeola (styes)
- acute/chronic papillary blepharoconjunctivitis
- dry eye
- inferior punctate epitheliopathy
- marginal keratitis
- phlyctenulosis
- bacteriology: Staph. aureus, Staph. epidermis.

Seborrhoeic blepharitis

- waxy and shiny lid margins
- greasy lashes
- non-adherent, soft greasy scales all over the lid margins
- seborrhoea (foamy tear meniscus)
- meibomitis
- meibomian gland duct plugging
- chalazia (see Figure 10)
- chronic papillary blepharoconjunctivitis
- interpalpebral punctate epitheliopathy
- tear film instability
- seborrhoeic dermatitis
- rosacea
- bacteriology: diphtheroids, corynebacteria, Pityrosporum ovale.

Exam questions

Question: *What is the commonest cause of 'dry eye' in the United Kingdom?*

Answer: Blepharitis.

Question: *What is madarosis?*

Answer: Loss of lashes. This is common in patients with chronic staphylococcal blepharitis.

Question: *What is poliosis?*

Answer: Whitening of hair including lashes. This is common in patients with chronic staphylococcal blepharitis. It is also a sign of albinism and Vogt–Koyanagi–Harada (VKH) syndrome.

Question: *How should patients with blepharitis be treated?*

Answer: Management of blepharitis is dependent on the type and severity of the condition. The mainstay of treatment is regular eyelid hygiene both to remove crusts/scales and to unplug blocked meibomian gland orifices. This can be achieved with cotton buds soaked in sodium bicarbonate solution or baby shampoo (which doesn't sting). With seborrhoeic blepharitis and significant meibomian gland dysfunction, warm compresses and massage of the eyelids can restore the flow of meibomian gland lipid. Topical lubricants may provide symptomatic relief and prevent corneal epitheliopathy, but will not cure the cause. Topical antibiotics (drops to the conjunctiva, ointment to the lid margins) are indicated if lid and/or conjunctival bacteriology have shown significant infection, and are most useful in staphylococcal blepharitis. Long-term, low dose systemic antibiotics (oxy-tetracycline or doxycycline) are indicated in severe cases of seborrhoeic blepharitis, particularly if accompanied by seborrhoeic dermatitis, although their mode of action in this situation remains unclear. Topical steroid therapy should be avoided if possible, although short courses are indicated when there is papillary conjunctivitis, marginal keratitis or phlyctenulosis. Epilation, electrolysis or cryotherapy may be required to treat any associated trichiasis.

Question: *How are patients with chalazia managed?*

Answer: Chalazia should be managed with eyelid hygiene, warm compresses, massage and prophylactic topical antibiotics in the first instance. A persistent, uninfected chalazion may require incision and curettage through a tarsal incision. It is important to remember that the rare condition of a meibomian gland carcinoma may masquerade as a recurrent chalazion.

22. Pterygium

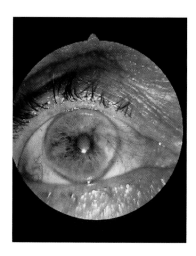

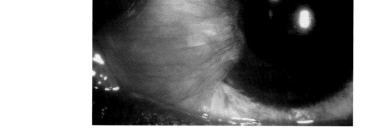

a   b

Figure 11 a: A moderate-sized right pterygium (courtesy of Gordon Douglas MD); b: A prominent left pterygium (courtesy of the Department of Medical Illustration, Moorfields Eye Hospital).

Definition

A characteristic triangular-shaped fibrovascular growth of conjunctival and subconjunctival tissue, which invades the cornea between the epithelium and Bowman's zone at its apex.

Clinical features

Pterygia occur within the interpalpebral space, and are more common on the nasal rather than the temporal side. An early pterygium can be difficult to differentiate from a pingueculum, but the latter never invades the cornea.

Exam questions

Question: *What is a Stocker's line?*

Answer: A curvilinear deposit of iron within the corneal epithelium anterior to the advancing head of a pterygium.

Question: *How are patients with pterygia managed?*

Answer: Many patients with pterygia require no active treatment. However, treatment may be indicated for relief of discomfort, if the visual axis is threatened or for improved cosmesis. Discomfort may be relieved with artificial tear supplementation. If definitive treatment is required, the lesion should be excised. In order to reduce the significant risk of recurrence following simple excision, an additional free conjunctival autograft (superior bulbar, with or without the limbus, to excised pterygium bed), a pedicle flap of conjunctiva, or amniotic membrane transplantation have been shown to be effective. Local β-irradiation and topical thiotepa or mitomycin-C as adjuncts to excision have been used to reduce the rate of recurrence, but severe, late complications have been reported. With large pterygia, a lamellar corneal graft may be required.

Question: *What is the aetiology of a pterygium?*

Answer: Pterygia tend to occur in patients who live or have lived in a hot and dry climate. It has therefore been suggested that they develop in response to chronic dryness or excessive ultraviolet (UV) light exposure. One theory advocates that internal reflection from the orbital margin and nose focuses UV light onto the medial limbus ('albedo'), where it affects stem cells or otherwise induces the formation of a pterygium.

Question: *What are the histopathological features of a pterygium?*

Answer: These include:

- conjunctival epithelial thinning
- a fibrovascular subepithelial mass
- elastoid degeneration of stromal collagen
- destruction of Bowman's zone of the cornea
- corneal epithelial iron deposition (Stocker's line).

Question: *What is a pseudopterygium?*

Answer: Unlike a true pterygium, a pseudopterygium is not adherent to underlying tissues throughout its length, but solely at its base and apex. Pseudopterygia develop following adhesion between a fold of conjunctiva and a peripheral corneal ulcer.

23. Vernal keratoconjunctivitis (VKC)

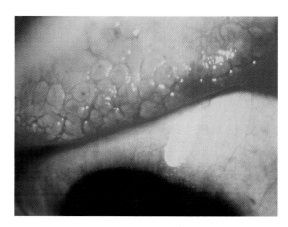

Figure 12 Vernal keratoconjunctivitis: cobblestone papillae seen by everting the upper eyelid (courtesy of Gordon Douglas MD).

Definition

A recurrent, bilateral, allergic form of papillary conjunctivitis, more common in spring and summer or in the tropics.

Classification

1. Limbal
2. Palpebral
3. Mixed.

Clinical features

The patient is usually a child or young adult, more commonly male, who frequently has a positive family or personal history of atopy. Occasionally, non-atopic individuals develop VKC.

Signs

1. *Limbal*:

   - limbal follicles
   - Trantas' dots
   - limbitis, hyperaemia, oedema
2. *Palpebral*:
   - affects superior tarsal conjunctiva
   - cobblestone papillae
   - ptosis
3. *Keratitis*.

Exam questions

Question: *What are the major symptoms of VKC?*

Answer: The symptoms include:

- itch (eyes and skin)
- foreign body or burning sensation
- lacrimation
- thick stringy mucous discharge
- photophobia
- ptosis.

Question: *What are Trantas' dots?*

Answer: These are discrete white superficial spots found in some cases of limbal VKC, and should not be confused with the larger limbal follicles with which they are associated. They are situated at the apex of follicles, and are composed predominantly of eosinophils.

Question: *How do the cobblestone papillae of VKC differ from those of giant papillary conjunctivitis (GPC)?*

Answer: Cobblestone papillae are usually large, but careful examination reveals that they are of varying size and shape. Giant papillae, which by definition are greater than 3 mm in diameter, tend to be all of similar size and shape.

Question: *How may VKC affect the cornea?*

Answer: There are various types of vernal keratitis (Buckley classification):

1. Superior punctate epithelial micro-erosions
2. Epithelial macro-erosions
3. Plaque (shield-ulcer)
4. Subepithelial 'ring' scarring
5. Pseudogerontoxon 'Cupid's bow'.

Superior punctate epithelial micro-erosions rarely present major problems, but can progress to macro-erosions. If the base of a macro-erosion becomes coated by the exudate of high mucus content, a non-wetting area develops and re-epithelialization fails to occur, forming the classical shield-ulcer. In severe, untreated cases, subepithelial scarring occurs around the ulcer forming a ring-scar. A pseudogerontoxon forms in some cases of limbal VKC as an outline of a previously inflamed sector of limbus – it may be confused with a corneal arcus.

Question: *How are patients with VKC managed?*

Answer: The pathogenesis of VKC is thought to involve an IgE mediated allergic response in which mast cells play a major role. Thus the mainstay of treatment is with topical mast cell stabilizers (sodium cromoglycate or lodoxamide), which are useful prophylactically and in mild cases. In more severe, acute exacerbations, topical steroids are required. Other topical medications such as lubricants and/or mucolytic agents may help. Corneal plaques (shield ulcers) sometimes require debriding. Some patients show improvement with systemic therapy in the form of oral antihistamines and/or aspirin.

24. Pars planitis

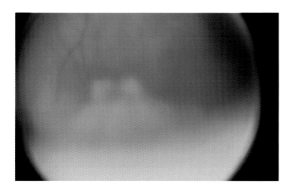

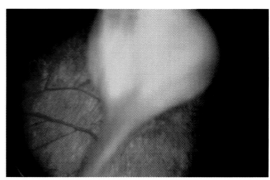

a   b

Figure 13   a: A snowbank in an eye with pars planitis or intermediate uveitis (courtesy of Robert Nozik MD and Carlos Pavesio MD); b: A toxocara granuloma should be considered in the differential diagnosis of a snowbank (courtesy of Robert Nozik MD and Carlos Pavesio MD).

Definition

A relatively common form of chronic (intermediate) uveitis, of unknown aetiology, characterized by vitritis, cyclitis, pars plana exudate and mild peripheral retinal periphlebitis.

Also known as:

- Intermediate Uveitis (a subtype of)
- Chronic Cyclitis
- Peripheral Uveitis.

Clinical features

The patient

- usually a young adult
- males and females are affected equally
- may be HLA-DR2 +ve
- there may be evidence of associated multiple sclerosis.

Signs

- bilateral in 80% (eventually)
- white eye(s)
- band keratopathy

- anterior chamber flare with a few cells
- keratic precipitates (small and rare)
- peripheral anterior synechiae
- posterior synechiae (very rare)
- vitritis
- anterior vitreous opacities and/or sheets
- peripheral periphlebitis (especially inferior)
- white granulomatous exudates ('snowballs') close to the pars plana (especially inferior)
- coalesced white exudates with collapsed vitreous gel and proliferating retinal astrocytes ('snow-banks') at the pars plana (especially inferior), which may become vascularized
- cystoid macular oedema
- peripapillary retinal oedema/swollen disc
- neovascularization (peripheral or disc); rare
- secondary cataract
- secondary glaucoma.

Exam questions

Question: *What is the most common presenting symptom of pars planitis?*

Answer: Floaters. The symptom is due to the presence of anterior vitreous opacities.

Question: *Is the presence of a snow-bank essential for the diagnosis of pars planitis?*

Answer: There is some confusion between the terms 'pars planitis' and the more general term of 'intermediate uveitis'. However, most ophthalmologists understand the term pars planitis to be the presence of vitritis in association with a snow-bank, whereas the latter is not required for the diagnosis of intermediate uveitis. In a patient with bilateral disease, a snow-bank may be present in only one eye despite the presence of vitritis in both eyes. In this situation, the patient is deemed to have bilateral pars planitis.

Question: *How are patients with pars planitis managed?*

Answer: Many patients with mild disease require no treatment, and the condition eventually resolves with no sequelae apart from persistent floaters. Treatment with either systemic or peri-ocular steroids should be avoided unless vision is reduced due to inflammation or macular oedema. If unilateral treatment only is indicated, first line therapy is with a peri-ocular depot-steroid injection, which may have to be repeated. Oral steroids are indicated if this fails or if there is bilateral disease. In severe and non-steroid-responsive cases, other immunosuppressive agents such as cyclosporin or cyclophosphamide may be required. Cryotherapy to the retinal periphery and surgical vitrectomy are playing an increasing role in the management of severe cases.

Question: *What is the prognosis for pars planitis?*

Answer: The disease tends to run one of three possible courses. About 10–20% of patients have a benign, self-limiting type, about 50–60% have a prolonged course without exacerbations, and about 30% have a course with multiple exacerbations. In all cases most patients retain good visual acuity, with over 70% maintaining 6/12 or better.

Question: *What are the possible complications of pars planitis?*

Answer: A relatively common complication is cystoid macular oedema, and this is the most common cause of reduced visual acuity in patients with pars planitis. Chronic cases may be complicated by epiretinal membrane, cataract, band keratopathy and/or glaucoma. In very severe cases, snow-banks become vascularized and extension can result in the formation of a retrolenticular cyclitic membrane. This itself may be complicated further by vitreous haemorrhage and/or traction retinal detachment. Fortunately, the latter complications are rare.

Question: *What is the differential diagnosis of intermediate uveitis?*

Answer: Vitritis with peripheral 'snowballs' may be a feature of toxoplasmosis, sarcoidosis, tuberculosis, syphilis, Crohn's or Whipple's disease, Lyme disease, collagen vascular disease, or multiple sclerosis. One should also think of Fuchs' heterochromic iridocyclitis (although careful examination should exclude this), reticulum cell sarcoma and amyloidosis. A toxocara granuloma may have the appearance of 'snow-banking'.

Question: *Is pars planitis more common in the winter months?*

Answer: No. Despite the presence of 'snowballs' and/or 'snow-banking', the condition shows no seasonal variation in incidence!

25. Vogt–Koyanagi–Harada (VKH) syndrome

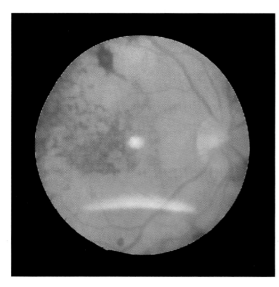

Figure 14 Mottled retinal pigment epithelium change (a late feature of Vogt–Koyanagi–Harada syndrome) (courtesy of Gordon Douglas MD).

Definition

A rare, multisystem disorder of unknown aetiology, characterized by a bilateral panuveitis, cerebral manifestations and skin and/or hair depigmentation.

Also known as:

Uveoencephalitis.

Clinical features

The patient is usually between the ages of 30 and 50 years, and commonly Japanese or from another oriental population. By definition, signs from at least three of the following four groups have to be present before a diagnosis of VKH syndrome can be made:

1. *Dermatological signs* (tend to develop a few weeks after the onset of the disease)
   - alopecia (loss of scalp hair)
   - poliosis (whitening of hair)
   - vitiligo (patchy skin depigmentation)
2. *Neurological signs* (tend to develop early)
   - meningeal irritation (headache, neck stiffness)
   - encephalopathy (fits, cranial nerve palsies, nystagmus, hemiparesis)
   - auditory (deafness, tinnitus, vertigo)
3. *Anterior uveitis* (develops early)
   - bilateral
   - granulomatous
   - often severe
4. *Posterior uveitis* (develops early)
   - bilateral
   - vitritis
   - multiple foci of elevated cloudy patches of choroid and retina (early)
   - patches coalesce to form oval-shaped exudative retinal detachments (later)
   - mottled retinal pigment epithelium (RPE) change (mixed focal atrophy and hyperpigmentation) (late, after resolution of retinal detachments)
   - macular oedema
   - disc hyperaemia/papillitis
   - subfoveal (retinal) neovascular membranes.

NB: Vogt–Koyanagi syndrome = anterior uveitis + dermatological/hair features; Harada's disease = posterior uveitis + neurological features.

Exam questions

Question: *What is the HLA association with VKH syndrome?*

Answer: HLA-B22, although this is not present in over 50% of cases. The condition is also relatively common among American Indians of the Cherokee nation, the majority of whom demonstrate HLA-DRW52.

Question: *What is the aetiology of VKH syndrome?*

Answer: Essentially this remains unknown, although it is suspected to be a complex T-cell mediated immunological or autoimmune reaction, perhaps triggered by a viral infection, in a genetically predisposed individual. Immunocytological findings have included mainly T-lymphocytes in the uveal infiltrates together with HLA-DR +ve macrophages. CD1 +ve, non-dendritic cells have been identified in the choroid in close proximity to melanocytes.

Question: *How are patients with VKH syndrome treated?*

Answer: Treatment requires high doses of topical, peri-ocular and systemic corticosteroids. If the response is inadequate, additional immunosuppressive agents may be required.

Question: *Is the CSF in patients with VKH syndrome normal or abnormal?*

Answer: In some patients who exhibit neurological features the CSF has been shown to have lymphocytosis.

Question: *What are the ocular complications of VKH syndrome?*

Answer: Failure or lack of response to treatment may result in failure of resolution, persistent inflammation and retinal detachment with resultant blindness. All the complications of uveitis may occur in patients with VKH syndrome; these include glaucoma, cataract, band keratopathy, hypotony and phthisis bulbi. In addition subretinal neovascular membranes may form, and these have a predilection for the sub-foveal region and hence have a poor visual prognosis. The ocular problems associated with 3rd, 4th, 6th and 7th cranial nerve palsies and nystagmus may also complicate VKH syndrome.

26. Sympathetic ophthalmitis

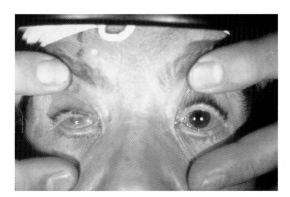

Figure 15 Sympathetic ophthalmitis of the right eye. The left eye had suffered previous penetrating trauma (courtesy of Gordon Douglas MD).

Definition

A rare, bilateral, granulomatous panuveitis, which can occur after penetrating ocular trauma, a perforating corneal ulcer or intra-ocular surgery to one eye, which have usually involved uveal prolapse.

Terms

- 'traumatized eye' = 'exciting eye'
- 'fellow eye' = 'sympathizing eye'.

Clinical features

Bilateral uveitis usually occurs one to two months after ocular penetration, but can occur after only nine days or after as much as 50 years. Early symptoms include blurring of vision (loss of accommodation), photophobia and red eye.

Sympathizing eye signs (tend to develop in the following order, although may start with posterior signs)

- ciliary flush
- vitritis
- iris Koeppe nodules
- posterior synechiae
- low grade anterior and intermediate uveitis
- retinal oedema
- Dalen–Fuchs nodules
- papillitis
- severe granulomatous panuveitis.

Exciting eye signs

- signs of trauma, perforation or surgery
- severe granulomatous panuveitis.

The condition has been considered as the traumatic counterpart of VKH syndrome, and some patients develop systemic and ocular features similar to those seen in VKH syndrome.
NB: Sympathetic ophthalmitis can be simulated by lens-induced endophthalmitis, which in very rare instances can affect the fellow eye. It is important that this is considered, since this responds to removal of released lens matter.

Exam questions

Question: *What is the pathogenesis of sympathetic ophthalmitis?*

Answer: Sympathetic ophthalmitis is thought to have an autoimmune basis, and has many features consistent with it being a Type IV hypersensitivity reaction. However, identification of a specific antigen has proved difficult. Initially, retinal S-antigen (present in the outer segments of the photoreceptors) was suspected. More recently, another retinal S-antigen-'like' 48-kD molecule, which has been identified in rod photoreceptor outer segments, choroidal plexus, cerebro-spinal fluid (CSF) and the pineal gland, has been suspected. The possibility of immunological cross-reactivity between the eye and the nervous system involving this antigen may be important in the aetiology of both VKH syndrome and sympathetic ophthalmitis. There is some evidence that individuals who are HLA-A11 positive are predisposed to sympathetic ophthalmitis.

Question: *What are Koeppe's nodules?*

Answer: These are a feature of granulomatous uveitis, and are adhesive iris aggregates consisting mainly of macrophages. They are situated at the pupillary border and tend to be smaller and more common than Busacca's nodules, which are located away from the pupil.

Question: *What are Dalen–Fuchs nodules?*

Answer: These are nodules of ciliary epithelial cells and epithelioid macrophages beneath and between the pigmented and non-pigmented layers of the ciliary body epithelium and also scattered throughout the fundus at a level above Bruch's membrane, where they appear at fundoscopy as multiple yellow-white spots. Dalen–Fuchs nodules are most common in sympathetic ophthalmitis, but may be present in eyes with tuberculosis or VKH syndrome.

Question: *How is sympathetic ophthalmitis managed?*

Answer: Treatment should be aggressive because of the risk of potential (bilateral) blindness, and initially involves high doses of topical, peri-ocular and systemic steroids. Once the inflammation has been controlled, the dosage can be reduced to a maintenance level of systemic steroids. Steroids may be used in combination with cyclosporin, azathioprine or chlorambucil when steroids alone have not been adequately effective.

Question: *Is enucleation of the exciting eye of value in the management of sympathetic ophthalmitis?*

Answer: Enucleation of a potential 'exciting eye' within 10 days of the 'trauma' almost invariably protects the fellow eye from developing sympathetic ophthalmitis. Enucleation after onset of sympathetic ophthalmitis does not halt progress of the inflammation, although there is some evidence that it may reduce the degree of inflammation. Thus, if the 'exciting eye' has no visual potential, enucleation should be considered. Even if enucleation is performed, the patient still requires therapy with steroids with or without other immunosuppressants.

27. Bird-shot retinochoroidopathy

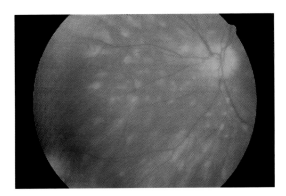

Figure 16 The fundus of an eye with bird-shot retinochoroidopathy (courtesy of Robert Nozik MD and Carlos Pavesio MD).

Definition

A rare, bilateral, symmetrical uveitic retino-choroidopathy of presumed autoimmune aetiology, characterized by multiple discrete cream-coloured areas of depigmentation scattered diffusely across the fundus.

Clinical features

The patient is usually over 40–50 years of age, and females are more commonly affected than males. The condition is characterized by multiple, distinct depigmented chorioretinal lesions scattered in a pattern reminiscent of bird shot scatter from a shotgun. There is an associated vitritis.

Exam questions

Question: *What is the HLA association with bird-shot retinochoroidopathy?*

Answer: HLA-A29 is strongly associated and has an estimated sensitivity of 96% and specificity of 93%.

Question: *What are the clinical signs of bird-shot retinochoroidopathy?*

Answer: The eye is white and there is usually only mild anterior chamber flare with a few cells. A vitritis usually involves both anterior and posterior vitreous, and there may be a degree of retinal vasculitis, particularly in the peri-foveal region. There may be associated cystoid macular oedema and swollen optic discs. The characteristic lesions, however, are the multiple, small, distinct depigmented spots at the level of the RPE, which are scattered throughout the fundus.

Question: *What are the fluorescein angiographic features of bird-shot retinochoroidopathy?*

Answer: The choroidal lesions characteristically show early hypofluorescence and late hyper-fluorescence. Early angiograms may, in addition, reveal dilated retinal capillaries at the optic disc and throughout the posterior pole together with background choroidal hyperfluor-escence. There may be evidence of cystoid macular oedema, even if this is not apparent clinically. In some cases the creamy-coloured spots may show no early hypofluorescence or late hyperfluorescence, thus giving a relatively normal appearance compared to the clinical appearance.

Question: *What is the natural history of bird-shot retinochoroidopathy?*

Answer: The condition tends to have a chronic course, with exacerbations and remissions. The patient usually complains of floaters, blurred vision (especially if there is cystoid macular oedema) and, in longstanding cases, may suffer poor night vision.

Question: *How is bird-shot retinochoroidopathy treated?*

Answer: There is no specific treatment, although systemic steroids may help reduce the ocular inflammation, macular oedema or optic disc oedema. There is some evidence that use of low dose steroid-sparing agents alone, such as cyclosporin, is as effective as steroid therapy.

Question: *What is the differential diagnosis of bird-shot retinochoroidopathy?*

Answer: This includes:

- multifocal choroiditis
- punctate inner choroidopathy (PIC)
- presumed ocular histoplasmosis syndrome (POHS)
- sarcoidosis
- syphilitic chorioretinitis
- multiple evanescent white dot syndrome
- reticulum cell sarcoma (lymphoma)
- Lyme disease.

28. Acute multifocal placoid pigment epitheliopathy (AMPPE)

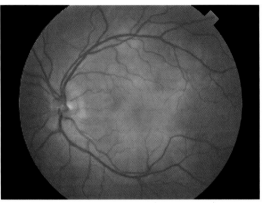
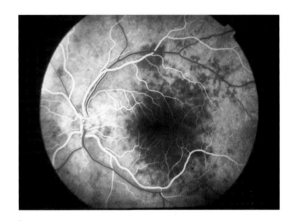

a   b

Figure 17 a: The fundus of a patient with acute multifocal placoid pigment epitheliopathy (AMPPE). Note the pallor at the level of the RPE; b: The associated fluorescein angiogram (early phase). There are areas of hypofluorescence corresponding to the areas of fundus pallor (courtesy of Philip Hykin MD FRCS FRCOphth).

Definition

A rare, bilateral condition of unknown aetiology, characterized by vitritis and characteristic multiple chorioretinal lesions affecting the posterior pole.

Clinical features

The patient is generally less than 25 years old. One eye is usually affected a few days before the other.

Ocular signs

1. *Early*:
   - one or several flat, deep whitish-grey/ opalescent plaque-like lesions, of between a quarter to a half a disc diameter in size, are seen at the posterior pole
   - if the fovea is involved, visual acuity is reduced to 6/60 or worse

   - vascular sheathing/papillitis/serous retinal detachments (rare)
   - there may be mild episcleritis, anterior chamber activity and/or vitritis
2. *Late*:
   - extensive pigmentary change throughout the posterior pole.

Exam questions

Question: *Does AMPPE only affect the eyes?*

Answer: No. The ocular condition is frequently preceded by a flu-like prodromal syndrome, and may be accompanied by various systemic features including:

- thyroiditis
- regional enteritis
- erythema nodosum
- cerebral vasculitis.

Question: *What is the possible aetiology of AMPPE?*

Answer: The aetiology is unknown, but is thought to have either an inflammatory/ischaemic basis characterized by obstruction of feeder vessels to segments of the choriocapillaris, or an immunological basis with a response directed against the RPE. Since 50% of patients present with flu-like symptoms, a viral aetiology has been proposed but not proved.

Question: *What are the fluorescein angiographic features of AMPPE?*

Answer: The lesions of early/active disease block out background choroidal fluorescence during the early stages of angiography, and subsequently leak and stain. Sometimes large choroidal vessels can be seen filling, in the absence of choriocapillaris filling, providing further evidence for the theory that the pathogenesis involves occlusion of a lobule feeder vessel. In late/inactive disease there is early transmission of the background choroidal fluorescence through the areas of depigmentation, reflecting extensive pigmentary disturbance.

Question: *How is AMMPE treated?*

Answer: No treatment has been shown to be of any benefit. However, there is often a dramatic return of vision within a few weeks of onset, and visual acuity may continue to improve over several months. Recurrence is very rare.

Question: *What is the differential diagnosis of AMPPE?*

Answer: Serpiginous choroidopathy may be confused with AMPPE, although it tends to affect older patients (over 40 years of age) and the lesions are characteristically geographic, starting around the optic disc and extending in all directions in a serpentine manner, rather than being isolated placoid lesions. The lesions of resolved AMPPE may also be confused with inactive foci of presumed ocular histoplasmosis.

29. Axenfeld–Rieger syndrome

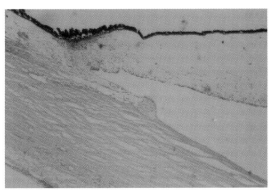

a

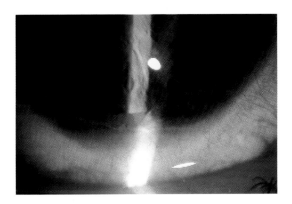

b

Figure 18 a: A histological section of an angle showing posterior embryotoxon; b: Axenfeld's anomaly (courtesy of Gordon Douglas MD).

Definition

A spectrum of congenital disorders characterized by abnormal development of the anterior segment and, in particular, the irido-corneal angle.

Old classification

1. – Posterior embryotoxon
   – Axenfeld's anomaly
   – Rieger's syndrome
   – Iridogoniodysgenesis
2. – Posterior keratoconus
   – Peters' anomaly
   – Anterior chamber cleavage syndrome.

Clinical features

Posterior embryotoxon

(Greek: toxon = bow)

- prominent Schwalbe's line
- occurs in 15% of the population
- no pathological significance.

Axenfeld's anomaly

- prominent Schwalbe's line
- iris strands to Schwalbe's line (i.e. large peripheral anterior synechiae [PAS])

Axenfeld–Rieger's syndrome

(Bilateral ocular signs)

- prominent Schwalbe's line
- iris strands to Schwalbe's line
- hypoplasia of anterior iris stroma (a featureless appearance of the iris)
- ectropion uveae, pseudopolycoria and pupil distortion
- peripheral corneal opacification
- glaucoma (50% of cases)

and

- abnormal dentition
- maxillary hypoplasia
- inguinal hernia
- hypospadias.

Iridogoniodysgenesis (outdated term)

- iris strands to Schwalbe's ring
- hypoplasia of anterior iris stroma
- glaucoma (50% of cases).

Posterior keratoconus (outdated term)

- posterior corneal depression.

Peters' anomaly (outdated term)

(Bilateral ocular signs in 80%)

- posterior corneal defect in Descemet's membrane
- central posterior corneal stromal opacity (leucoma)
- iris adhesions to leucoma margins
- glaucoma (50% of cases)
- may be associated with other anomalies such as sclerocornea or microphthalmos.

Anterior chamber cleavage syndrome (outdated term)

- prominent Schwalbe's ring
- hypoplasia of anterior iris stroma
- posterior corneal defect in Descemet's membrane
- central posterior corneal stromal opacity (leucoma)
- iris adhesions to Schwalbe's ring and leucoma margins
- lens apposition to the leucoma
- glaucoma (>50% of cases).

Exam questions

Question: *What is Schwalbe's line or ring?*

Answer: Schwalbe's line is the peripheral edge of Descemet's membrane where it terminates at the anterior aspect of the trabecular meshwork.

Question: *What is the nature of inheritance of Axenfeld–Rieger's syndrome?*

Answer: Autosomal dominant. The disorder has been mapped to chromosome 4 (4q25–26) by linkage in some points.

Question: *When does the glaucoma associated with Axenfeld–Rieger's syndrome tend to present?*

Answer: Glaucoma is not always a feature of these congenital disorders, but does occur in about 50% of cases of Rieger's syndrome, iridogoniodysgenesis, Peters' anomaly and the full anterior chamber cleavage syndrome. Although the glaucoma may present at birth, it usually presents within the fist three decades of life.

Question: *What are the systemic features of Axenfeld–Rieger's syndrome?*

Answer: Dental abnormalities include microdontia (small teeth) and hypodontia (a reduction in the number of teeth). Large gaps between the teeth are thus evident. Maxillary hypoplasia produces a flat face, and this is often associated with a protruding lower lip and a receding upper lip. Other features include hypertelorism, empty sella syndrome, inguinal and umbilical hernias and heart defects.

30. Ptosis

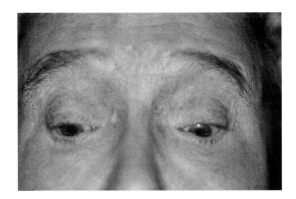
a

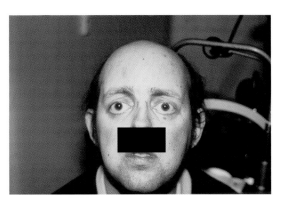
b

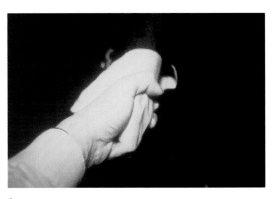
c

Figure 19 a: Blepharophimosis – a rare cause of ptosis (courtesy of Jane Gardiner MD); b: A patient with dystrophia myotonica showing frontal balding, an abnormal head posture with neck extension secondary to ptosis (courtesy of Peng Khaw PhD MRCP FRCS FRCOphth); c: The persistent handshake of a patient with dystrophia myotonica (courtesy of Peng Khaw PhD MRCP FRCS FRCOphth).

Definition

An abnormal drooping of the upper eyelid(s).

Clinical features

When minimal, detection of ptosis can be difficult, particularly if bilateral. It is important before assessing ptosis to exclude causes of pseudoptosis, such as:

1. *Same eye*:
   - small globe (microphthalmos, phthisis bulbi)
   - hypertropia
   - cornea plana
2. *Other eye*:
   - lid retraction
   - hypotropia
   - proptosis.

See Assessment of ptosis.

Exam questions

Question: *What are the causes of ptosis?*

Answer: Ptosis may result from neurogenic, myogenic, aponeurotic or mechanical causes, and may be congenital or acquired.

Neurogenic causes include Horner's syndrome, third cranial nerve palsy, aberrant third cranial nerve regeneration syndrome, tabes dorsalis and Marcus Gunn jaw-winking syndrome.

Congenital myogenic ptosis is usually due to levator dystrophy and rarely blepharophimosis syndrome.

Acquired myogenic ptosis, which is often bilateral, may be due to myasthenia gravis, dystrophia myotonica, ocular myopathy or oculopharyngeal muscular dystrophy.

Aponeurotic ptosis, usually involutional in nature, also occurs as a temporary post-operative complication. A rare cause is blepharochalasis.

Mechanical ptosis may be due to excessive weight of the upper eyelid (tumour, dermatochalasis) or conjunctival scarring (cicatricial ptosis).

All four elements can be involved in a traumatic ptosis.

Question: *How can ptosis be managed?*

Answer: Depending on the cause and degree of ptosis, management can be conservative, medical or surgical.

Conservative management includes doing nothing, spectacle ptosis props, haptic contact lenses or corneal lubrication.

Medical treatment of myasthenia gravis can improve ptosis.

Various surgical techniques are available. These include procedures on the:

- levator – resection
- aponeurosis – strengthening
- tarsus/conjunctiva – resection
- frontalis – brow suspension.

Question: *What are potential indications for brow suspension surgery?*

Answer: Brow suspension surgery is required for:

- a ptosis with less than 4 mm of levator function
- prevention of amblyopia in an infant with a severe congenital ptosis, when assessment of levator function is impossible
- following a levator excision (e.g. for Marcus Gunn jaw-winking syndrome).

Question: *What is the aetiology of the Marcus Gunn jaw-winking syndrome?*

Answer: There is linked movement (synkinesis) between the levator palpebrae superioris and the ipsilateral pterygoid muscle. This may be due to a brainstem abnormality. The result is a retraction of the ptotic eyelid when the ipsilateral pterygoid muscle is stimulated, usually during chewing or opening the mouth.

Question: *What is dermatochalasis, and how does this differ from blepharochalasis?*

Answer: Dermatochalasis is a common involutional change, which can produce a mechanical ptosis. There is excessive upper eyelid skin, and fat may protrude through an atrophic orbital septum. It is thus the cause of the frequently seen baggy eyelids of the elderly. In contrast, blepharochalasis is rare and most commonly seen in young women. Recurrent eyelid oedema of unknown aetiology can produce an aponeurotic ptosis due to stretching or disinsertion of the levator aponeurosis.

31. Xanthelasma

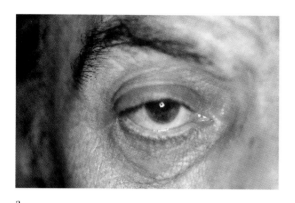 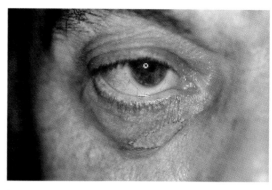

a   b

Figure 20   Xanthelasma. a: Pre-laser therapy; b: Post-laser therapy (courtesy of Jane Gardiner MD).

Definition

Plaques of deposited lipid (predominantly cholesterol) in the subcutaneous tissue of the eyelids.

Clinical features

The deposits are sharply circumscribed, flat and yellow in colour. They are usually found at the medial end of both upper eyelids.

Exam questions

Question: *What specific ophthalmic signs may be found in a patient with xanthelasma?*

Answer: Since some patients with xanthelasma have a primary hyperlipidaemia, there may be corneal arcus or lipaemia retinalis.

Question: *What general clinical signs are indicative of primary hyperlipidaemia?*

Answer: There may be evidence of vascular disease, but the specific feature is of xanthomata.

Tendon xanthomata, found in the extensor tendons of the hands, in the buttocks or in the Achilles or patellar tendons, are found in familial hypercholesterolaemia. Some of these may be nodular or tuberous xanthomata.

Eruptive xanthomata are yellow/orange papules (which may be tender) found on extensor surfaces, especially over joints, on the dorsal surface of the limbs and on the back and buttocks. They are found in patients with hypertriglyceridaemia. These patients are prone to develop pancreatitis. Palmar xanthomata appear as yellowish palmar and digital creases. They are most commonly associated with Type III hyperlipoproteinaemia.

Question: *How can causes of secondary hyperlipidaemia affect the eyes?*

Answer:

1. Diabetes mellitus – ocular complications of diabetes
2. Obstructive jaundice – yellowish appearance to sclera
3. Myxoedema – periorbital puffiness, loss of lateral third of eyebrow
4. Nephrotic syndrome – periorbital oedema
5. Alcoholism – toxic optic neuropathy.

Question: *What is the histology of a xanthelasma?*

Answer: The epidermal lesion is seen to contain numerous lipid laden macrophages (foam cells), the cells having small round nuclei and extensive foamy cytoplasm which appears empty in routine sections.

Question: *How are xanthelasma managed?*

Answer: It is important to identify and treat causes of secondary hyperlipidaemia. Primary hyperlipidaemia should be treated by diet and, if this fails, with lipid-lowering drugs. Surgical excision of xanthelasma can be performed, but recurrence occurs in 60% of cases. More recently laser therapy is showing promise.

32. Corneal arcus

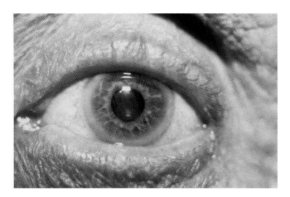

Figure 21 Corneal arcus (courtesy of Peng Khaw PhD MRCP FRCS FRCOphth).

Definition

Lipid (predominantly cholesterol and phospholipid) deposition starting in the peripheral inferior corneal stroma and eventually involving the whole corneal circumference.

Clinical features

The deposition, in the form of a whitish opacity, lies at all levels of the stroma, parallel to the limbus but separated from it by a zone of clear cornea. It often involves only a sector of the cornea.

Exam questions

Question: *What is arcus senilis?*

Answer: This is the commonest type of corneal arcus, being very common in all middle-aged and elderly people. It is symptomless, invariably idiopathic and requires no treatment. It is also referred to as gerontoxon.

Question: *What is arcus juvenilis?*

Answer: This refers to corneal arcus found in youth. It is usually secondary to chronic inflammation but can be a sign of a hyperlipidaemia (particularly common or familial hypercholesterolaemia). It is more commonly seen in smokers. In the absence of local ocular disease patients under the age of 40 years with arcus should be referred for vascular and lipid assessment.
A rare association of arcus juvenilis is osteogenesis imperfecta.

Question: *Is a corneal arcus always circular?*

Answer: No. In the presence of a corneal pannus for example the lesion is situated parallel to the 'false' limbus.

Question: *What are the causes of secondary hyperlipidaemia?*

Answer: There are many causes, including diabetes mellitus, alcoholism, myxoedema, obstructive jaundice, iatrogenic (steroid or oral contraceptive administration), nephrotic syndrome, myelomatosis and acute porphyria.

Question: *Are there any racial differences associated with corneal arcus?*

Answer: Yes. Arcus senilis develops more commonly in black patients, and at an earlier age than in white patients.

33. Eyelid basal cell carcinoma (BCC)

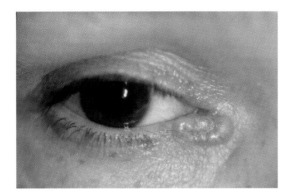

Figure 22 A medial canthal basal cell carcinoma (courtesy of Jane Gardiner MD).

Definition

A common malignant tumour of eyelid skin, originating from the basal layer of the epidermis or a hair follicle.

Clinical features

Clinical appearance is variable, but there are two main types.

1. The nodulo-ulcerative type appears as a pearly nodule or as a 'rodent' ulcer with the classical rolled edge and fine surface vessels which may bleed with minor trauma.
2. The fibrosing/sclerosing type originates in the epidermis but may invade and spread radially within the dermis, giving it an indistinct flat scar like appearance without telangiectatic vessels.

Exam questions

Question: *Is a patient with a BCC likely to present with local lymphadenopathy?*

Answer: No. These tumours are non-metastasizing, slow-growing, locally invasive and destructive. If an ulcer becomes secondarily infected there may be a reactive lymphadenopathy.

Question: *Where are these tumours most commonly found?*

Answer: The commonest sites are on the lower eyelid and at the medial canthus. They are more commonly seen in fair skinned men over the age of 50 years.

Question: *What treatment modalities are suitable for a BCC?*

Answer: Treatment can be successful with surgical excision (+/− frozen section control), cryotherapy (using a −30°C freeze-thaw-refreeze technique) or radiotherapy. The choice is dependent on tumour size/site and clinician/patient choice.

Question: *Which form of treatment is considered ideal for a small medial lower eyelid BCC, and why?*

Answer: Cryotherapy, because the lacrimal drainage apparatus is relatively resistant to cryo-damage.

Question: *What are the disadvantages of cryotherapy treatment?*

Answer: Skin depigmentation occurs at −10°C and madarosis (loss of eyelashes) occurs at −20°C. The recurrence rate is about 10%, but this is similar to that after surgical excision or radiotherapy.

Question: *What is the classical histological feature of a BCC?*

Answer: The histology of a BCC can be of 4 types; solid, cystic, adenoid or morpheic (fibrosing). The commonest type is solid, the classic feature of which is a regular palisading (fencing) of basal cells surrounding islands of haphazardly arranged cells.

34. Proptosis

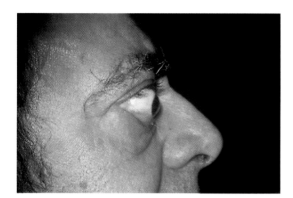

Figure 23   Proptosis secondary to dysthyroid eye disease (courtesy of Duncan Anderson MD).

Definition

An abnormal prominence of one or both eyes produced by a retrobulbar mass. The term exophthalmos refers to proptosis secondary to dysthyroid eye disease.

Clinical features

Scleral show (above the lower eyelid margin and below the upper eyelid margin) is a useful initial sign in cases of proptosis not immediately obvious. This sign can, however, also occur with eyelid retraction in the absence of proptosis.

The normal distance between the apex of the cornea and the lateral orbital rim is 16–21 mm. This value can be measured using an exophthalmometer. Anything above the normal range indicates proptosis. An asymmetry of more than 2 mm between the two eyes, with values within the normal range, is suggestive of unilateral proptosis and warrants further investigation.

Proptosis can be axial or non-axial, depending on whether the retrobulbar mass is respectively intra- or extra-conal (i.e. within or outside the cone formed by the extra-ocular muscles). This aspect of proptosis can simply be assessed using a clear plastic ruler.

(See Assessment of Orbital Disease, p. 28.)

Exam questions

Question: *What is pseudoproptosis, and what causes it?*

Answer: This is the simulation of prominence of one or both globes, or a true prominence not caused by a retrobulbar mass.

Apparent prominence may occur in the presence of contralateral enophthalmos, or may occur when there is asymmetry of palpebral aperture size, such as with ipsilateral lid retraction or contralateral ptosis.

True prominence, not due to proptosis, may arise if a globe is enlarged (high axial myopia, buphthalmos) or if the orbit is shallow (congenital, post-irradiation or post-surgical).

Question: *Why might visual acuity be reduced in a proptosed eye?*

Answer: Vision can be affected by:

- optic nerve compression
- exposure keratopathy
- posterior pole choroidal folds
- pseudohypermetropia

There is no relationship between the degree of optic nerve compression and proptosis. In some situations the proptosis 'relieves' the compression.

If a child presents with a mild proptosis and poor visual acuity, one should suspect an optic nerve glioma.

Question: *What is the commonest cause of bilateral proptosis in an adult?*

Answer: Dysthyroid eye disease. This results in an axial proptosis in most cases.

Question: *What is the commonest cause of unilateral proptosis in an adult?*

Answer: Dysthyroid eye disease. At least 80% of cases of axial proptosis are due to this, particularly during the early stages of thyrotoxicosis. Non-axial proptosis can also result from this condition. However, since over 90% of orbital tumours are extraconal these should always be considered in cases of non-axial proptosis.

Question: *What are the less common causes of proptosis in adults?*

Answer: Bilateral proptosis can occur in association with a cavernous sinus thrombosis or a carotico-cavernous fistula (pulsating proptosis).

Unilateral proptosis can complicate orbital cellulitis, orbital myositis (pseudotumour), a retrobulbar haemorrhage, vascular abnormality or an orbital tumour.

Question: *What are the causes of proptosis in children?*

Answer: Proptosis in childhood may arise secondary to:

- orbital cellulitis
- rhabdomyosarcoma
- orbital pseudotumour
- optic nerve glioma
- retrobulbar haemorrhage
- vascular abnormality

and rarely due to

- thyroid ophthalmopathy
- neuroblastoma
- histiocytosis.

35. Dysthyroid eye disease

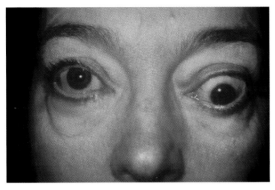

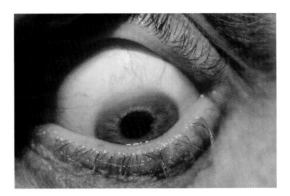

a   b

Figure 24   a: Severe ocular misalignment secondary to dysthyroid eye disease (courtesy of Gordon Douglas MD); b: Superior limbic keratoconjunctivitis (courtesy of Peng Khaw PhD MRCP FRCS FRCOphth).

Definition

Ophthalmic disease, which is associated with a disorder of the thyroid gland in most cases.

Clinical features

There are numerous potential clinical signs.

Eyelid signs:

- Eyelid retraction (Dalrymple's sign) – look for scleral show
- Upper lid-lag on downgaze (von Graefe's sign)
- Eyelid oedema/puffiness
- Fine tremor of closed eyelids (Rosenbach's sign)
- Reduced blink rate (Stellwag's sign)
- Increased eyelid pigmentation (Jellinek's sign)
- Increased upper lid resistance to downward traction (Grove's sign).

Other soft tissue signs:

- Conjunctival injection
- Chemosis
- Superior Limbic Keratoconjunctivitis (SLK)
- Palpable lacrimal gland and inferior rectus muscles
- Orbital fat extrusion.

Proptosis (Exophthalmos):

- usually bilateral and axial, but can be unilateral and non-axial. Dysthyroid eye disease is the commonest cause of proptosis in adults
- there may be an associated rise in intra-ocular pressure on upgaze and signs of corneal exposure. With unilateral proptosis a rise in pressure on upgaze in the non-affected eye is suggestive of dysthyroid eye disease.

Signs of optic neuropathy:

- reduced visual acuity
- reduced colour vision
- visual field defects

- relative afferant pupillary defect
- retinal vascular congestion
- chorioretinal folds
- optic nerve head swelling or atrophy.

Restrictive strabismus:

- contractures most commonly involve the inferior rectus and then the medial rectus.

Involvement of the superior rectus is rare and the lateral rectus is very rarely involved.

Exam questions

Question: *What is the likely thyroid status of a patient with dysthyroid eye disease?*

Answer: Many patients will have had hyperthyroidism at some stage. However, the eye disease is unrelated to thyroid hormone levels; indeed, treatment of hyperthyroidism can make proptosis worse. Patients may thus be hyper-, hypo- or eu-thyroid, both clinically or biochemically.

Question: *What is the HLA association with dysthyroid eye disease?*

Answer: HLA-DR3.

Question: *What are the pathological changes that occur in the orbit to produce proptosis?*

Answer: Extraocular muscle enlargement occurs due to hypertrophy, oedema and infiltration by inflammatory cells, especially lymphocytes. In addition there is an apparent increase in the amount of orbital fat and connective tissue associated with accumulation of fluid, glycosaminoglycans and lymphocytes. The number of orbital mast cells is also increased.
The increased mass of orbital contents results in the proptosis. Later there is degeneration of muscle cells, fibrosis and contracture.

Question: *How can acute optic nerve compression due to dysthyroid eye disease be treated?*

Answer: Some clinicians prefer a medical, others a surgical approach. Medical (immunosuppressive) decompression involves treatment with a high dose systemic steroid regimen (with or without adjunctive radiotherapy). Surgical decompression has a high success rate providing that the posterior third of the orbit is decompressed. Post-operatively treatment can be augmented with a short period of steroid therapy and radiotherapy which is effective after a lag period.

Question: *What is the most commonly performed squint operation for restrictive dysthyroid eye disease?*

Answer: Inferior rectus recession. The commonest eye movement defect affecting patients with dysthyroid eye disease is an elevator palsy due to a fibrotic contracture of the inferior rectus muscle. Once the deviation is static, a recession using adjustable sutures is ideal. An associated conjunctival recession may be required. Post-operative sub-conjunctival steroid injections may improve results.

Question: *What is superior limbic keratoconjunctivitis (SLK)?*

Answer: This is a condition which usually affects middle aged women with dysthyroid eye disease but which may occur following intraocular surgery or viral keratoconjunctivitis. The main features, confined to the superior part of both eyes, are bulbar conjunctival injection, limbitis, filamentary keratitis and tarsal papillary hypertrophy. The condition is chronic and is managed with topical lubricants and acetylcysteine. Use of soft contact lenses may provide symptomatic relief.

36. Keratoconjunctivitis sicca (KCS)

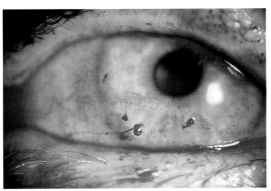

a

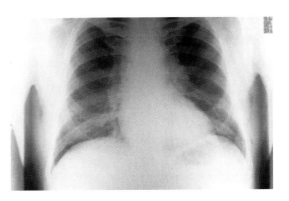

b

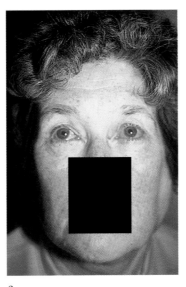

c

Figure 25 Keratoconjunctivitis sicca. a: Corneal mucous plaques stained with rose bengal stain (courtesy of Jack Kanski MD MS FRCOphth); b: A rare cause of KCS is sarcoidosis. This chest X-ray shows hilar lymphadenopathy in a patient with Mikulicz syndrome (courtesy of Robert Nozik MD and Carlos Pavesio MD); c: Red eyes and a swollen parotid gland in a patient with Mikulicz syndrome (courtesy of Peng Khaw PhD MRCP FRCS FRCOphth).

Definition

A dry eye syndrome due to deficient production of the aqueous component of the pre-corneal tear film.

Clinical features

1. the lower lid tear meniscus is reduced to less than 0.2 mm
2. non-adherent mucus threads

3. adherent corneal epithelial filaments
4. interpalpebral:
   - punctate epithelial erosions
   - Rose Bengal staining
   - corneal opacification
5. reduced tear secretion as measured by the Schirmer's test
6. evidence of secondary infective keratitis or conjunctivitis.

Exam questions

Question: *If a patient complains of dry eyes, what is the most likely diagnosis?*

Answer: Blepharitis.

Question: *What are the causes of KCS?*

Answer: Causes include the autoimmune conditions of pure KCS or Sjögren's syndrome. Other causes include sarcoidosis (including Mikulicz syndrome), blockage of the lacrimal glands excretory ducts by conjunctival scarring and absence of the lacrimal gland. Familial dysautonomia (Riley–Day syndrome) is a very rare cause. KCS is also found more commonly in patients with psoriasis or inflammatory bowel disease.

Question: *What is Sjögren's syndrome?*

Answer: Primary Sjögren's syndrome, also known as the 'sicca syndrome', is an autoimmune disorder, usually affecting middle-aged women, characterized by destruction of the lacrimal and salivary glands resulting in dry eyes and a dry mouth (xerostomia). In addition there may be dryness of the nose, pharynx, tracheo-bronchial tree, stomach, vagina or skin. Associated autoantibodies include (in order of frequency), ANA, RhF, anti-Ro(SS-A) and anti-La(SS-B). Histopathological examination of involved glands reveals an infiltration of lymphocytes and plasma cells in early disease and fibrosis in late disease.

Secondary Sjögren's syndrome is the sicca complex in association with a connective tissue disorder such as rheumatoid arthritis.

Question: *Are patients with Sjögren's syndrome at increased risk of any malignancy?*

Answer: Yes. These patients have a 40-fold increased risk of developing a non-Hodgkin's lymphoma.

Question: *Is the tear film lysozyme concentration affected in KCS?*

Answer: Yes, it is reduced. This is partly responsible for the increased risk of secondary infections which patients with KCS experience.

37. Xerophthalmia

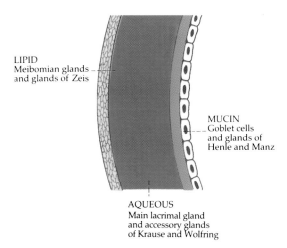

LIPID
Meibomian glands
and glands of Zeis

MUCIN
Goblet cells
and glands of
Henle and Manz

AQUEOUS
Main lacrimal gland
and accessory glands
of Krause and Wolfring

Figure 26   The three layers of the normal pre-corneal tear film (reproduced, with permission, from *Clinical Ophthalmology*, third edition by Jack Kanski MD MS FRCOphth).

Definition

A dry eye syndrome due to deficient production of the mucin component of the pre-corneal tear film.

Clinical features

- areas of non-wetting on the ocular surface
- a reduction in the tear film break-up time, often to <10 sec.
- a normal Schirmer's test (cf KCS)
- Bitot spots may be present. These superficial, refractile masses, with a silvery colour and foamy texture are found on exposed bulbar conjunctiva, usually temporally within the palpebral fissure.

Exam questions

Question: *What are the causes of xerophthalmia?*

Answer: Primary xerophthalmia is due to Vitamin A deficiency which can occur due to:

- dietary deficiency
- malabsorption syndromes (coeliac disease, cystic fibrosis, post-small bowel resection etc.).

Xerophthalmia can also occur secondary to conditions which result in conjunctival scarring and goblet cell dysfunction or destruction. Conjunctival scarring of a sufficient degree can occur with:

- Stevens–Johnson syndrome
- ocular cicatricial pemphigoid
- chemical burns
- irradiation
- trachoma.

If the conjunctival scarring is associated with scarring of the lacrimal gland ducts, an element of KCS is superimposed.

Question: *When, and in whom, are Bitot spots found?*

Answer: Bitot spots are found mainly in children (especially boys) with an acute deficiency in dietary Vitamin A. In association with dryness of the conjunctiva (xerosis conjunctivae) they are an early surface sign of the deficiency. Night blindness is invariably an associated finding. Similar spots can also be seen in eyes with a tear film disturbance or in association with contact lens wear.

Question: *How can a deficiency of Vitamin A adversely affect vision?*

Answer: Anterior segment changes can occur due to xerophthalmia (dry eye) or keratomalacia (corneal softening), these, in association with concurrent infection, being a leading cause of worldwide blindness.

Loss of photoreceptor sensitivity occurs due to the loss of a photopigment component (retinal). This is initially manifest by night blindness.

Rare causes include bone growth abnormalities resulting in optic nerve compression and foetal abnormalities due to maternal vitamin deficiency.

Question: *Where is the pre-corneal tear film mucin produced?*

Answer: Mucin is produced by conjunctival goblet cells, by corneal and conjunctival epithelial cell microvilli and by the lacrimal gland. The lacrimal gland in fact possesses twice the number of mucin acini as aqueous acini.

Question: *Which part of the pre-corneal tear film does the mucin component form?*

Answer: The innermost of the three layers. The middle layer, which is the thickest is formed by the aqueous components and the outermost layer is the lipid layer.

Question: *What is the treatment for xerophthalmia?*

Answer: High doses of Vitamin A.

38. Follicular conjunctivitis

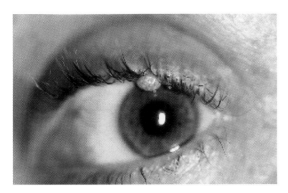

Figure 27 Follicular conjunctivitis. Molluscum contagiosum (courtesy of Jane Gardiner MD).

Definition

Conjunctival inflammation characterized by conjunctival follicles.

Clinical features

Follicles

These are small elevated swellings of lymphoid tissue, which often have the appearance of small subconjunctival grains of rice (0.5–5 mm in size). They are encircled by blood vessels, which aids distinguishing them from papillae which have a central core of blood vessels.
It is important to examine the inferior fornix where follicles are most commonly found but in the examination situation a candidate should ask the patient and examiner before everting the upper eyelid.

Exam questions

Question: *Are conjunctival follicles always of clinical significance?*

Answer: No. In an asymptomatic young patient a moderate degree of lymphoid hyperplasia can be normal, requiring no investigation or treatment.

Question: *What pathological state can a follicular conjunctivitis represent?*

Answer: Follicles represent lymphoid hyperplasia. They are particularly indicative of conditions in which cell-mediated immune mechanisms are involved. These include viral, chlamydial and drug-hypersensitivity disorders.

Question: *What are the causes of an acute follicular conjunctivitis?*

Answer: This is usually due to a viral or chlamydial infection. The commonest causes are adenoviral, primary herpetic and chlamydial (trachomatis and oculogenitalis) infections. Rare causes are epidemic haemorrhagic conjunctivitis (enterovirus-70; a picorna-virus infection) and Newcastle disease.

Question: *What conditions could cause a chronic follicular conjunctivitis in a child?*

Answer: Molluscum contagiosum and adenoviral infections are the commonest cause in the UK, but trachoma causes the most cases worldwide.
In all cases of follicular conjunctivitis it is important to examine the eyelids for evidence of the pale, waxy, umbilicated, elevated nodules specific to molluscum contagiosum.

Question: *Is neonatal inclusion conjunctivitis (a chlamydial infection) follicular in nature?*

Answer: No. Follicles, which are lymphoid tissue, do not form in infants less than three months of age. The conjunctivitis is acute, mucopurulent and papillary in nature.

39.   Cicatricial conjunctival disease

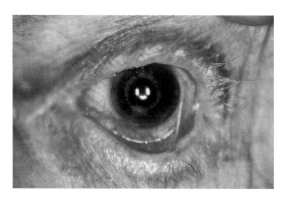

Figure 28   Ocular cicatricial pemphigoid (courtesy of Jane Gardiner MD).

Definition

A group of disorders associated with scarring and shrinkage of the conjunctiva.

Classification

1. *Trauma*
   - Physical
   - Burns
   - Ionising radiation
2. *Infection*
   - Trachoma
   - Membranous conjunctivitis
3. *Drug-induced*
   - Systemic
   - Topical (pseudopemphigoid)
4. *Oculocutaneous disorders*
   - Mucous membrane/ocular pemphigoid
   - Stevens–Johnson syndrome (Erythema multiforme)
   - Toxic epidermal necrolysis
   - Linear IgA disease
   - Epidermolysis bullosa
   - Dermatitis herpetiformis
   - Pemphigus
   - Chronic atopic keratoconjunctivitis (AKC)
5. *Other*
   - Paraneoplastic syndromes
   - Rosacea
   - Sjögren's syndrome
   - Inflammatory bowel disease
   - Immune complex diseases
   - Graft-versus-host disease.

Clinical features

It is important to not only observe the conjunctival scarring and shrinkage, but in addition to notice the associated ocular complications. These include:

- symblepharon (adhesions between palpebral and bulbar conjunctiva)
- ankyloblepharon (adhesions between eyelids)
- eyelid deformity (entropion, trichiasis, lagophthalmos)
- KCS (keratoconjunctivitis sicca) (see p. 127)
- xerophthalmia (see p. 129)
- corneal involvement (exposure, opacification, ulceration, pannus, pseudopterygium).

Additional clues can aid the making of a diagnosis:

1. If unilateral, then trauma, irradiation, a chemical burn or hypersensitivity/toxicity to a topical drug are more likely to be involved in the aetiology.
2. If bilateral and associated with skin or mucous membrane lesions, a mucocutaneous bullous disorder should be considered. These include:
   - cicatricial pemphigoid
   - Stevens–Johnson syndrome
   - pemphigus
   - drug-induced
3. An early subtle sign of ocular cicatricial pemphigoid is loss of medial canthal architecture.

Exam questions

Question: *What drugs can cause cicatricial conjunctival disease?*

Answer: Systemic use of the β-blocker Practolol can cause the oculomucocutaneous syndrome, which is characterized by conjunctival scarring, a psoriasis like rash, peritoneal and retroperitoneal fibrosis. Chronic, topical administration of antiglaucomatous medications (such as adrenaline and pilocarpine), phospholine iodide or anti-viral agents such as trifluorothymidine (F₃T) may also induce conjunctival scarring. The preservatives present in these topical preparations may play a significant role in their adverse effect.

In addition, Stevens–Johnson syndrome can be a complication of certain drugs such as sulphonamides.

Question: *What is the aetiology of Stevens–Johnson syndrome (Erythema multiforme)?*

Answer: This is an acute Type III hypersensitivity reaction to sulphonamides, including acetazolamide; non-steroidal anti-inflammatory drugs (NSAIDs); barbiturates; penicillin; tetracycline or certain bacteria and viruses. An immune vasculitis occurs secondary to the deposition of circulating antigen with complement-fixing antibody (immune complex deposition).

Question: *Which HLA type is associated with cicatricial pemphigoid?*

Answer: HLA-B12 and HLA-DQw7.

Question: *Are the skin blisters of pemphigoid more or less likely to rupture than those of pemphigus?*

Answer: Less. The blisters of pemphigoid form at the level of the basement membrane between the epidermis and dermis. They are thus thicker, and less likely to rupture than those of pemphigus which form within the epidermis.

Question: *How do the symblephara of ocular cicatricial pemphigoid and Stevens–Johnson syndrome differ?*

Answer: The symblephara of pemphigoid tend to be broad and those of Stevens–Johnson syndrome tend to be narrow.

40. Conjunctival melanosis

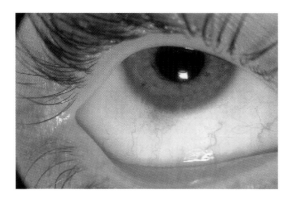

Figure 29 Inferior limbal/bulbar conjunctival melanosis (courtesy of Gordon Douglas MD).

Definition

Increased pigmentation of the conjunctiva (diffuse or localized) due to hyperplasia and/or hypertrophy of conjunctival melanocytes. Lesions can be classified into the following types:

1. naevus
2. ephilis (freckle)
3. lentigo
4. primary acquired melanosis:
   - (simple/racial)
   - (with moderate atypia)
   - (with marked atypia, superficial spreading melanoma)
5. malignant melanoma
6. sub-epithelial melanosis:
   - (episcleral melanosis)
   - (congenital melanosis oculi)
   - (oculodermal melanocytosis or naevus of Ota).

Clinical features

On clinical examination it can be difficult to distinguish a benign, pre-malignant or frankly malignant lesion. Certain features can however, be helpful.

Naevi or freckles are usually single, well demarcated, flat or only slightly elevated lesions. They are usually situated at the limbus and tend to move with the conjunctiva.

Lentigo lesions are usually multiple macules of irregular shape and size seen in areas exposed to sunlight in elderly subjects.

Simple or racial epithelial melanosis presents as a flat lesion which moves freely over the sclera, but it is characteristically patchy. The pigmentation is usually most prominent at the limbus and around the perforating branches of the anterior ciliary arteries close to where they pierce the sclera.

Primary acquired (epithelial) melanosis, which histologically can show a full range in degree of atypia, may appear like a naevus, but when a degree of radial spread has occurred the lesion tends to be less well demarcated and/or more extensive than the typical naevus. Deep spread frequently occurs with the lesions that histologically show marked atypia. This can be associated with immobility of the conjunctiva over the sclera.

Primary malignant melanoma of the conjunctiva, which can arise 'de novo' or within a naevus or area of primary acquired melanosis, often shows conjunctival immobility, may be raised and is frequently associated with feeder vessels.

Sub-epithelial melanosis of whatever type tends to have a bluish tinge. In cases of ocular melanocytosis there will be evidence of other ocular melanocytic lesions and with the naevus of Ota an ipsilateral, periorbital dermal naevus will be evident.

The degree of pigmentation is variable with all these lesions and should not be used alone to predict the likelihood of malignancy. A malignant melanoma can be completely non-pigmented. The two most important aspects are the **history** and the **histology**, neither of which may be available in a short case examination.

Exam questions

Question: *How should a case of primary acquired melanosis of the conjunctiva be managed?*

Answer: This is dependent on the extent of the lesion, any reported or noted change within the lesion, the age of the patient and if a previous biopsy has been taken, on the degree of histological atypia. If, for example the lesion is multicentric, flat and superficial having developed in old age, observation (± photography) is sufficient. A suspicious area should be biopsied. If a lesion has changed (in degree of pigmentation, increase in size, thickness or nodularity, development of tethering, feeder vessels, etc.) or the patient is relatively young, a simple excision should be performed. If a biopsy shows a moderate or marked degree of atypia it should be excised since the risk of frank malignant change is up to 50–60%.

Question: *When may the degree of pigmentation of a conjunctival naevus change?*

Answer: An increase in the degree of pigmentation often occurs at puberty or during pregnancy. Malignant transformation within a naevus, although rare, can occur with junctional or compound naevi and may be associated with either an increase or decrease in the degree of pigmentation.

Question: *How does conjunctival malignant melanoma spread?*

Answer: Local spread within the conjunctiva can be radial and/or deep. Local spread beyond the conjunctiva can involve the eyelids, orbit and globe.
Lymphatic spread is to the pre-auricular and/or sub-mandibular nodes.
Blood borne metastases are most common in the liver, lung or bone.

Question: *What potentially curative methods of treatment are suitable for conjunctival malignant melanoma?*

Answer: Surgical excision is ideal for non-metastatic lesions. This may be simple or may require lamellar corneo-scleral resection, enucleation if invasion is through the sclera or exenteration if spread has involved the orbit or eyelids. Radiotherapy is at present only used as adjuvant therapy and the role of cryotherapy has yet to be fully evaluated. In cases of metastatic disease there may be a role for regional lymph node dissection and/or chemotherapy.

Question: *Is there an association between the naevus of Ota and conjunctival malignant melanoma?*

Answer: No. However, these patients are at an increased risk of developing a uveal melanoma for which annual follow up appointments should be arranged.

Question: *At which site does a conjunctival malignant melanoma, which has arisen in an area of primary acquired melanosis, have the worst prognosis?*

Answer: A melanoma of the palpebral conjunctiva which has arisen in an area of pre-existing primary acquired melanosis has the worst prognosis of all conjunctival melanomas, with a 5 year survival rate of 50%. This compares with 80% for limbal tumours and almost 100% for those arising in bulbar conjunctiva. There is more likely to be a delay in diagnosis of palpebral tumours and this may partially explain the lower survival rate.

Malignant melanoma of the caruncle carries the same prognosis as that of palpebral conjunctival tumours. The caruncle is derived from skin and thus should not be classified as a 'conjunctival' melanoma.

41. Corneal dystrophies

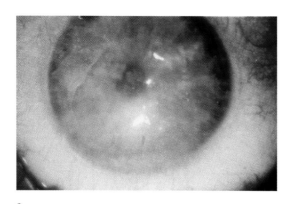

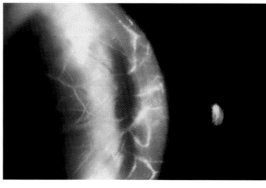

a   b

Figure 30 a: Macular dystrophy (courtesy of Gordon Douglas MD); b: Lattice dystrophy (courtesy of the Department of Medical Illustration, Moorfields Eye Hospital).

Definition

A corneal dystrophy is a primary corneal change unaccompanied by systemic disease, which is slowly progressive and not associated with vascularization.

There are many types and only the more common dystrophies will be dealt with here, since these are more likely to appear in examinations. These can be classified as anterior, stromal, posterior or ectatic. Although the pathology is bilateral, the signs can be significantly asymmetrical.

Anterior

1. *Epithelial*:
   – Meesman's Epithelial Dystrophy
   – Hereditary Epithelial Dystrophy
2. *Bowman's*:
   – Cogan's Microcystic Dystrophy
   – Reis-Bucklers' Dystrophy.

Stromal

1. Lattice Dystrophy
2. Granular Dystrophy

3. Macular Dystrophy
4. Combined granular-lattice (Avellino) Dystrophy.

Posterior

1. Corneal Guttata
2. Fuchs' Endothelial Dystrophy
3. Posterior Polymorphous Dystrophy.

Ectatic

1. Keratoconus
2. Pellucid marginal degeneration.

Clinical features

Meesman's Epithelial Dystrophy

The epithelium is diffusely studded with very small opacities, which on retro-illumination may appear as collections of opaque material within clear spherical microcysts (10–15 µm). The opacities are of variable density and distribution and can be difficult to distinguish from the microcysts of early corneal oedema.

Hereditary Epithelial Dystrophy

Minute transparent epithelial droplet lesions have a predilection for the central cornea. These are best seen by retro-illumination, but remain difficult to distinguish from the lesions of Meesman's Dystrophy.

Cogan's Microcystic Dystrophy

This dystrophy includes dot, cystic, fingerprint and map variants, any one of which, over a long period of time, can change to another. The lesions can be found in the epithelium or within Bowman's zone and are best seen by retro-illumination.

1. Dot lesions are round or comma shaped, greyish and found in the epithelium. They have been referred to as 'putty-marks'.
2. Cystic lesions are transparent cysts within the epithelium which are larger than the microcysts of the epithelial dystrophies.
3. Fingerprint lesions are groups of curvilinear lucent opacities present on the anterior surface of Bowman's zone, which can look somewhat like a fingerprint.
4. Map lesions are large polymorphic, faintly grey opacities found between the epithelium and Bowman's zone. They represent abnormal basement membrane.

Reis-Bucklers' Dystrophy

This condition is characterized by a central 'honeycomb' lesion based around Bowman's zone with crescentic or hoop-like opacities which project into both the epithelium and the anterior stroma. The anterior corneal surface may be distorted and there may be diffuse anterior scarring. The peripheral cornea is spared and corneal sensation is decreased.

Lattice Dystrophy

In the younger patient the spiders-web like deposits which characterize this dystrophy are only seen in the anterior stroma. These may be confused with prominent corneal nerves. In older patients the branching filaments are seen to be radially arranged, interlacing and overlapping at all levels, with a predilection for anterior stroma. Dot or stellate opacities may be present between the filaments. The peripheral cornea is spared and corneal sensation is decreased.

Granular Dystrophy

The characteristic feature of this condition is the presence of discrete whitish granules in the anterior axial corneal stroma. The lesions have been described as 'crumb-like'. In older patients the lesions may be seen in the mid-stroma but the peripheral cornea is always spared. Corneal sensation is normal.

Macular Dystrophy

In young patients this condition is characterized by a diffuse clouding of the central cornea with most involvement in the anterior stroma. The older patient shows superimposed, poorly defined, greyish opacities at all stromal levels and spread to the limbus may be evident. The peripheral lesions tend to be deeper. Corneal sensation is impaired.

Corneal Guttata

These are focal accumulations ('warty excrescences') of collagen on the posterior surface of Descemet's membrane. They are commonly seen in the older patient. Characteristic features include disruption of the regular endothelial mosaic, dark-spots on specular reflection, a beaten-metal appearance when advanced and occasionally associated melanin pigment deposits. If the peripheral cornea is involved the guttata are referred to as Hassall-Henle bodies and they represent an age related change. If the periphery is spared, the lesions may indicate early Fuchs' endothelial dystrophy.

Fuchs' Endothelial Dystrophy

An early feature is of corneal guttata with peripheral sparing. In more advanced cases there is evidence of endothelial decompensation, which may result in bullous keratopathy if severe. Frequent complications or associations include peripheral corneal vascularization, cataract and open angle glaucoma.

Posterior Polymorphous Dystrophy

This dystrophy is characterized by blisters and diffuse polymorphous opacities situated at the level of Descemet's membrane and the endothelium. The opacities can be vesicular, curvilinear or map like and may project into the posterior corneal stroma and/or the anterior chamber. Descemet's membrane is usually generally thickened. Curvilinear lesions may be confused with breaks in Descemet's membrane.

Keratoconus (conical cornea)

This condition is characterized by many clinical signs and is thus commonly seen in examinations. The main features are due to distortion of the normal symmetrical curvature of the cornea, induced by a thinning of its central and paracentral areas.

1. *Early signs*:
   - irregular myopic astigmatism
   - an irregular retinoscopy reflex (oil-drop sign)
   - abnormal keratoscopic figures
   - abnormal keratometric mires
   - abnormal keratometry
   - an irregular reflection with Placido's disc
   - Vogt's striae (vertical deep stromal and Descemet's membrane folds)
   - prominent corneal nerves
2. *Late signs*:
   - axial corneal thinning and high curvature (a cone shaped cornea)
   - reticular scarring in Bowman's zone
   - Fleischer's ring (epithelial iron deposits surrounding the cone base)
   - Munson's sign (a bulging of the lower eyelid on downgaze)
   - Descemet's membrane ruptures (acute hydrops).

A number of associated ocular anomalies have been described as occurring with greater frequency in patients with keratoconus in comparison with the normal population. These include:

- allergic eye disease
- blue sclera
- ectopia lentis
- cataract
- aniridia
- retinitis pigmentosa
- optic atrophy
- microcornea
- Leber's congenital amaurosis
- contact lens wear.

NB: Don't risk bad grace with an examiner by not asking if he/she would like you to test a patient's corneal sensation before you launch-in!

Exam questions

Question: *By what mode are the corneal dystrophies inherited?*

Answer: Most of the corneal dystrophies are inherited in an autosomal dominant manner. Exceptions include Macular Dystrophy, which has an autosomal recessive inheritance and keratoconus which only rarely has a recognized pattern of inheritance.

Question: *What do the deposits which form the opacities of the stromal corneal dystrophies consist of?*

Answer: In Lattice Dystrophy the deposits are extracellular and consist of amyloid-like material. In Granular Dystrophy the deposits are also extracellular and consist of non-collagenous protein. In Macular Dystrophy there is deposition of glycosaminoglycans (mucopolysaccharides) both extra- and intra-cellularly.

Question: *Can stromal corneal dystrophies recur after penetrating keratoplasty?*

Answer: Lattice and Macular Dystrophies can both recur in donor cornea, usually after about five years. Patients with Granular Dystrophy rarely require corneal grafting, but should this prove necessary recurrence does not occur.

Question: *What are the causes of the recurrent corneal erosion syndrome?*

Answer: The commonest cause of this is trauma, particularly corneal scratches or abrasions caused by sharp instruments or often from the edge of a piece of paper. Of the corneal dystrophies, the strongest association is with Cogan's Microcystic Dystrophy, but recurrent erosions are also a feature of Reis-Bucklers', Lattice and Macular dystrophies. Recurrent erosions can also affect the upper cornea in patients with rosacea.

Patients who also have diabetes mellitus tend to suffer a more severe form of the condition.

Question: *When and how does Reis-Bucklers' Dystrophy usually present?*

Answer: Presentation is usually in early childhood with recurrent corneal erosions.

Question: *How can patients with Fuchs' Endothelial Dystrophy be managed?*

Answer: The appropriate type of management is dependent on the severity of the condition. If mild and asymptomatic no treatment is required. If severe, and cataract extraction is contemplated, consideration should be given to performing a penetrating keratoplasty at the same time as cataract surgery. If endothelial decompensation has caused epithelial oedema, this may respond to topical hypertonic agents. Intra-ocular pressure reduction (e.g. with topical β-blockers) can reduce both epithelial and stromal oedema, although use of topical carbonic anhydrase inhibitors (e.g. dorzolamide) should be avoided. For painful bullous keratopathy soft bandage contact lenses can provide relief. Penetrating keratoplasty, which has a high success rate, is at present the only means of definitive treatment.

Question: *How do patients with Posterior Polymorphous Corneal Dystrophy usually present?*

Answer: This condition is usually asymptomatic, innocuous and non-progressive and thus usually presents as an incidental finding.

Question: *What systemic diseases or syndromes are associated with keratoconus?*

Answer: Keratoconus, in comparison with the normal population, occurs with a greater frequency in patients with various conditions such as:

- atopy
- Down's syndrome
- Turner's syndrome
- Ehlers–Danlos syndrome
- Marfan's syndrome
- Apert's syndrome
- Addison's disease
- neurofibromatosis.

Question: *Patients with prominent corneal nerves may be misdiagnosed as having a corneal dystrophy. In what conditions can prominent corneal nerves sometimes be seen?*

Answer: Prominent corneal nerves can in fact be seen in association with one of the corneal dystrophies, namely keratoconus. Other associated conditions include leprosy, neurofibromatosis and type II multiple endocrine adenomatosis (MEA II, Sipple Syndrome). In most cases no cause is ever identified.

Question: *Can treatment with contact lenses halt the progression of keratoconus?*

Answer: No. Although hard contact lenses can neutralize the irregular myopic astigmatism of early keratoconus, they have no effect on disease progression.

Question: *Is the success rate of penetrating keratoplasty good or bad in patients with keratoconus?*

Answer: Very good. The result of grafting is not compromised by pre-existing vascularization and the patients tend to be young, fit and well motivated.

Question: *What is acute hydrops?*

Answer: This condition, which can occur with keratoconus, is secondary to ruptures in Descemet's membrane. The ruptures allow an acute influx of fluid into the corneal stroma and epithelium. This is seen clinically as gross corneal oedema affecting mainly the axial cornea, resulting in pain and a rapid fall in visual acuity.

42. Band keratopathy

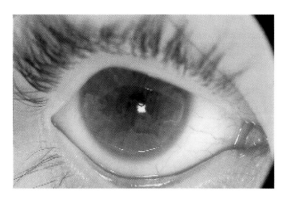

Figure 31 Right corneal band keratopathy secondary to previous long-standing childhood uveitis (courtesy of Gordon Douglas MD).

Definition

Deposition of calcium salts in the inter-palpebral region of the cornea.

Clinical features

Deposition is mainly in the sub-epithelial space and anterior part of Bowman's zone of the inter-palpebral region of the cornea. A clear space separates the lesion from the limbus. The lesion starts in both the 3 and 9 o'clock positions and progression occurs centrally, the lesion becoming a single plaque. Small holes within the plaque may represent channels within Bowman's zone which transmit corneal nerves. In the more advanced case deposition may extend posteriorly into the corneal stroma and anteriorly to produce an irregular epithelial surface which can break down causing pain.

Exam questions

Question: *What are the causes of band keratopathy?*

Answer: Band keratopathy is most commonly seen in elderly patients and in most cases is idiopathic. As a general principle the band forms when the concentrations of calcium and phosphate exceed the level at which they are soluble (i.e. due to factors that alter pH, tear evaporation or concentration of the salts). In a fair number of cases there is a history of chronic uveitis of childhood and in rare cases prolonged hypercalcaemia is the cause. A band is commonly seen in association with phthisis bulbi and has also been found with a higher frequency in patients with posterior polymorphous corneal dystrophy.

Question: *What are the indications for treatment of band keratopathy?*

Answer: Treatment may be required for visual or cosmetic reasons or to remove the cause of an irregular epithelial surface which has broken down and produced a painful lesion.

Question: *How can band keratopathy be removed?*

Answer: After mechanical debridement of the corneal epithelium application of a chelating agent (sodium edetate or versenate) aids band debridement. Excimer laser removal of band keratopathy is proving promising.

Question: *With what might early band keratopathy be confused?*

Answer: Vogt's limbal girdle or an incomplete corneal arcus.

43. Lipid keratopathy

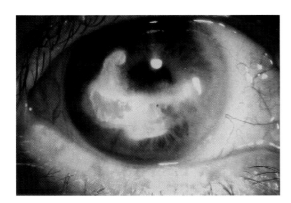

Figure 32 Lipid keratopathy (courtesy of the Department of Medical Illustration, Moorfields Eye Hospital).

Definition

Plaques of lipid (mainly cholesterol and fatty acids) within the corneal stroma resulting from haemorrhage or exudation of plasma from stromal vessels.

Clinical features

Plaques of yellow-white intra-stromal lipid are associated with corneal neovascularization. Other signs of the cause of corneal neovascularization may be evident.

Exam questions

Question: *What are the causes of lipid keratopathy?*

Answer: Corneal neovascularization secondary to any cause may be associated with lipid keratopathy and this is particularly likely if the cornea has previously been inflamed. Herpetic corneal disease is a common cause in the UK and USA. Disorders of fat metabolism which can produce such a keratopathy are rare.

Question: *Is surgery the only possible method of treating lipid keratopathy?*

Answer: No. Argon laser photocoagulation of the corneal vessels may be followed by resorption of the fat but this is usually very slow.

Question: *What are the histopathological features of lipid keratopathy?*

Answer: Corneal specimens prepared by a standard method will show empty clefts representing lipid dissolved during preparation, a granulomatous inflammatory reaction and stromal blood vessels.

Question: *Is spheroidal degeneration of the cornea a type of lipid keratopathy?*

Answer: No. This condition, which has also been called corneal elastosis, Labrador keratopathy, climatic droplet keratopathy or Bietti's nodular dystrophy is a degenerative condition probably related to excessive ultraviolet radiation exposure. Small, amber coloured, drop-like lesions are present in the interpalpebral anterior corneal stroma. These are associated with variable corneal opacification. The lesions do not consist of lipid but represent elastoid degeneration of collagen and other proteins containing tryptophan, tyrosine, cysteine and cystine.

Question: *What other ocular condition is spheroidal degeneration often associated with?*

Answer: Conjunctival pingueculae are frequently seen in association with spheroidal degeneration of the cornea. These are also thought to be related to ultraviolet radiation exposure.

44. Corneal opacification

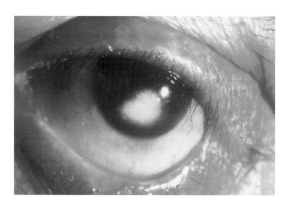

Figure 33 Corneal leucoma (courtesy of Gordon Douglas MD).

Definitions

Leucoma:

(Gk. white) the involved part of the cornea is totally opaque. A 'localized leucoma' is surrounded by normal cornea, whereas with a 'generalized' leucoma the whole cornea is white. An 'adherent' leucoma is a corneal opacity complicated by attachment of ocular tissue posterior to the cornea, such as the iris.

Macular:

(Lat. spot) the corneal opacity is dense and circumscribed but more transparent than a leucoma.

Nebula:

(Lat. cloud) the opacification is slight and diffuse.

Causes can be congenital or acquired. Acquired causes include trauma, inflammation (including infection), degeneration or dystrophy.

Clinical features

The clinical signs are highly variable depending on the cause of the opacification. Even if the cause remains obscure credit can be obtained in the exam situation for fully describing the opacification. The candidate should describe the extent, depth, density and nature of the opacification and in addition any associated features such as neovascularization or irregularity of the corneal surface. It is important to look for clues which may indicate an aetiology and in particular the eyelids, eyelashes, conjunctiva and anterior chamber should be examined carefully.

Exam questions

Question: *What are the possible causes of corneal opacification in a newborn infant?*

Answer: Congenital corneal leucoma may occur secondary to embryonic dysgenesis, oedema, in-born errors of metabolism, inflammation or chromosomal defects.

With embryonic dysgenesis opacification may occur because the lens vesicle fails to fully separate from the surface ectoderm (anterior chamber cleavage syndrome), the endothelium fails to form (congenital hereditary endothelial dystrophy) or the cornea fails to differentiate from the sclera (sclerocornea).

In addition to endothelial dystrophy, oedema producing corneal opacification may occur with congenital glaucoma or Descemet's membrane ruptures secondary to birth trauma.

In-born errors of metabolism which can be associated with corneal opacification include the mucopolysaccharidoses, mucolipidosis, gangliosidosis, cystinosis, Lowe's and Riley–Day syndromes and von Gierke's disease.

Post-inflammatory opacities of the cornea can be present with the rubella syndrome, interstitial keratitis or congenital herpes simplex infection.

Chromosomal defects which may be associated with corneal opacification include the trisomies 13, 14, 15, 18 and 21.

Question: *What is the importance of involvement of Bowman's zone or deeper parts of the cornea in traumatic lesions?*

Answer: Traumatic epithelial defects heal without scarring. Deeper lesions, however, involving Bowman's zone and below heal with permanent opaque scarring.

Question: *What are recipient adverse prognostic factors for penetrating keratoplasty?*

Answer: These include:

- stromal vascularization
- corneal anaesthesia
- thinning of the proposed host-graft junction
- uncontrolled glaucoma
- anterior synechiae
- conjunctival inflammation
- epithelial abnormality
- stem cell deficiency

- tear film dysfunction
- eyelid malposition
- infancy
- poor post-operative care.

Question: *What are the major problems with a corneal graft greater than 8.5 mm in diameter?*

Answer: There is a high risk of peripheral anterior synechiae formation, graft vascularization, raised intra-ocular pressure and graft failure.

Question: *What is the major problem with a corneal graft less than 7.5 mm in diameter?*

Answer: An increased risk of post-operative corneal astigmatism. If penetrating keratoplasty is considered appropriate treatment for a small corneal opacity it is better to remove some normal surrounding cornea, making the graft about 7.5 mm in diameter, rather than performing a small graft which is likely to cause irregular astigmatism. A rotational autograft may be appropriate for treatment of a small corneal opacity.

45. Peripheral corneal ulceration

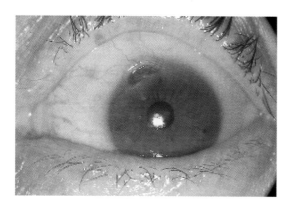

Figure 34 Peripheral corneal ulceration. A Mooren's ulcer (courtesy of Gordon Douglas MD).

Definition

Peripheral corneal ulceration or melting secondary to one of an unrelated group of ocular and systemic conditions.

Ocular conditions:

1. dellen
2. marginal keratitis
3. phlyctenulosis
4. Terrien's marginal degeneration
5. Mooren's ulcer.

Systemic conditions:

1. rosacea
2. connective tissue disorders:
   - sero +ve rheumatoid arthritis
   - systemic lupus erythematosis (SLE)
   - scleroderma
   - polyarteritis nodosa (PAN)
   - giant cell (temporal) arteritis (GCA)
   - Wegener's granulomatosis
   - relapsing polychondritis

3. other rare associations:
   - acute leukaemia
   - gold toxicity
   - bacillary dysentery
   - influenza.

Clinical features

These conditions are characterized by, or associated with, either peripheral corneal thinning or frank ulceration. The peripheral corneal changes show certain specific characteristics with some of the conditions and associated non-corneal signs can aid making a diagnosis.

Dellen

There is a peripheral saucer-like thinning of the cornea usually associated with a raised limbal lesion.

Marginal keratitis

A marginal ulcer is preceded by sub-epithelial infiltrate separated from the limbus by a clear zone of cornea. Common sites are at the 2, 4, 8 and 10 o'clock positions. With time the lesions spread circumferentially and become complicated by corneal vascularization. A common associated feature is chronic blepharoconjunctivitis. An acute ulcer is unlikely to be seen in the exam situation but the scars produced may be seen, even if only in a patient with multiple pathology.

Phlyctenulosis

A corneal phlycten starts as a cystic lesion and becomes a fleshy nodule which lies astride the limbus. If this fails to resolve, extension further onto the cornea associated with a leash of fine vessels can form a fascicular ulcer. Again, the acute lesion is unlikely to be seen as a short case, particularly since this usually occurs in childhood. However, a resulting scar may be evident. These are classically triangular limbal-based scars.

Terrien's marginal degeneration

Although rare this is seen more commonly in exams than in the clinic. An established lesion is seen as a peripheral opacification associated with localized corneal thinning forming a gutter. The outer slope of the gutter shelves gradually whereas the inner slope is steep, often being demarcated by lipid deposits. It is separated from the limbus by a clear zone of cornea which is commonly bridged by vessels which come to lie in the floor of the gutter. The clear peripheral cornea may show signs of ectasia. The lesion is not a true ulcer since the epithelium remains intact and the condition is usually bilateral, occurring in quiet white eyes.

Mooren's ulcer

This is a rare and painful condition and is thus not likely to be seen in exams. In its limited form the condition is unilateral, whereas the progressive type is bilateral. The key features of the established lesion are a gutter with an overhanging advancing (innermost) edge, epithelial loss (a true ulcer), vascularization of the base and thin peripheral corneal scarring. The sclera is never involved, unlike with peripheral ulcers associated with some systemic conditions.

Peripheral corneal ulceration secondary to systemic disease

(see also Rosacea, p. 149)
Any peripheral corneal ulcer that appears to be unexplained by ocular disease may be secondary to systemic disease. It is therefore important to look for the general features of conditions such as rosacea, rheumatoid arthritis, SLE or scleroderma.

Exam questions

Question: *What is the aetiology and pathology of a dellen?*

Answer: A dellen is a localized area of corneal stromal dehydration and the pathological change is thus of compaction of corneal lamellae producing a localized excavation. The aetiology usually involves a raised limbal lesion associated with localized pre-corneal tear film instability. Causative limbal lesions include a dermoid, conjunctival chemosis or haemorrhage, a large or hooded trabeculectomy bleb, a pterygium, a phlycten or an episcleritis nodule.

Question: *How can early marginal keratitis be distinguished from a peripheral herpes simplex virus (HSV) ulcer and why is this important?*

Answer: This can be difficult unless the condition is seen in its earliest stage. A marginal ulcer is preceded by sub-epithelial infiltration whereas an HSV ulcer starts as an epithelial defect which only later becomes associated with such infiltration. Corneal sensation may be decreased with HSV disease but is normal with marginal keratitis. Marginal keratitis is frequently associated with chronic staphylococcal blepharoconjunctivitis, but this alone cannot exclude HSV disease.
The importance of distinguishing these two conditions lies in the fact that should HSV disease be treated for marginal keratitis, namely with topical steroids, it would progress and may result in corneal perforation.

Question: *What are the symptoms and complications of Terrien's marginal degeneration?*

Answer: Recurrent episodes of pain and inflammation are rare but the patient may complain of mild irritation. A gradual fall in visual acuity occurs due to progressive corneal astigmatism which is a common complication. Other complications are rare but include pseudo-pterygia formation and spontaneous perforation.

Question: *What type of patient typically presents with Terrien's marginal degeneration?*

Answer: Over 70% of patients are male and over 70% are over 40 years of age.

Question: *What is the prognosis for a corneal graft in a patient with Mooren's ulcer?*

Answer: Poor. Both lamellar and penetrating keratoplasty donor tissue often melts or becomes vascularized in patients treated for a Mooren's ulcer.

46. Acquired corneal pigmentation

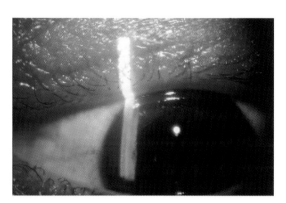

Figure 35 Acquired corneal pigmentation. A Kayser–Fleischer ring associated with Wilson's disease (courtesy of Jane Gardiner MD).

Definition

An unrelated group of conditions characterized by abnormal pigmentation of the cornea or deposition of drugs or metals within the cornea.

Local causes:

- Hudson-Stähli line
- foreign bodies
- adrenaline
- haemorrhage.

Associated with systemic disease and drugs:

- Wilson's disease
- verticillata
- haemolytic anaemia
- mercurial preservatives
- argyrosis
- chrysiasis.

Associated with ocular disease:

- Fleischer's ring
- Stocker's line
- Ferry's line
- Krukenberg's spindle.

Clinical features

Pigments can be deposited in any region of the cornea and at any depth, depending on the pigment type and the cause. In a short case examination it is best to fully describe the pigmentation before suggesting an aetiology. Don't forget to examine the rest of the eye (and patient) for additional clues.

Hudson-Stähli line

This is a deposition of iron (derived from tears) in the epithelium, which occurs in a line corresponding to that of lid closure.

Foreign bodies (FB)

Local stromal pigmentation can be seen around sites or previous sites of metallic FB. With iron FB there may be other signs of siderosis and with copper FB signs of chalcosis. In all cases the candidate should look for other signs of trauma.

Adrenaline

Dark sub-epithelial and Bowman's zone adrenochrome deposits may be seen in patients who have had prolonged use of topical adrenaline. The candidate should look for conjunctival adrenochrome deposits which are more common and for evidence of glaucoma for which the patient has received adrenaline therapy.

Haemorrhage

After long-standing hyphaema deep stromal staining with iron can occur. This may also be seen in patients with haemolytic anaemia.

Wilson's disease

In chronic cases of this disease copper deposits are located in the peripheral part of Descemet's membrane where they form a Kayser–Fleischer ring. At different levels of illumination the deposits alter in colour. The condition is bilateral. A rare associated ocular feature are 'green sun-flower' cataracts. Systemic features include CNS disorders and cirrhosis.

Verticillata

These are grey/gold epithelial deposits which occur bilaterally and symmetrically and appear in a vortex pattern or whorl-like fashion based on a point in the lower half of the cornea.

Mercurial preservative use, argyrosis, chrysiasis

Mercury or silver deposition (grey/black in colour) occurs at a level based around Descemet's membrane. In cases of argyrosis conjunctival staining is more obvious. Prolonged administration of gold may be associated with red/purple deposits in the anterior stroma.

Fleischer's ring (see also p. 138)

This is epithelial deposition of iron at the base of the cone in keratoconus. In an early case a full ring may not have formed.

Stocker's line and Ferry's line

These are epithelial depositions of iron seen respectively in association with a pterygium and a trabeculectomy bleb.

Krukenberg's spindle (see also p. 167)

This is deposition of melanin pigment occurring as a vertical spindle on the corneal endothelium. The candidate should look for other features of pigment dispersion.

Exam questions

Question: *What are the causes of verticillata?*

Answer: Verticillata (not an Italian wine or cheese!) may be congenital, drug-induced or associated with systemic disease. The congenital form is very rare. Causative drugs include amiodarone, chloroquine, indomethacin and the phenothiazines. The characteristic pattern of corneal deposition is also seen in Fabry's disease.

Question: *What is the cause and what are the features of Fabry's disease?*

Answer: This is an X-linked recessively inherited glycosphingolipidosis (also called angiokeratoma corporis diffusum universale!) due to a deficiency of α-galactosidase A.
Systemic features include excruciating pain of the extremities, fever, angiokeratomata (purple telangiectatic skin lesions) and renal lesions/disease (most common cause of death).
Ocular features include corneal verticillata, tortuous conjunctival and retinal veins, spoke-like sub-capsular cataracts and myopia. There may be signs of previous central retinal vein or artery occlusion.

Question: *What are the features of amiodarone keratopathy?*

Answer: The characteristic corneal verticillata are usually only seen in patients on a relatively high dose of this anti-arrhythmic (>400 mg/day). The extent is proportional to dose and duration and the keratopathy is reversible upon stopping the drug.

Question: *How can chloroquine affect the eye?*

Answer: Use of chloroquine may cause keratopathy, retinopathy and/or myopathy. The latter is rare but may affect the extra-ocular muscles. In addition upon starting the drug there may be a transient reduction in accommodative power. Chloroquine keratopathy is in the form of verticillata and its occurrence is not dependent on dosage or duration. It is usually reversible upon stopping the drug, but can in some cases clear even when the drug is continued. Symptoms are rare but in severe cases include a slight fall in visual acuity with glare or haloes.

In contrast, chloroquine retinopathy is dose and duration dependent and only affects patients on long-term high dose therapy. Most patients with this retinopathy have had a total dose of over 300 g. The pigmentary degeneration can be severe and blinding. Progression of the condition passes through a reversible pre-maculopathy and an established maculopathy before the characteristic bull's eye maculopathy develops.

Question: *What causes Wilson's disease?*

Answer: Kinnier Wilson disease, or hepatolenticular degeneration, is an autosomal recessive disorder of copper excretion due to a deficiency of ceruloplasmin (the copper carrying α_2-globulin) which results in the deposition of copper within, and subsequent degeneration of, the liver, brain, kidneys, joints and eyes.

47. Rosacea

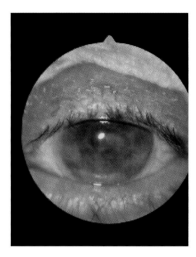

Figure 36 Keratitis secondary to rosacea (courtesy of Gordon Douglas MD).

Definition

A relatively common condition of unknown aetiology which primarily affects the skin with sebaceous gland hyperplasia and vasomotor instability. Ocular rosacea is a potentially serious complication.

Clinical features

The condition is commonest amongst fair-skinned middle-aged females, but since the disease tends to be more severe in males either could easily be seen in an exam (or in the clinic!).

Skin signs

1. chronic facial hyperaemia, usually involving the nose, upper cheeks and central forehead
2. telangiectasis
3. papules, pustules and excessive sebum production (the pustules tend to heal without scarring, unlike those of acne vulgaris and are not associated with comedones)
4. rhinophyma (sebaceous gland hyperplasia with periglandular fibrosis of the nose).

Ocular signs

1. blepharoconjunctivitis (the blepharitis is usually of the seborrhoeic type)
2. chalazia
3. keratitis:
   a) peripheral vascularization
   b) corneal thinning (and risk of perforation)
   c punctate epithelial erosions (lower cornea)
   d recurrent epithelial erosions (upper cornea)
   e) map or dot sub-epithelial opacities
   f) pannus and eventual neovascularization of whole cornea
4. nodular episcleritis.

Exam questions

Question: *In rosacea keratitis where in the cornea is the peripheral vascularization usually seen?*

Answer: In early disease the vessels are most frequently found in the lower temporal and lower nasal quadrants. In severe chronic cases an extensive inferior pannus may be evident.

Question: *Is ocular rosacea only seen in patients with clinically obvious rosacea of the skin?*

Answer: No. Ocular rosacea occurs in up to 20% of cases before skin disease becomes apparent. Most patients with the skin disease develop ocular rosacea of some sort, usually blepharoconjunctivitis and less than 10% develop keratitis.

Question: *Are topical corticosteroids of use in the management of rosacea?*

Answer: Short-term, low dose therapy with topical ocular steroid is very effective in reducing the inflammatory processes of rosacea keratitis. However, steroid therapy should be limited because of a high risk of corneal melting and perforation.

Topical hydrocortisone skin ointment (with sulphur) can relieve skin discomfort. Potent or fluorinated topical steroids should be avoided since these can aggravate established lesions.

Question: *What facial dermatoses may be confused with rosacea?*

Answer: The differential diagnosis includes acne vulgaris, contact dermatitis, systemic lupus erythematosis (SLE), peri-oral dermatitis and light sensitivity.

Question: *In which patients are systemic tetracyclines contra-indicated?*

Answer: Pregnant women and children should not be prescribed tetracyclines since they are deposited in growing bones and teeth (being bound to calcium) which can result in staining of teeth, dental hypoplasia or rarely defective bone growth in a child or foetus. In addition, because most tetracyclines exacerbate renal failure, they should be avoided in patients with compromised renal function. This includes about 60% of patients with SLE, hence the importance of not confusing the butterfly rash of SLE with the skin disease of rosacea for which tetracyclines can be beneficial.

48. Blue sclera

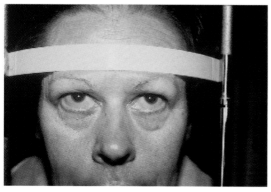

a

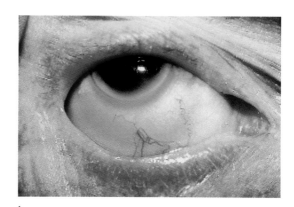

b

Figure 37   a: Particularly vivid blue sclera of a patient with osteogenesis imperfecta; b: Another eye of a patient with osteogenesis imperfecta showing the classic blue colour of inferior sclera (courtesy of Peng Khaw PhD MRCP FRCS FRCOphth).

Definition

An unrelated group of conditions characterized by an apparent blue discolouration of the sclera. The cause is scleral thinning which allows choroidal pigment to become partially visible with a bluish hue.

Clinical features

The candidate should note if the blueness is bilateral, unilateral, generalized or localized and if the patient is young or old. A general examination or more detailed ocular examination may give clues to the cause. In particular, observe the patient's stature and look for skin or joint disease, deformity due to poor fracture healing and note if the patient wears a myopic correction.

Exam questions

Question: *What are the causes of bilateral generalized 'blue sclera'?*

Answer: This can be a normal finding in infants or in the elderly, or can be a sign of a generalized disorder, when it may appear more vividly. Causative conditions include osteogenesis imperfecta, Marfan's syndrome, Ehlers–Danlos syndrome, Lowe's syndrome, high myopia and keratoconus (rare).

Question: *What is osteogenesis imperfecta?*

Answer: Osteogenesis imperfecta is an inherited disorder which can be transmitted in either an autosomal dominant or recessive manner. The bones are fragile and fracture easily (especially in the recessive form) and due to poor healing may cause deformity. Associated ocular features include thinning of the sclera giving it a slatey-blue appearance and thinning of the cornea making it susceptible to perforation.

Question: *What can produce unilateral or localized 'blue sclera'?*

Answer: Any cause of unilateral or localized scleral thinning can produce blue sclera. Causes include long-standing uveal or scleral inflammation (including rheumatoid arthritis), trauma and unilateral myopia (anisometropia).

Question: *Is alkaptonuria a cause of 'blue sclera'?*

Answer: No. The sclera is not thinned. However, greyish-black discolouration, due to abnormal deposits within the sclera, does occur. Due to an absence of the enzyme homogentisic acid oxidase, involved in phenylalanine and tyrosine metabolism, homogentisic acid accumulates and is deposited in connective tissue including the cornea, sclera and conjunctiva. Clinically there are bilateral, slate-grey, oval deposits just anterior to the horizontal recti insertions. In addition there may be small round, golden brown deposits in Bowman's zone of the cornea.

Question: *Is the sclera pigmented in patients with jaundice?*

Answer: No. The sclera only appears to be yellow because of the high level of bilirubin in the conjunctiva.

49. Interstitial keratitis

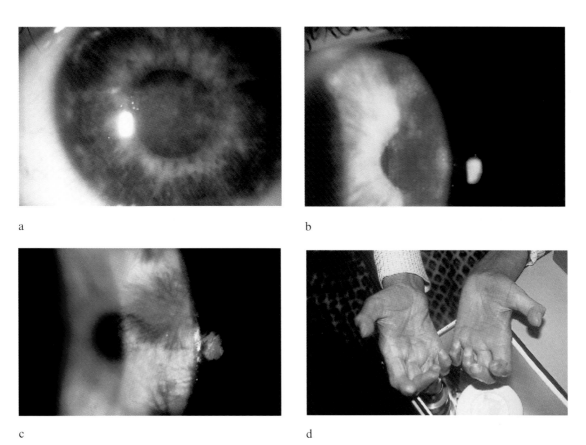

a   b

c   d

Figure 38   a and b: Interstitial keratitis secondary to congenital syphilis (courtesy of Robert Nozik MD and Carlos Pavesio MD); c: Interstitial keratitis secondary to leprosy (courtesy of Peng Khaw PhD MRCP FRCS FRCOphth); d: Claw hands in a patient with leprosy due to multiple nerve palsies (courtesy of Peng Khaw PhD MRCP FRCS FRCOphth).

Definition

Deep stromal keratitis, probably due to an immune reaction, which although classically associated with syphilis has several causes.

Clinical features

In the exam setting a candidate will only encounter 'old' interstitial keratitis. On general examina-tion the cornea has a ground-glass opacification. The characteristic feature of this is a feathery appearance of ghost vessels in the corneal stroma. Ghost vessels are empty vessels which with slit-lamp biomicroscopy appear as faint grey double-lines. The condition is invariably asso-ciated with many guttata. The condition is usually bilateral and the candidate should therefore be careful to exclude a corneal dystrophy. If inter-stitial keratitis is suspected the candidate should look for other signs of congenital syphilis.

(Remember that use of the word 'syphilis' within earshot of a patient can result in another period of intense revision in 6 months time! Thus use the term leuetic disease or 'VDRL positive'.)

Exam questions

Question: *What are the causes of interstitial keratitis?*

Answer: The classic cause is congenital syphilis, but the keratitis can also be a feature of acquired syphilis and various other infections including leprosy, tuberculosis, herpes simplex, varicella, mumps, onchocerciasis, lympho-granuloma venereum, malaria, brucellosis and trypanosomiasis.

Question: *What is Hutchinson's triad?*

Answer: This is a triad of clinical signs characteristic of congenital syphilis. The signs, all sequelae of focal inflammation, involve the nose, teeth and eyes:

1. The bridge of the nose is flattened (saddle-nose)
2. The upper incisor teeth are widely spaced, peg shaped and have a crescentic notch at the cutting edge (Hutchinson's teeth, not to be confused with Moon's mulberry molars), and
3. Interstitial keratitis.

Question: *Can you describe the natural history of syphilitic interstitial keratitis?*

Answer: Clinical onset is usually between the ages of 5 and 25 years (although it has been seen at birth, treponemes being isolated from the corneas of the affected newborn). Initially there is deep stromal and endothelial oedema associated with reduced visual acuity, pain, lacrimation, photophobia, blepharospasm and circumcorneal injection. This is followed by a deep stromal cellular infiltration, an increasing corneal haze and an anterior uveitis. As the acute inflammatory reaction resolves peripheral neovascularization occurs. This extends to form a pinkish colour to the central cornea (salmon patch). After a few months the corneal oedema and opacification reduce and the vessels, empty of blood, remain as ghost vessels. In addition to these, deep stromal opacities and guttata are present. Old interstitial keratitis remains static, although the ghost vessels can refill should the eye subsequently become inflamed for whatever reason.

Question: *How may congenital syphilis affect the eye?*

Answer: Early congenital syphilis (in infants under 2 years) can affect the eye in the form of conjunctivitis and/or chorioretinitis. The commonest form of chorioretinitis is characterized by widespread, small, yellow-white exudates which after resolution leave a 'salt and pepper fundus'. A less common variety is seen as isolated well-circumscribed areas of peripheral chorioretinal atrophy which resolves leaving a 'bone-spicule' pigmentary retinopathy. Late congenital syphilis can affect the eye with interstitial keratitis and if neurosyphilis develops there may be optic atrophy and/or Argyll-Robertson pupils.

Question: *Is penetrating keratoplasty a good form of treatment for old interstitial keratitis?*

Answer: At present this is the only way that corneal transparency can be restored. However there is an increased risk of graft rejection mainly because the ghost vessels can refill with blood resulting in all the problems of a vascularized cornea. It should be remembered that there may be an element of optic atrophy or amblyopia, not curable by grafting!

50. Presumed ocular histoplasmosis syndrome (POHS)

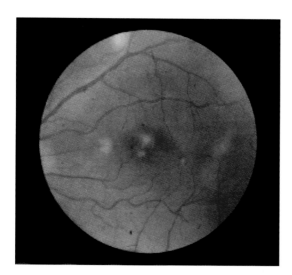

Figure 39 Presumed ocular histoplasmosis syndrome. Histo-spots and disciform maculopathy (courtesy of Gordon Douglas MD).

Definition

Histoplasmosis is a fungal infection endemic in the mid-west USA. Over 99% of these infections are asymptomatic and benign. Symptomatic infection is most commonly due to pulmonary disease but can also be due to posterior uveitis. Although the fungus (Histoplasma capsulatum) is not found in Europe, the specific ocular clinical signs of the condition can be seen in patients who have never lived in an endemic area and have no clinical or serological evidence of systemic histoplasma infection. The syndrome has thus been prefixed by the word 'presumed'. The syndrome may be a hypersensitivity reaction rather than a primary infection.

Clinical features

There are 4 specific features to established POHS:

1. *Histo-spots*
   - These multifocal atrophic choroidal lesions, caused by disseminated choroiditis, tend to occur behind the equator. A variable number may be seen in each eye (bilateral in two thirds of cases), the average number being about 10. For an unknown reason they are more commonly found in left eyes. Each spot is roundish (0.2–0.7 disc diameters in size), yellow and may have a pigmented border.
2. *Peripapillary chorioretinal atrophy*
   - This is indistinguishable from that of high myopia but is due to a resolved chorioretinitis.
3. *Disciform maculopathy*
   - This is a late feature of the syndrome, usually starting between the ages of 20 and 40 years. At an early stage the lesion is seen as a detachment of the pigment epithelium and sensory retina surrounded by a pigmented ring. A subretinal neovascular membrane may be visible. Eventual haemorrhage and fibrosis results in disciform scarring. The latter lesion is more likely to be seen in an exam.
4. *Peripheral linear streaks of chorioretinal atrophy*
   - These are not always present.

An important negative finding is that the vitreous appears normal and clear.

Exam questions

Question: *Is POHS associated with any particular HLA-type?*

Answer: Yes. HLA-B7.

Question: *What is the cause of POHS maculo-pathy?*

Answer: A posterior pole histo-spot damages Bruch's membrane allowing the development of a subretinal neovascular membrane from the choroid. Leakage of fluid causes pigment epithelial and sensory retinal detachment. Haemorrhage and subsequent fibrosis produce the disciform lesion.

Question: *What conditions should be considered in the differential diagnosis of POHS?*

Answer: High myopia may cause a similar fundal appearance with peripapillary atrophy, a Fuchs' spot maculopathy and peripheral retinal degeneration. The maculopathy can also be simulated by a senile disciform lesion or a maculopathy associated with angioid streaks. A haemorrhagic peripapillary lesion can occur in both POHS and in association with optic disc drusen.

Question: *How should cases of POHS be diagnosed and managed?*

Answer: The diagnosis is best made on clinical grounds although histoplasma skin testing which is positive in most cases can be useful. Histoplasma complement fixation testing is only positive in 30% of cases and is thus of limited value. Fluorescein angiography should be performed in pre-disciform cases to identify and assess sub-retinal neovascular membranes. Treatment is difficult, although systemic steroids can help in some cases. Complete laser photocoagulation of extra-foveal sub-retinal neovascular membranes should be performed as early as possible. Surgical excision of the Type II, sub-foveal membranes associated with POHS may restore useful vision in some patients.

Question: *Is amphotericin-B useful in treating patients with POHS?*

Answer: No. Although useful in treating active systemic histoplasmosis, anti-fungal drugs are of no value in the management of POHS.

51. Toxoplasma retinochoroiditis

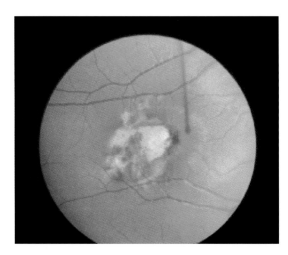

Figure 40 A characteristic retinochoroiditis scar secondary to toxoplasmosis (courtesy of Gordon Douglas MD).

Definition

A condition secondary to infestation by the obligatory intracellular protozoan parasite, Toxoplasma gondii, which can be congenital or acquired.

Ocular involvement in acquired cases only occurs in immunocompromised patients. Congenital toxoplasmosis, however, is the commonest proved cause of retinochoroiditis worldwide and recurrences are commonly seen in ophthalmic clinics or casualty departments. Congenital infection with toxoplasma is usually subclinical. Healed chorioretinal scars presumed to be due to toxoplasmosis may be an incidental finding or may be identified in patients who develop recurrence. It is patients with healed chorioretinal scars who are most likely to appear in exams.

Clinical features

Typical quiescent toxoplasma scars are sharply circumscribed chorioretinal lesions of variable size with associated areas of pigmentation (dark brown) and pigment epithelial atrophy (yellow-white). The scars are usually between 1–3 disc diameters in size, single (with or without satellite lesions), situated in the posterior poles of both eyes and may be associated with visible nerve fibre defects.

Macular involvement apart from reducing visual acuity may be associated with strabismus. Other ocular features of severe congenital toxoplasmosis include microphthalmos and cataract.

General clinical features of severe congenital toxoplasmosis (in those who survive) reflect the organism's predilection for the central nervous system:

- mental retardation
- hydrocephalus
- encephalitis
- epilepsy
- intracranial calcification.

Remember the 'C's of Congenital toxoplasmosis:

1. Chorioretinitis (although strictly a retinochoroiditis)
2. Calcification (intraCranial)
3. Convulsions (epilepsy)
4. Cataract.

Exam questions

Question: *What maternal factors are important in congenital toxoplasmosis?*

Answer: If a pregnant woman is infected with toxoplasma the foetus has approximately a 40% risk of acquiring the disease in utero. The chance of trans-placental transmission is greatest when the infection is acquired during the last trimester, but the disease is most severe if acquired early in pregnancy. Infection acquired in the first few months may result in stillbirth.

Question: *What is the life cycle of Toxoplasma gondii?*

Answer: The sexual phase occurs in the intestinal tract of a cat and the oocysts are shed in the faeces. The oocysts reach man by one of 3 routes:

- direct ingestion,
- via flies, onto food or,
- via an intermediate host (such as a herbivore) and subsequent ingestion of inadequately cooked meat from this host.

The asexual phase can occur in an intermediate host or in man. Sporozoites hatch, penetrate the gut wall and may parasitize any nucleated cell where they develop into trophozoites. These multiply and either cause cell rupture and dissemination or tissue-cyst formation. The parasites can remain dormant in cysts for years.

Question: *What are the clinical features of recurrent ocular toxoplasmosis?*

Answer: The primary lesion is a necrotizing retinitis, secondary features including a choroiditis, a vitritis and in some cases an associated optic neuritis and/or anterior granulomatous uveitis. The characteristic retinal lesion is usually a satellite to an old toxoplasma scar and is thus most commonly seen at the posterior pole. Such lesions are usually single, about 1 disc diameter in size, pale yellow in colour and slightly raised with an indistinct outline. The secondary vitritis can be extensive and in severe cases has been described as having the appearance of 'grapevines covered in wet snow'!

Question: *How are patients with recurrence of toxoplasma retinochoroiditis managed?*

Answer: The diagnosis is usually made on clinical grounds alone, although negative toxo-serology is helpful in excluding the condition. Spontaneous resolution can occur and specific treatment involves toxic drugs so should only be instigated when a lesion involves the macula or papillo-macular bundle, threatens or involves the optic nerve head or is associated with a severe vitritis and/or uveitis. Treatment regimens vary from centre to centre but many clinicians use systemic corticosteroids in conjunction with at least one anti-toxoplasma drug such as pyrimethamine, clindamycin or a sulphonamide. Lesion photocoagulation or cryotherapy has been used in refractory cases.

Question: *What laboratory tests may be useful in the management of suspected cases of toxoplasma retinochoroiditis?*

Answer: Appropriate serological tests include an indirect fluorescent antibody (IFA) test, an enzyme-linked immunosorbent assay (ELISA) or a haemagglutination test. These have replaced the previous gold-standard dye test which had the disadvantage of requiring maintenance of live Toxoplasma organisms in the laboratory with a subsequent risk of infection to the microbiologist. In atypical cases, obtaining specimens of aqueous, vitreous or retina/choroid may be indicated. These specimens can be processed for culture and subsequent isolation of the organism, histology, immunohisto-chemistry or polymerase chain reaction (PCR) analysis. PCR has the potential to be the most sensitive and specific of the tests since it is designed to amplify and detect even minute quantities of Toxoplasma gondii DNA.

Question: *What is Jensen's choroiditis?*

Answer: This refers to a focal area of toxoplasma 'retinitis' adjacent to the optic disc.

52. Fuchs' heterochromic iridocyclitis

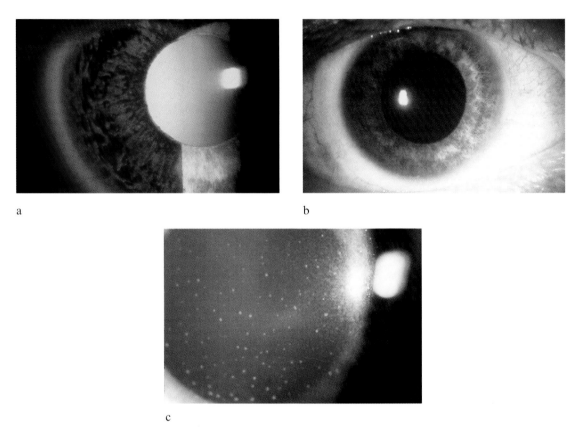

Figure 41 a: Iris transillumination with Fuchs' heterochromic iridocyclitis, in an eye; b: which otherwise looks essentially normal (courtesy of the Department of Medical Illustration, Moorfields Eye Hospital); c: The keratic precipitates characteristic of Fuchs' heterochromic iridocyclitis (courtesy of Robert Nozik MD and Carlos Pavesio MD).

Definition

A specific condition of unknown aetiology which may be a manifestation of anterior segment ischaemia, inflammation or both.

Clinical features

Although the condition is frequently seen as a unilateral disease in a young adult, with long-term follow-up it is seen that the fellow eye becomes involved in 10% of cases. A candidate should not therefore exclude the diagnosis because it appears to be bilateral. The disease features include:

- keratic precipitates
- minimal anterior chamber activity
- an absence of posterior synechiae
- iris heterochromia
- abnormal angle vessels

- a posterior subcapsular lens opacity (70%)
- anterior vitreous precipitates
- evidence of open angle glaucoma (20%).

The keratic precipitates are round or stellate, and are scattered over the whole corneal endothelium. They stay single and unpigmented, and thin filaments are often present between them forming a 'syncytium'.

The anterior chamber may have a faint flare, but few inflammatory cells are present and posterior synechiae do not form.

The iris is atrophic, and in established unilateral or asymmetrical cases there is obvious heterochromia. This is best seen in daylight, a brown iris becoming less brown and a blue iris becoming more saturated blue. Iris transillumination may be evident.

Vitreous precipitates are white, of moderate size and are adherent to the anterior vitreous framework.

Exam questions

Question: *How do patients with Fuchs' heterochromic iridocyclitis present?*

Answer: Many patients present complaining of floaters, which are due to the presence of vitreous precipitates. Others complain of poor vision, which is due to the development of a posterior subcapsular cataract. Some are referred by opticians who have detected glaucomatous changes, and a minority of patients present having noticed iris heterochromia.

Question: *What is Amsler's sign?*

Answer: Abnormal angle vessels are commonly seen at gonioscopy in patients with Fuchs' heterochromia. These often bleed at anterior chamber paracentesis (e.g. at cataract extraction). Haemorrhage from these vessels at gonioscopy is Amsler's sign.

Question: *Are topical corticosteroids and mydriatics useful in the management of Fuchs' heterochromic iridocyclitis?*

Answer: No. Corticosteroids are usually of no benefit, and may increase intraocular pressure or make a cataract worse. Since posterior synechiae never form, mydriatics are not required either. Topical anti-glaucoma treatment is required in some patients, although the glaucoma is often very resistant to topical therapy.

Question: *If a patient with Fuchs' heterochromic iridocyclitis requires a cataract extraction, should an intraocular lens be implanted?*

Answer: Yes, unless there are other contraindications. There is no evidence that the results of lens implantation are worse than for 'normals'.

Question: *What is the evidence suggesting that anterior segment ischaemia may, at least in part, be involved in the aetiology of Fuchs' heterochromia?*

Answer: Anterior segment fluorescein angiography demonstrates perfusion defects and histopathology shows hyalinization of iris blood vessels. The presence of fine angle vessels may be a response to local ischaemia, although rubeosis and neovascular glaucoma have only rarely been seen in these patients.

Question: *What are the other causes of iris heterochromia?*

Answer: Common causes of iris heterochromia are idiopathic, hereditary and secondary to unilateral atrophy, of which the common causes are inflammation and trauma (including surgery).

Rare causes of heterochromia include a congenital Horner's syndrome, siderosis and melanoma. Two very rare conditions associated with iris heterochromia are the Waardenburg and Parry–Romberg syndromes.

53. Primary open angle glaucoma (POAG)

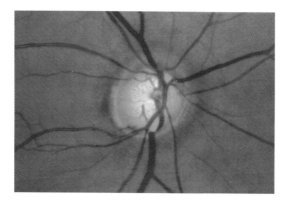

a

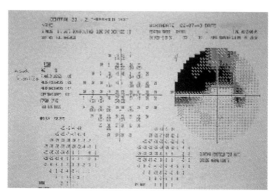

b

Figure 42 Primary open angle glaucoma. a: A right glaucomatous optic nerve head with an inferior haemorrhage, and; b: the associated visual field defect (courtesy of Stephen Drance MD OC).

Definition

A common ocular condition characterized by an open angle and an intraocular pressure (IOP) sufficiently high to result in a progressive optic neuropathy usually associated with disc cupping and resultant, characteristic visual field defects.

Yes, patients with simple glaucoma do appear in exams! Even if the diagnosis is clear, the answer to an examiner's question can be far from obvious!

The classical criteria for diagnosis are:

- an IOP >21 mmHg
- an open iridocorneal angle at gonioscopy
- pathological optic disc cupping and an associated glaucomatous visual field defect.

POAG should not be confused with ocular hypertension (OH) or a subgroup of POAG called 'normal tension glaucoma' (NTG).

In OH there is raised IOP (>21 mmHg) in the absence of disc cupping or a field defect; in NTG, the IOP is normal (⩽21 mmHg), the angle is open, but there is optic disc cupping and a glaucomatous visual field defect.

NB: There is some evidence that optic disc changes and axonal loss occur before detectable visual field defects develop, and these may be such that the diagnosis of glaucoma cannot rely on visual field analysis alone.

Clinical features

Pathological optic disc changes

- an increased cup:disc ratio (a normal ratio is <0.3, but it is often difficult to distinguish a pathological cup from a large physiological cup, and the ratio tends to increase with age. Remember that assessment of the disc neuroretinal rim is more important than the cup itself. Be aware of small discs – a relatively small cup in these discs may represent a large amount of neural tissue loss)
- asymmetry of the left and right cup:disc ratios of >0.2
- disc neuroretinal rim notching (reflects more focal neural loss cf. generalized cupping)

- disc pallor (an area of the disc lacking visible microvasculature)
- nasal shift of major vessels on the disc
- baring of neuroretinal rim vessels
- disc or disc margin haemorrhages (particularly common in NTG)
- saucerization of the disc (senile sclerotic change)
- peripapillary atrophy.

Features of glaucomatous visual field defects

Visual field loss can be diffuse and/or focal. Relatively specific focal visual field defects include:

- a paracentral scotoma 10–20° from the blind spot
- a nasal step which respects the horizontal meridian (Rœnne scotoma)
- a temporal wedge defect
- the classical arcuate scotoma, a comma-shaped extension of the blind spot (Seidel's scotoma)
- an arcuate scotoma with peripheral breakthrough
- generalized constriction.

Other signs

- retinal nerve fibre layer atrophy or bundle defect (best seen in red-free light)
- miosis (if patient treated with topical miotic)
- mydriasis (if patient treated with topical sympathomimetic)
- signs of previous filtration surgery (if a candidate fails to lift the upper eyelid a superior peripheral iridectomy or trabeculectomy bleb may not be noticed, and this is a serious error).

Exam questions

Question: *What histopathological features may be evident in an eye with POAG?*

Answer: Pathological features may be evident in the trabecular meshwork, at the optic nerve head and in the retina.
Examination of the meshwork may show:

- endothelial cell loss
- fusion and thickening of trabeculae
- hyperpigmented meshwork cells
- a reduced number of giant vacuoles in the drainage wall of Schlemm's canal
- an increase of altered extracellular matrix material within the meshwork.

Examination of the optic nerve head and retina may show:

- compression, posterior bowing and/or collapse of the lamina cribrosa
- swollen axons (early)
- selective axonal loss (late)
- retinal atrophy.

Question: *Is optic disc ischaemia important in the pathogenesis of POAG?*

Answer: This is a highly debated issue. Some investigators consider that the glaucomatous optic neuropathy occurs due to mechanical injury of axons as they pass through the lamina cribrosa. Others believe that it results from ischaemia, which may be either a primary event or secondary to an abnormal intraocular pressure. Evidence is growing to suggest that altered blood flow to the optic nerve head may have a role in the pathogenesis, particularly in normal tension glaucoma (NTG) and certain subgroups of patients with POAG. It remains unknown, however, whether this is a primary feature or whether it secondarily increases the susceptibility of the axons to an abnormal intraocular pressure. Indirect evidence for a vascular component to the pathogenesis comes from the association between POAG and NTG and other systemic conditions with a vascular component such as hypertension, diabetes, migraine, vasospastic peripheral vascular disease and diseases associated with raised blood viscosity.

Question: *What ocular conditions are associated with an increased risk of developing POAG?*

Answer: Patients with high myopia, retinitis pigmentosa, Fuchs' endothelial dystrophy and retinal vein occlusion may have a slightly increased risk. In addition, patients with retinal detachment are more prone to developing open angle glaucoma but this may, at least in part, be due to the association between myopia and retinal detachment.

Question: *What is the role of psychophysical and electrophysiological testing in glaucoma?*

Answer: Routine perimetry is capable of detecting established glaucomatous visual field defects. However, by the time that such defects are detectable a significant amount of neuronal loss has occurred. New tests, based on a psychophysical and/or electrophysiological basis, are currently undergoing assessment in an attempt to develop simple tests capable of detecting glaucomatous damage at an early stage. Development of tests based on colour vision and contrast sensitivity, motion sensitivity and the pattern electroretinogram continues, but at present these are not used in routine practice. The shortwave-sensitive mechanisms in central and peripheral vision have been shown to be damaged early so that blue-on-yellow perimetry is more sensitive than conventional white-on-white. Testing for a reduction in motion sensitivity is based on the fact that in glaucoma there is preferential early loss of the larger ganglion cell axons, which are associated with the magnocellular system and are involved in motion processing. Use of the pattern electroretinogram (PERG) requires hospital-based technical facilities and is unlikely to become useful as a screening test. However because early ganglion cell loss occurs in glaucoma, the PERG, which is a response of inner retinal layers to pattern (stripe or checkerboard) reversal, has proved sensitive in detecting damage in both ocular hypertension and POAG.

Question: *In general, how are patients with POAG managed, and how do the various treatment modalities work?*

Answer: The aim of management is to preserve as much vision as possible for patients for the remainder of their lives. This relates to visual acuity as well as visual field. The treatment has to be tailored to the individual patient and the risks/side-effects of the various forms of therapy should be taken into account. The overall quality of life is important, and aggressive therapy may not be indicated in an elderly patient with mild glaucoma.

At present the mainstay of treatment is reduction of IOP, which can be achieved with topical or systemic drugs, laser trabeculoplasty, surgical filtration and partial cycloablation. Topical agents include β-blockers (e.g. betaxolol, timolol, levobunolol or carteolol), miotics (e.g. pilocarpine), sympathomimetics (e.g. adrenaline or dipivefrin), α-agonists (e.g. apraclonidine), carbonic anhydrase inhibitors (e.g. dorzolamide) and prostaglandins (e.g. latanoprost [$PgF_2\alpha$-ester]). Systemic carbonic anhydrase inhibitors include acetazolamide, metazolamide and dichlorphenamide. β-blockers, carbonic anhydrase inhibitors and α-agonists reduce IOP by reducing production of aqueous. Miotics increase conventional outflow, and the prostaglandin, latanoprost, increases non-conventional outflow (uveoscleral). Sympathomimetics have multiple effects, the balance of which results in a lowering of IOP. They are non-selective α- and β-adrenergic agonists which cause an indirect decrease in aqueous formation (α), a direct increase in formation (β), an increase in uveoscleral outflow (β) and trabecular meshwork outflow (β). Successful laser trabeculoplasty increases aqueous outflow, but the mechanism of action remains unknown. Routine filtration surgery is achieved by trabeculectomy or insertion of silicone tubes (e.g. a Molteno implant), which result in diversion of the aqueous into the subconjunctival space. In certain cases IOP reduction can only be achieved by trans-scleral partial cycloablation (e.g. using the diode or YAG laser or cryotherapy), which can significantly reduce aqueous production.

Question: *How does latanoprost lower intraocular pressure, and what are the known side-effects of its use?*

Answer: Latanoprost increases aqueous outflow via the non-conventional outflow (uveoscleral) pathway. Known side-effects include: discomfort upon instillation, red eye and benign increased iris pigmentation (irides heterogenous in colour can become noticeably darker), and lengthening/thickening/darkening of eyelashes has been reported.

Question: *What is the ideal treated IOP level required to prevent visual field deterioration in patients with POAG?*

Answer: This is unknown, although there is some evidence that a pressure of <15 mmHg is ideal if patients with glaucoma are considered as a group. It is most likely that different patients require a different degree of IOP reduction (i.e. a different 'target pressure').

Question: *What are the possible complications of trabeculectomy?*

Answer: Complications include:

- hyphaema
- a flat anterior chamber
- hypotony
- choroidal detachments and folds
- malignant glaucoma
- cataract
- altered refraction (including corneal astigmatism)
- immediate visual field deterioration
- Tenon's capsule cyst formation
- bleb dysaesthesia (e.g. due to an excessive sized conjunctival bleb)
- endophthalmitis
- side-effects of adjunctive therapy (e.g. 5-flourouracil, mitomycin-C, steroids)
- failure.

Question: *What groups of patients are considered to be at an increased risk of failure of filtration surgery?*

Answer: The actual evidence for at risk groups is rather weak, but it is thought that an exaggerated wound-healing response causing filtration failure occurs with:

- black patients
- patients with secondary glaucoma (e.g. uveitic, traumatic)
- young patients
- patients who have undergone previous ocular surgery
- patients who have undergone previous laser trabeculoplasty
- patients who have been treated for many years with multiple topical antiglaucomatous medications, particularly if including a sympathomimetic.

Question: *What is the van Herick test?*

Answer: This is a method by which an estimate of angle configuration can be made without a gonioscope. A thin slit-beam of light is focused onto the peripheral AC and cornea, at and perpendicular to the limbus. The beam is viewed at 60°. The likely gonioscopic appearance of the angle can then be classified:

Grade	Angle	van Herick feature
0	closed	iris touches corneal endothelium
1	closeable	Peripheral AC depth $< \frac{1}{4}$ of corneal thickness
2	closeable	Peripheral AC depth $= \frac{1}{4}$ of corneal thickness
3	open	Peripheral AC depth $= \frac{1}{2}$ of corneal thickness
4	wide open	Peripheral AC depth $>$ corneal thickness

The van Herick assessment of an angle is not a substitute for gonioscopy, but is useful in providing additional clues before gonioscopy is performed and in cases when a gonioscopic view is precluded by corneal oedema, scarring etc. When gonioscopy can be performed it is superior, because the angle is viewed 'directly'. The van Herick method cannot be used to diagnose angle recession, plateau iris, PAS, rubeosis, angle pigmentation, angle tumour or cyclodialysis cleft, or to identify foreign material within the angle (e.g. blood, silicone oil, foreign bodies).

Question: *What is a cyclodialysis cleft? What are the causes of such a cleft and do they require treatment?*

Answer: A cyclodialysis cleft is a detachment of the ciliary body from the scleral spur, which is often associated with hypotony. Causes include as a planned surgical procedure (used in the past to treat glaucoma), as an inadvertent surgical complication, or as a result of trauma. Management is only required if there is symptomatic hypotony. Closure can happen spontaneously, but if this does not occur, an attempt to close the cleft using trans-scleral cryotherapy, direct argon laser photocoagulation or surgery should be made if the hypotony is causing a reduction in vision.

54. Pseudoexfoliation syndrome

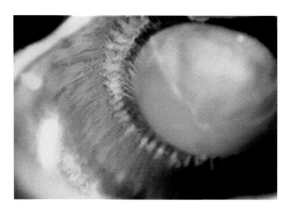

Figure 43 Pseudoexfoliation syndrome. A pathological specimen showing PXF material on the ciliary processes and zonules (courtesy of Gordon Douglas MD).

Definition

An ocular condition due to the deposition of pseudoexfoliation material within the eye, which can be associated with glaucoma. The specific source of the material remains unknown.

Clinical features

The patient is most likely to be elderly. Clinically obvious bilateral involvement occurs in about half of the cases; however, the true incidence of bilateral involvement may be higher, since signs can be very subtle and may be missed if the pupil is not dilated. Signs may be seen to develop if follow-up is sufficient. The important features are:

- deposits of pseudoexfoliation material
- iris transillumination defects
- Sampoelesi's line
- evidence of open angle glaucoma.

The dandruff-like deposits may be found on the anterior lens capsule (except in a mid-peripheral zone, where the iris is thought to rub it off), at the pupillary margin, in the angle and sometimes on the corneal endothelium. Occasionally the deposits may be seen on the ciliary processes and zonules, on the anterior vitreous face and in association with conjunctival vessels.

Iris transillumination defects occur adjacent to the pupil margin as a result of rubbing against material deposited on the anterior lens capsule. The dispersed pigment can be seen in the angle, forming Sampoelesi's line (a pigmented line at Schwalbe's line), in the anterior chamber, on the anterior iris surface and on the corneal endothelium.

Exam questions

Question: *How do the iris transillumination defects of pseudoexfoliation differ from those of the pigment dispersion syndrome?*

Answer: In pseudoexfoliation the defects are adjacent to the pupil margin, whereas in pigment dispersion they are classically in the mid-periphery of the iris.

Question: *What is glaucoma capsulare?*

Answer: This is the combination of pseudo-exfoliation and secondary open angle glaucoma due to the presence of pseudoexfoliation material and pigment in the trabecular meshwork. These physically block the meshwork and/or alter angle function by destroying trabecular meshwork cells, resulting in a decreased facility of outflow. Glaucoma capsulare develops in over 60% of clinically affected eyes and, interestingly, an open angle glaucoma also occurs in 20% of fellow ('unaffected') eyes, indicating subclinical disease. The intraocular pressure tends to be higher in patients with glaucoma capsulare in comparison with primary open angle glaucoma. Treatment is as for POAG, and although often resistant to medical therapy, it may respond to filtration surgery.

Question: *Should all patients with pseudo-exfoliation undergo lens extraction if possible?*

Answer: No. Lens extraction is of no specific benefit for these patients, although if a cataract should develop, cataract extraction is not contraindicated. However, the surgeon should be aware that the zonules tend to be weaker in patents with pseudoexfoliation, and there is an increased incidence of zonular dehiscence with the potential of vitreous loss.

Question: *What is pseudoexfoliation material?*

Answer: Histochemical analysis has found the material to be a proteoglycan gel with a fibrillary structure similar to that of amyloid (but it shows no reaction with Congo red). The fibres are 35–40 nm in width and have 50 nm cross-bands. The material also has some features of basement membrane, being eosinophilic and weakly PAS positive. The source of material remains unknown.

Question: *In which race of people is pseudo-exfoliation syndrome most common?*

Answer: Although observed in all races, it is most commonly seen in Scandinavians. The syndrome also shows regional variation in its incidence throughout the British Isles, and is thought to be more common in East Anglia and in Ireland.

Question: *Can pseudoexfoliation syndrome be associated with acute large increases in IOP?*

Answer: Yes. Patients with pseudoexfoliation syndrome are more prone than average to acute rises in IOP following pupil dilation, without pupil block/angle closure. The IOP may rise to levels above 40 or 50 mmHg. It is thought that an already compromised trabecular meshwork is acutely and further compromised by release of iris pigment as the pupil dilates, with a resultant rise in IOP.

55. Pigment dispersion syndrome

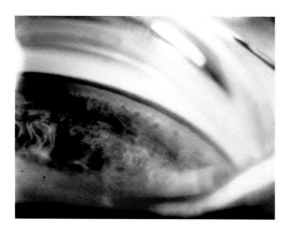

Figure 44 Pigment dispersion syndrome. Gonioscopic view of heavy angle pigmentation secondary to PDS (courtesy of Gordon Douglas MD).

Definition

An ocular condition produced by dispersion of iris pigment throughout the anterior segment. Mid-peripheral iris concavity and iris trauma from the lens zonules or abnormal ciliary processes (large and/or anteriorly positioned) may be involved in the aetiology.

Clinical features

The patient is typically a young (20–40 year old) male myope, so it is worth examining the patient's glasses if they are available. Affected female patients tend to be older than their male counterparts. The condition is bilateral, but can be asymmetrical. Other features include:

- Krukenberg's spindle
- a deep AC
- circulating AC pigment
- deposition of pigment on the anterior iris surface (in circumferential troughs)

- Sampoelesi's line
- a 360° hyperpigmented band within the trabecular meshwork
- radial mid-peripheral iris transillumination defects
- posterior bowing of mid-peripheral iris (in some cases only)
- pigment deposition on the posterior lens equator, on the anterior surface of the iris and in the retinal periphery
- evidence of (secondary) open angle glaucoma (50%)
- wide fluctuations in IOP in those patients who develop glaucoma.

Corneal pigmentation occurs in the form of a Sampoelesi's line (as with pseudoexfoliation, see p. 165) and in a vertically orientated spindle-shaped scatter of pigment on the central part of the endothelium (Krukenberg's spindle).

Exam questions

Question: *Is the glaucoma associated with pigment dispersion acute or chronic in nature?*

Answer: It can be either or, rather, both. The glaucoma is usually chronic and similar to POAG, although in some patients a degree of improvement (or at least stability) can occur with time. However, wide fluctuations in intraocular pressure can occur, with acute crises of raised pressure sufficient to cause corneal epithelial oedema and the symptom of haloes. These crises can be induced by exercise or after pupil dilation. Thus the differential diagnosis includes acute angle closure glaucoma.

Question: *What is the cause of glaucoma in the pigment dispersion syndrome?*

Answer: Although a significant amount of pigment is deposited in the angle, the glaucoma is not thought to be due to simple mechanical meshwork blockage alone. Pigment has been demonstrated within phagosomes of trabecular meshwork cells, and it has been suggested that this causes their death and/or migration to the endothelial (juxtacanalicular) part of the meshwork where they block the narrowest passages and raise resistance to flow. In addition, denuding of the trabeculae of the uveal and corneoscleral parts of the meshwork allows them to adhere to one another, so causing blockage throughout the whole meshwork.

Question: *How is pigmentary glaucoma treated?*

Answer: Treatment is basically as for POAG, although it tends to be more resistant to medical therapy. At the stage of pigment dispersion, laser iridotomy may reverse posterior bowing of the peripheral iris, if this has been clearly demonstrated. This therapy is controversial, but may reduce the dispersion of pigment and prevent development or progression of the glaucoma. Laser trabeculoplasty has been advocated, but the effect of this is often only short-lived and these young patients frequently require filtration surgery when they have developed established glaucoma.

Question: *Are miotics such as pilocarpine useful in the treatment of pigmentary glaucoma?*

Answer: Pigment dispersion syndrome tends to affect young patients, and since tolerance of miotics is often low they should be avoided in such cases. Prophylactic use of pilocarpine has, however, been found to help in preventing the pressure rise associated with severe exercise, and can therefore be useful for patients who wish to exercise in this way. The induced miosis is associated with flattening of the iris and also reduces iris movement, trauma and pigment dispersion.

Question: *Why is it thought that the deposition of corneal pigment occurs in a spindle-shaped pattern?*

Answer: A Krukenberg spindle is thought to occur due to the pattern of aqueous convection currents within the anterior chamber and subsequent phagocytosis of the circulating pigment by corneal endothelial cells.

56. Rubeosis iridis

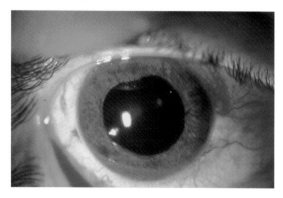

Figure 45 Rubeosis in a diabetic eye with neovascular glaucoma (courtesy of Gordon Douglas MD).

Definition

Neovascularization of the iris.

Clinical features

Iris neovascularization occurs in the form of an irregular network of fine surface and stromal new vessels. If extensive, these give the iris a pinkish hue. At slit-lamp examination the vessels are seen to be markedly tortuous and to possess many anastomoses. Rubeosis can be localized or generalized, depending on the cause and its duration. Generalized rubeosis usually starts at the pupil margin as small buds from iris capillaries and venules. If progressive, extension often occurs radially towards the angle:

1. *Stage 1*:
   – Rubeosis between the pupil margin and the iris collarette
2. *Stage 2*:
   – Rubeosis extending across the whole iris with involvement of the angle, which remains open

3. *Stage 3*:
   – Rubeosis extending across the whole iris with involvement of the angle, associated peripheral anterior synechiae (PAS) and angle closure. The pupil may show distortion and ectropion.

Not all cases of rubeosis follow this pattern, and angle neovascularization may occur in the absence of clinically obvious iris surface rubeosis.

If a sufficient amount of angle is involved, Stage 2 rubeosis is a cause of secondary open angle glaucoma and Stage 3 is a cause of secondary closed angle glaucoma (neovascular glaucoma). With neovascular glaucoma the intraocular pressure (IOP) can be markedly raised, the globe congested and the patient in obvious pain; thus patients with acute neovascular glaucoma are unlikely to be seen in exams.

Exam questions

Question: *What are the causes of rubeosis?*

Answer: By far the most common causes are ischaemic central retinal vein occlusion (CRVO) and diabetic retinopathy. All the causes, however, can be classified into three groups; ischaemia, neoplasia and other.

Ischaemic causes include causes of retinal ischaemia (CRVO, diabetes, sickle cell anaemia, retinopathy of prematurity (ROP), Eales disease, sarcoidosis and (rarely) central retinal artery occlusion (CRAO)) and anterior segment ischaemia (postoperative, local atherosclerosis, carotid artery occlusive disease, vasculitis).

Neoplastic causes include malignant melanoma, juvenile xanthogranuloma (JXG), metastases, retinoblastoma and haemangioma.

Other causes include POAG, chronic uveitis and trauma.

Question: *How should the eye of a diabetic with Stage 1 rubeosis be treated?*

Answer: With adequate pan-retinal laser photo-coagulation, as soon as possible. This can halt progression and, in most cases, induce regression of the rubeosis.

Question: *How should the eye of a diabetic with Stage 2 rubeosis be treated?*

Answer: Again, adequate pan-retinal photo-coagulation (PRP) should be performed as soon as possible. In addition, any associated glaucoma should be medically treated.

Question: *What is thrombotic glaucoma?*

Answer: This term refers to neovascular glaucoma secondary to a central retinal vein occlusion (i.e. due to 'thrombotic' occlusion of the central retinal vein). A better name would be post-thrombotic glaucoma. This type of glaucoma has also been called 100 day or 3 month glaucoma, since it usually occurs after such a lag period.

Question: *If a patient requires a vitrectomy for advanced diabetic eye disease, how can the surgeon minimize the chance of postoperative rubeosis or of extension of pre-existent rubeosis?*

Answer: This can often be very difficult, but there are a number of principles that should be adhered to. Adequate PRP should be performed either preoperatively or during surgery (endophotocoagulation). Retinal reattachment should be achieved whenever possible, and this alone can induce regression of rubeosis. In addition, the surgeon should avoid prophylactic 360° cryotherapy, 360° circumferential buckles, gas tamponade and lensectomy at the time of vitrectomy.

57. Aniridia

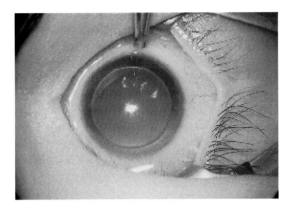

Figure 46 Aniridia. The whole lens with its zonules is clearly visible (courtesy of Gordon Douglas MD).

Definition

A congenital disorder characterized by bilateral under-development of the iris, other ocular abnormalities and, in some cases, systemic abnormalities.

Clinical features

The iris (although not totally absent) is rudimentary, in the form of a peripheral stump (seen at gonioscopy), and the eye through the cornea appears jet black (i.e. all pupil). Associated ocular abnormalities include:

- progressive stem cell deficiency
- epibulbar dermoids
- congenital ptosis
- degenerative corneal pannus (apparent microcornea)
- congenital cataract
- ectopia lentis (especially lens subluxation)
- angle anomalies and evidence of glaucoma (50%)
- macular hypoplasia (correlates well with poor visual acuity, nystagmus and photophobia)

- retinopathy (small peripheral yellow dot lesions)
- optic nerve hypoplasia or aplasia
- strabismus.

Systemic associations include:

- Wilms' tumour (there may be evidence of previous surgery, chemotherapy or [renal] dialysis)
- digital abnormalities
- body hemihypertrophy
- hypogonadism
- mental retardation.

Exam questions

Question: *How is aniridia inherited?*

Answer: Aniridia can be inherited as an autosomal dominant trait or can present sporadically. Aniridia can be associated with deletion of the short arm of chromosome 11, in which case the aniridia is more likely to be associated with systemic features. Wilms' tumour develops in 20% of the sporadic cases, and only very rarely in autosomal dominant cases.

Question: *Is the glaucoma associated with aniridia usually present at birth?*

Answer: No. Glaucoma, which occurs in about 50% of cases, is not present at birth but develops as adhesions between the rudimentary iris and the trabecular meshwork form. These tend to take a few years to develop, resulting in infantile glaucoma rather than congenital glaucoma.

Question: *What is Miller's syndrome?*

Answer: This refers to the association between aniridia and Wilms' tumour (nephroblastoma). Miller's syndrome occurs in 20% of sporadic aniridia cases. Upon diagnosing aniridia in an infant with no family history, investigations should be performed to exclude or identify a renal tumour. The urine should be tested for the presence of blood and an ultrasound scan or (rarely) an intravenous urogram (IVU) should be performed. If negative, the investigations should be repeated six monthly or annually for a few years, the clinician checking carefully for any pelvicalyceal system distortion.

Question: *On which side is a Wilms' tumour most common?*

Answer: Left kidney involvement is more common than right, although the tumour is bilateral in 10% of cases.

Question: *How can patients with a unilateral Wilms' tumour be treated?*

Answer: A nephrectomy should be performed; this including removal of the ureter, local lymph nodes and any locally infiltrated tissue. The excised tissue should be sent to the histopathology department for staging. Survival is good for patients with Stage 1 or 2 disease. Patients with Stage 3 or 4 disease should also be treated with chemotherapy and/or radiotherapy, which in recent years has been shown to increase survival.

58. Irido-corneal endothelial (ICE) syndrome

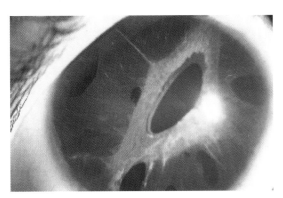

Figure 47 Irido-corneal endothelial (ICE) syndrome. The essential iris atrophy subtype of the ICE syndrome (courtesy of Gordon Douglas MD).

Definition

ICE syndrome is a proliferative endotheliopathy – a dysplasia of the corneal endothelium. Although classically divided into three types, the condition is probably a spectrum involving various clinical features but representing one disease.

The importance of the condition is that it can be associated with corneal endothelial dysfunction and, due to endothelial proliferation over the angle with PAS formation, is a cause of secondary glaucoma.

The three classic subtypes should be known, even if only for exam purposes!

1. Essential iris atrophy
2. Iris naevus (Cogan–Reese) syndrome
3. Chandler's syndrome.

Clinical features

ICE syndrome is usually unilateral, and is typically diagnosed in young/middle-aged women. The features of the three subtypes are as follows:

Essential iris atrophy

- progressive iris atrophy
- PAS formation (with extension anterior to Schwalbe's line)
- pupil distortion towards an area of PAS
- iris hole formation, opposite the site of PAS (pseudopolycoria)
- corneal endothelial dysfunction (mild)
- iris nodules (these are actually islands of normal iris tissue surrounded by sheets of endothelial cells) evidence of glaucoma (may be severe).

Iris naevus (Cogan–Reese) syndrome

- a diffuse iris naevus (involves the anterior iris)
- iris 'nodules'
- PAS formation (with extension anterior to Schwalbe's line)
- ectropion uveae
- corneal endothelial dysfunction (moderate)
- little (if any) iris atrophy
- evidence of glaucoma.

Chandler's syndrome

- corneal endothelial dysfunction (may be severe)
- PAS formation (mild)
- iris atrophy (mild) without hole formation
- corectopia (eccentric pupil)
- evidence of glaucoma (mild).

Although these subdivisions can be useful, it is important to remember that they are probably artificial.

Exam questions

Question: *Why is the glaucoma of ICE syndrome often more severe than the extent of PAS formation would imply?*

Answer: The glaucoma of ICE syndrome is not only secondary to PAS formation; in addition, there is proliferation of corneal endothelium across the angle and within the trabecular meshwork. Aqueous outflow is further compromised by the fact that the endothelial cells continue to produce Descemet's membrane-like material.

Question: *Has an HLA association with ICE syndrome been identified?*

Answer: No.

Question: *What is different about the PAS of ICE syndrome and those of other conditions?*

Answer: Unlike with other causes, the PAS of ICE syndrome tend to extend anterior to Schwalbe's line.

Question: *In general, how are PAS distinguished from iris processes?*

Answer: Iris processes are small and fine with a lacy character, whereas PAS are of any size and have a tented-up appearance.

Question: *Is surgery appropriate in the management of ICE syndrome?*

Answer: Yes. Filtration surgery is frequently required to manage the associated glaucoma. If a trabeculectomy is performed, the high risk of failure can be reduced somewhat by the use of peroperative mitomycin-C. Some surgeons prefer to insert silicone drainage tubes as the initial form of surgery. Maintenance of a low IOP can prevent corneal oedema when endothelial function is compromised. In some cases (at the Chandler's syndrome end of the spectrum), penetrating keratoplasty is required to restore corneal transparency.

Question: *Apart from ICE syndrome, what are the causes of iris atrophy?*

Answer: Generalized iris atrophy can occur as an ageing change, as a complication of anterior uveitis (especially if secondary to herpes zoster ophthalmicus), or due to anterior segment ischaemia, Fuchs' heterochromic iridocyclitis or trauma. Iris muscle atrophy can complicate diabetes, neurosyphilis and ciliary ganglion lesions. Sphincter atrophy or necrosis may occur following acute angle closure glaucoma. An atrophic pigmented epithelium can be a feature of pigment dispersion syndrome, pseudo-exfoliation syndrome, albinism, onchocerciasis and, for an unexplained reason, in association with phacolytic glaucoma.

Question: *Does the ICE syndrome have a genetic component?*

Answer: If it does, it remains to be discovered.

Question: *Are there any other possible aetiologies for ICE syndrome?*

Answer: Herpes simplex virus has been implicated, based on polymerase chain reaction studies for HSV DNA in ICE corneas.

59. Lens ectopia

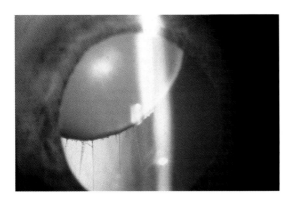

Figure 48 Lens subluxation secondary to Marfan's syndrome (courtesy of Gordon Douglas MD).

Definition

An ectopic lens is a lens that is not in its normal position. It may be subluxed or dislocated, and the cause may be hereditary or acquired. A subluxed lens remains in the lenticular fossa, whereas a dislocated lens lies outside the lenticular fossa.

A subluxed lens may:

- remain supported by some (but not all) of the zonules which, acting as a hinge, allow the lens to move slightly out of position, or
- remain attached to the zonules, but since they are differentially stretched they allow the lens to move from its axis.

A dislocated lens has no zonular support and is thus free to move. It may:

- move posteriorly into the vitreous cavity
- move anteriorly to become incarcerated in the pupil or enter the AC.

Clinical features

Lens subluxation

The signs of mild subluxation can be quite subtle, but useful signs (if of a sufficient degree) are a deep AC and iridodonesis (a tremulous iris). If a lens is subluxed from its axis, the lens equator may be visible through the pupil.

Lens dislocation

A patient with an anteriorly dislocated lens is unlikely to be seen in an exam. A patient with a posteriorly dislocated lens, however, may be seen. The patient will be hypermetropic (unless previously highly myopic), and other signs of aphakia will be evident; a deep AC, iridodonesis and apparent absence of the lens. At ophthalmoscopy, however, the lens will be seen in the vitreous cavity.

In all cases both eyes should be fully examined, and a candidate should note if the ectopia is unilateral, bilateral, asymmetrical or symmetrical and, in the case of subluxation, its direction. A general examination can often help identify the cause.

Exam questions

Question: *What are the hereditary causes of lens ectopia, and by what mode are they transmitted?*

Answer: All such causes are rare, but the commonest is Marfan's syndrome. Other causes include homocystinuria, Weill–Marchesani syndrome, hyperlysinaemia, familial lens ectopia, aniridia, sulphite oxidase deficiency and Ehlers–Danlos syndrome. All these causes can be transmitted in an autosomal recessive manner except for Marfan's syndrome and aniridia, which usually have autosomal dominant inheritance. Ehlers–Danlos syndrome can be transmitted in an autosomal dominant, autosomal recessive or X-linked recessive manner.

Question: *Apart from lens ectopia, how can Marfan's syndrome affect the eye?*

Answer: Other ocular features include axial myopia, cornea plana (a flat cornea), a hypoplastic dilator pupillae (making pupil dilation difficult), angle anomalies, microspherophakia and lattice retinal degeneration. Glaucoma (either lens-induced or secondary to angle anomalies) is common, and rhegmatogenous retinal detachment is more common than normal due to associated myopia and lattice degeneration.

Question: *How does the lens subluxation of Marfan's syndrome differ from that of homocystinuria?*

Answer: Lens subluxation usually occurs upwards in Marfan's syndrome and because the zonule remains intact, although variably stretched, a degree of accommodation is retained. In contrast, the lens subluxation of homocystinuria is usually downwards and due to acquired zonular degeneration is associated with loss of accommodation.

Question: *What are the acquired causes of lens ectopia?*

Answer: Trauma is the commonest cause, others include anterior uveal tumours, hypermature cataract, syphilis and (rarely) chronic cyclitis. A large eye due to high myopia or buphthalmos is also more likely to be associated with an ectopic lens than an eye of normal size.

Question: *What are the indications for extraction of an ectopic lens, and why can this be particularly hazardous under general anaesthesia for some patients?*

Answer: Indications include anterior dislocation into the AC, lens-induced uveitis, secondary glaucoma and uniocular diplopia. Lens extraction under general anaesthesia is hazardous to patients with Marfan's syndrome who have regurgitant valvular heart disease, increased risk of cardiac arrhythmia and are prone to develop spontaneous pneumothorax. Patients with homocystinuria have increased platelet stickiness, and post-anaesthesia are at particular risk of thrombosis (including deep vein thrombosis with risk of pulmonary embolus).

Question: *What is Weill–Marchesani syndrome?*

Answer: This is an autosomal recessive hereditary disorder of connective tissue, which has both systemic and ocular features. Systemic features include short stature, broad hands with short stubby fingers, joint stiffness with poor mobility, carpal tunnel syndrome and mental retardation. The ocular features include high myopia, microphthalmos, microspherophakia and lens ectopia (usually inferior but may be posterior or anterior, when it may be associated with acute glaucoma).

60. Rhegmatogenous retinal detachment

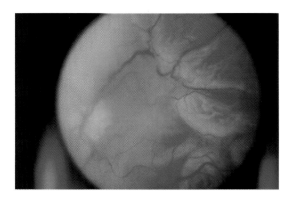

Figure 49 A temporal rhegmatogenous retinal detachment (courtesy of Peng Khaw PhD MRCP FRCS FRCOphth).

Definition

A detachment of the photoreceptor layer from the pigment epithelial layer of the retina secondary to a retinal break. Fluid accumulates between these layers and, progressively, the whole retina may detach.

A retinal break refers to any full thickness retinal defect, a retinal tear is a break caused by vitreous traction or trauma, and a retinal hole is a break caused by retinal degeneration or atrophy.

Clinical features

A fresh or untreated rhegmatogenous retinal detachment is unlikely to be seen in the exam setting, so the clinical signs will be simply listed.

Slit-lamp and/or ophthalmoscopy

1. Anterior uveitis
2. A low IOP (usually)
3. Posterior vitreous detachment (PVD)
4. Anterior vitreous pigment (tobacco dust)

5. Evidence of an aetiological factor (e.g. trauma or aphakia).

(NB: It is always important to exclude a retinal detachment in an eye in which the IOP falls suddenly.)

Ophthalmoscopy (direct and indirect)

1. Detached retina:
   - raised opaque retina with a corrugated appearance
   - loss of underlying choroidal details
   - darker appearance of retinal vessels
   - convex shape to the surface
   - undulations with eye movements
2. Retinal break(s)
3. Proliferative vitreoretinopathy (PVR)
4. Further evidence of an aetiological factor (e.g. myopia, retinal degeneration or traction retinal detachment).

In the exam situation, a candidate is more likely to encounter a patient with a treated detachment. Evidence of previous surgery includes:

- enophthalmos
- disturbed conjunctival anatomy
- external view of an explant
- cataract
- PVD
- intraocular gas or silicone oil (remember that oil floats on aqueous)
- cryotherapy or laser scars
- internal view of an explant or of explants
- closed breaks
- drainage and infusion site scars.

Enophthalmos can complicate encirclement and disturbed conjunctival anatomy may be seen after any conjunctival incision. A degree of explant extrusion may be evident on far gaze.

A PVD, seen as a collapsed vitreous body with or without an obvious Weis (hyaloid) ring, will be evident unless the patient has undergone a vitrectomy. Post-vitrectomy, the vitreous cavity may appear optically empty or there may be a gas bubble or silicone oil present. In aphakic patients, oil may be seen in the AC. Remember that oil floats on aqueous. In the eyes of some unfortunate patients there may be emulsification of the oil and reduced optical clarity.

For one or two days after cryotherapy the retina is locally oedematous. After four or five days (or longer in previously detached retina) a pigmented atrophic scar develops. A region of cryotherapy scarring may be seen overlying the raised profile of an explant (plomb). Closed breaks can be difficult to identify within cryo-scars, but isolated drainage or infusion site scars may be seen clearly.

A candidate should not perform scleral indentation without first asking the examiner and alerting the patient.

Exam questions

Question: *What are the predisposing factors for rhegmatogenous retinal detachment?*

Answer: There are two basic predisposing factors, vitreoretinal traction and retinal weakness. Either or both of these play a role in causing detachment in patients with vitreous degeneration (including PVD), myopia, aphakia, trauma, retinal degeneration, tractional retinal detachment, certain hereditary vitreoretinal disorders and necrotizing retinitis.

Question: *What peripheral retinal degenerations can predispose to retinal detachment?*

Answer: Lattice retinal degeneration is a relatively common condition, found in about 6% of otherwise normal eyes. Although most patients with lattice degeneration never suffer a detachment, it remains a definite risk factor and is found in up to 40% of eyes with non-traumatic rhegmatogenous detachments. Round holes, U-tears and giant tears may be associated with lattice.

Patients with snail-track degeneration show a pronounced predisposition to form large round retinal holes with subsequent retinal detachment. Traction tears may occur at the posterior aspect of cystic retinal tufts, and the rare juvenile type of retinoschisis should also be included in the group of predisposing degenerations.

Question: *What proportion of patients with rhegmatogenous retinal detachment present with the symptoms of 'flashes and floaters'?*

Answer: Only about 50% of patients with rhegmatogenous retinal detachment report these symptoms. Some patients complain of reduced visual acuity and/or a visual field defect, the latter indicating extension of the detachment posterior to the equator. A number of patients have no symptoms, the detachment being found incidentally.

Question: *What factors affect the spread of subretinal fluid and thus the extension of a rhegmatogenous retinal detachment?*

Answer: Spread of this fluid is dependent on retinal and vitreous factors. These include the size and position of the retinal break, the degree of adhesion between the RPE and the neuroepithelium and the state of the vitreous. Spread is faster with larger breaks and, due to gravity, occurs more rapidly if the break is sited in the upper half of the retina. If RPE – neuroepithelial adhesion is weak, as in aphakia, the RPE pump is less efficient and the fluid accumulates more rapidly, particularly if the vitreous gel is liquefied.

Question: *Why is it important to assess the depth of subretinal fluid beneath a rhegmatogenous retinal detachment?*

Answer: This is important in the preoperative assessment of the patient because it determines whether or not subretinal fluid drainage is required at operation. Scleral depression can help assess the depth. If shallow, gentle indentation will close a hole, but if deep this is impossible. Deep fluid requires drainage to make break localization possible and to aid cryo applications.

Question: *What are high-water marks?*

Answer: These are one of a number of fundal signs which indicate a long-standing retinal detachment. They form beneath flat retina in front of an advancing wall of subretinal fluid and appear as pigmented and fibrotic demarcation lines. Other signs of long-standing detachment include thinning of the detached retina, development of intraretinal cysts and telangiectatic vascular tufts.

Question: *What is PVR, and which patients are at particular risk of developing it?*

Answer: PVR (or proliferative vitreoretinopathy) is defined as the development of cellular membranes on either or both surfaces of the retina and/or within the vitreous cavity in an eye with a rhegmatogenous retinal detachment. PVR is particularly common in eyes with long-standing detachment; detachments secondary to penetrating trauma, large or giant tears; detachments associated with vitreous or choroidal haemorrhage, inflammation or hypotony, and also detachments that have failed to respond to surgical treatment. Surgery complicated by haemorrhage, inflammation, retinal incarceration, vitreous loss, excessive cryotherapy, intraocular gas injection or hypotony is more likely to result in PVR. Use of silicone oil may also increase the risk of PVR.

Question: *How is PVR classified?*

Answer: PVR is divided into four main groups; Grades A – minimal, B – moderate, C – marked and D – massive.
Grade A represents vitreous haze and/or pigment clumps; no membranes are seen.
Grade B is characterized by wrinkling of the retinal surface, a rolled edge to the break(s), vessel tortuosity and retinal stiffness; no membranes are seen clinically.
Grade C is characterized by fixed, full-thickness retinal folds and visible membranes, and is subdivided into C1, C2 and C3, the number indicating the number of involved quadrants.
Grade D is characterized by fixed, full-thickness retinal folds in all four quadrants. D1 indicates an open wide funnel; D2 a narrow funnel with a visible disc, and D3 a closed funnel, such that the disc is not visible.

Question: *What are the surgical principles which apply to the treatment of PVR?*

Answer: The most important aspect of surgical management of PVR is to close the retinal break(s). It is also important to remove fibrous tissue and relieve any traction on the retina. The closed intraocular microsurgical techniques required are often difficult and should only be undertaken by an adequately trained surgeon. Routine detachment and vitrectomy techniques are required and, in addition, membrane peeling and/or relieving retinotomy may be required.

Question: *What are the indications for subretinal fluid drainage?*

Answer: SRF drainage is indicated when the amount of fluid is sufficient to hinder break localization, the retina is immobile and/or the retinal detachment is long-standing. With long-standing detachments the SRF is viscous and post-operative absorption is slow, even if break closure is achieved without drainage. In cases requiring internal tamponade, drainage is often performed to provide sufficient room in the vitreous cavity. Drainage is also indicated when a potential rise in IOP carries too much risk. Scleral suturing of explants can raise IOP above 60–70 mmHg. In healthy eyes this rise would be short-lived, but such a rise should be avoided in patients with advanced glaucoma or a recently sutured anterior segment wound (surgical or traumatic); those in whom the optic disc cannot be seen, since central retinal artery pulsation has to be assessed; those with poor ocular perfusion and also patients with thin sclera to avoid suture cut-out.

Question: *What are the complications specific to subretinal fluid drainage?*

Answer: Choroidal haemorrhage is the most serious complication of drainage operations. Transillumination of the scleral incision before drainage reduces the risk of this. Other complications include retinal incarceration, iatrogenic retinal tear formation, vitreous loss, hypotony and intraocular infection.

Question: *What is a giant retinal break, and how should a patient with such a break be managed?*

Answer: A giant retinal break involves more than 90° of the retinal circumference, is usually sited in pre-equatorial retina and is characterized by independent mobility of its posterior flap. These breaks do not pass through the 6 o'clock meridian. Most are idiopathic, but they can occur secondary to trauma (including posterior segment surgery) or in association with collagen diseases including Stickler's syndrome. Treatment is controversial, and should be performed by an experienced vitreoretinal surgeon. Treatment usually requires vitrectomy and internal tamponade with silicone oil. External buckles are required for breaks extending below the horizontal meridian. In the past tilting operating tables were used to unravel the posterior flap, but new heavy liquids used as a peroperative tool may prove better for this job. Once unravelled, most giant tears can be treated with retinal laser therapy and an injection of long-acting gas. For relatively 'simple' giant tears, 'simple' retrovitreal injection of a long-acting gas (such as perfluoropropene) may prove the safest method of treatment.

Prophylactic treatment of the fellow eye is important in non-traumatic cases, but is controversial in eyes with an intact vitreous, since 360° cryotherapy may induce a PVD and subsequent giant tear. Prophylactic indirect laser treatment may reduce this risk in fellow eyes with no PVD.

Question: *What are considered the main indications for retinal prophylaxis?*

Answer: The indications for prophylaxis are controversial because the prevalence of retinal detachment is so much lower than that of predisposing lesions (0.01% vs. 10%), and because prophylaxis is not without potential side-effects. The main indications, however, include:

- all symptomatic breaks
- all breaks in high-risk eyes (e.g. aphakic and fellow eyes)
- some asymptomatic breaks (dialysis, U-tears, equatorial breaks and those within areas of lattice or snail-track degeneration)
- some breaks in certain myopes (especially in young, high myopes with breaks not within the vitreous base)
- the fellow eye of an eye with an atraumatic giant tear

- areas of lattice or snail-track degeneration in eyes with a detachment, in fellow eyes, or if a break is seen within the area of degeneration (as previously mentioned).

Question: *What are the complications of retinal cryotherapy?*

Answer: Numerous adverse effects of cryotherapy have been reported although fortunately most are minor or rare, unless treatment is excessive. Mild conjunctival chemosis, uveitis, local retinal haemorrhages and pigment dropout are common and usually insignificant. Potentially severe complications include choroidal haemorrhage, especially if cryo applications are made to vortex veins, or scleral rupture due to an attempt to remove an unthawed cryoprobe too early. With excessive retinal cryotherapy there is an increased risk of reactive choroidal hyperaemia, serous choroidal detachment, cystoid macular oedema, chorioretinal necrosis and PVR. In an eye without PVD there is a risk of inducing one, which may cause a break. Unless applications are made carefully there is a risk of eyelid freezing or external ocular muscle freezing, which causes transient diplopia. Mechanical distortion of the eye may cause dehiscence of recent anterior segment wounds and can produce dislocation of unstable intraocular lenses.

Question: *Have you read the paper by Lincoff and Gieser entitled 'Finding the retinal hole'? (Lincoff and Gieser, (1971). Finding the retinal hole. Arch. Ophthalmol., 85, 565–9.)*

Answer: Yes!

61. Lattice retinal degeneration

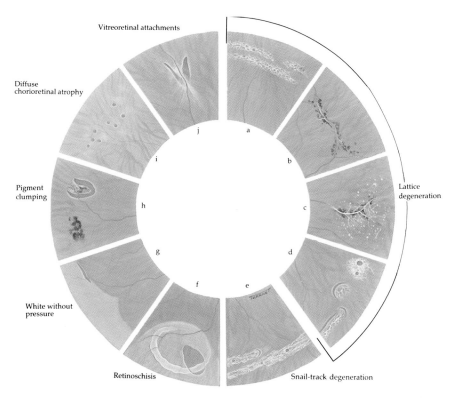

Figure 50 Peripheral retinal degenerations (Reproduced, with permission, from *Clinical Ophthalmology*, third edition by Jack Kanski MD MS FRCOphth)

Definition

A peripheral retinal degeneration which can predispose to retinal break formation and subsequent rhegmatogenous retinal detachment.

Clinical features

Areas of lattice degeneration usually appear as a spindle-shaped area of thinned retina with a network of fine white lines that are continuous with retinal vessels. Each region is sharply demarcated, circumferentially orientated and situated at or anterior to the equator. Lesions are seen bilaterally in 50% of cases. Associated features include overlying vitreous liquefaction, vitreous traction at the lesion margins and, in some cases, hyperplasia of the underlying RPE. The patient is more likely to have other retinal changes, including 'benign' snowflake degeneration, white with or without pressure and retinal erosions.

Exam questions

Question: *In which quadrant is lattice degeneration most common?*

Answer: Upper temporal. It is more common temporally compared with nasally and superiorly compared with inferiorly, making the upper temporal quadrant the most likely site.

Question: *In whom is lattice seen?*

Answer: Although present in about 40% of eyes with rhegmatogenous retinal detachment, it is seen in 5–10% of otherwise 'normal' eyes, and in most cases such an eye does not progress to develop a detachment. Lattice is more common in a myopic eye, and the combination of lattice and myopia makes detachment more likely than the separate risk factors would suggest. Patients with lattice are usually over 30 years old, and it is very rarely seen in children under 10 years.

Question: *What are the white lines seen in areas of lattice?*

Answer: Each line consists of a hyalinized retinal blood vessel.

Question: *Which types of retinal break may be seen associated with lattice lesions?*

Answer: Lattice degeneration predisposes to round holes, U-tears and giant retinal breaks. If present, round holes are usually seen at the end of a spindle shaped lesion. U-tears are caused by a PVD with vitreous traction on the weakened retina. If an operculum forms, the features of lattice may be evident within it. Giant tears can arise from the posterior edge of a long lattice lesion.

Question: *When should an area of lattice be treated prophylactically?*

Answer: This is controversial, but prophylactic treatment is invariably indicated in eyes with a detachment, in fellow eyes or if a break is seen within the lattice. Some ophthalmologists treat lattice in other high-risk eyes, such as the aphakic eye or an eye with high myopia, but others feel that this is unnecessary since such eyes are invariably associated with an established PVD.

62. Retinoschisis

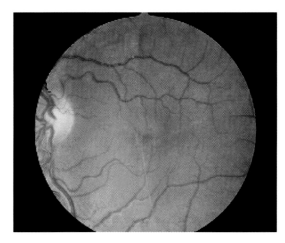

Figure 51 The macula of a patient with X-linked retinoschisis (courtesy of the Department of Medical Illustration, Moorfields Eye Hospital).

Definition

A retinoschisis is a splitting of the layers within the neurosensory retina. There are 3 types:

1. Senile
2. Juvenile
3. Secondary (to vitreous traction).

A candidate is most likely to encounter the senile variety.

Clinical features

Senile retinoschisis

The patient is commonly hypermetropic (70%) and the condition is most often peripheral and inferotemporal. It is bilateral in 33% of cases. The innermost layer of the split retina (i.e. nearest the vitreous) is referred to as the 'inner leaf' and the outermost layer as the 'outer leaf'. Features which aid distinguishing a schisis from a detachment include:

- a smooth, immobile dome-like elevation (the inner leaf) with an absence of retinal folding (probably the best sign)
- beaten metal appearance of the inner leaf
- white dots on the inner limiting membrane
- sheathing of peripheral retinal vessels
- peripheral microcystoid degeneration
- an absence of pigment demarcation lines (high water marks)
- blanching of the retina (outer leaf) on scleral depression, as with normal but not detached retina.

Retinal breaks are not always present. If present they may be seen in both inner and/or outer leaf. Inner leaf breaks are small and round. Outer leaf breaks can be large and tend to be irregular with rolled and scalloped edges. Retinal detachment occurs only if there are breaks in both inner and outer leaf.

Juvenile retinoschisis

This is very rarely seen but should not be missed (it may be the only case you ever see!). There is bilateral degeneration of both vitreous and retina, the latter having the appearance of Swiss cheese. The macula is involved to some extent in all cases. The ERG shows an abnormal b-wave.

Secondary retinoschisis

This is very difficult to distinguish from tractional retinal detachment. High water marks do not form and inner leaf breaks do not result in rhegmatogenous detachment, but in other respects the schisis has the features of a tractional retinal detachment. Fortunately the distinction is unimportant. It is more important to identify the cause of vitreous traction such as proliferative retinopathy or trauma.

Exam questions

Question: *From where is the term 'schisis' derived?*

Answer: Schisis is the Greek word for 'division'.

Question: *What symptoms are associated with acquired senile retinoschisis?*

Answer: Most patients have no symptoms and in many cases the diagnosis is made as an incidental finding. Acquired retinoschisis may be present in up to 5% of the adult population but since in most cases it is only the far retinal periphery that is involved no visual impairment is noticed. Extension of the schisis posterior to the equator results in a field defect which may be reported. Only 1% of cases progress to retinal detachment but if this occurs then the symptoms of detachment supervene.

Question: *At which level in the retina does the splitting of a retinoschisis occur?*

Answer: This is dependent on the type of schisis. Senile retinoschisis occurs when the cavities of cystoid degeneration become confluent and the split thus occurs in the outer plexiform layer. Juvenile retinoschisis is characterized by a split in the nerve fibre layer.

Question: *Who develops juvenile retinoschisis?*

Answer: Most cases are inherited in a x-linked recessive manner and so are diagnosed in boys usually before the age of 20 years. Autosomal recessive cases have also been seen, some of which are due to Goldmann–Favre's disease. Retinoschisis is also a feature of Wagner's disease which is inherited in an autosomal dominant manner.

Question: *How should a patient with retinoschisis be managed?*

Answer: In most cases management is conservative with periodic observation with or without visual field testing. Surgery is indicated should detachment occur, but in cases of juvenile retinoschisis the prognosis is very poor. In the rare situation when progression of a senile retinoschisis threatens the macula this can be prevented by treating the advancing edge or collapsing the schisis cavity with photocoagulation or cryotherapy. Additional scleral buckling may be required.

63. Asteroid hyalosis

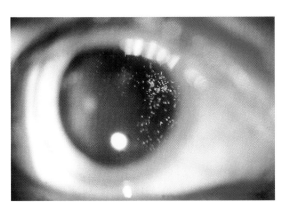

Figure 52 A slit-lamp view of asteroid hyalosis (courtesy of Jane Gardiner MD).

Definition

Also known as Benson's disease this is a condition of the vitreous characterized by fixed vitreous opacities composed of calcium soaps (palmitate and stearate).

Clinical features

The multiple opacities seen in one eye are solid, round or discoid and usually white in colour. They are suspended in otherwise clinically normal vitreous. The opacities may be seen throughout the whole gel or confined to a part of it.

Exam questions

Question: *How do patients with asteroid hyalosis present?*

Answer: The condition is usually asymptomatic and the diagnosis made as an incidental finding. It is relatively common being seen in 0.5% of healthy eyes.

Question: *Do the opacities of asteroid hyalosis settle at rest?*

Answer: No. The opacities are fixed to the vitreous fibrils and thus do not settle unless there is a PVD.

Question: *With what could asteroid hyalosis be confused?*

Answer: A number of other vitreous opacities could be misdiagnosed as asteroid hyalosis without an adequate history or full examination of both eyes. These include muscae volitantes (flying flies), which are remnants of the hyaloid system; syneretic or myopic opacities; chronic vitreous haemorrhage or synchysis scintillans; inflammatory opacities, including those of Fuch's heterochromia, neoplastic opacities and the very rare condition of vitreous amyloidosis.

Question: *Is asteroid hyalosis associated with any systemic diseases?*

Answer: There is no strict association with a systemic disease but the condition is more common in patients with diabetes mellitus.

Question: *How is asteroid hyalosis treated?*

Answer: No treatment is required in the majority of cases. If the patient has troublesome symptoms and a cataract extraction is also indicated some surgeons advocate a primary posterior capsulorrhexis and anterior vitrectomy. However, this is controversial.

64. Vitreous haemorrhage

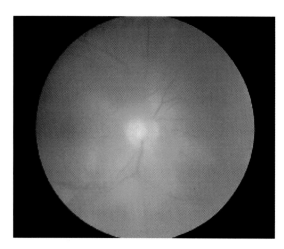

Figure 53 The obscured fundus of an eye with a vitreous haemorrhage (courtesy of the Department of Medical Illustration, Moorfields Eye Hospital).

Definition

Haemorrhage into the vitreous.

Clinical features

These are highly variable and depend on the cause, source, extent and degree, state of the vitreous and on how long after the bleed the patient is seen.

Acutely the blood is red and may be localized or spread diffusely throughout the gel. In a young patient resorption is often rapid but with the older patient persistence of the blood leaves collections of yellow/white debris or fibrous membranes, usually seen inferiorly. In addition, there may be yellowish discolouration (xanthochromia) in the anterior chamber, or if a drainage bleb is present, of the conjunctiva.

A candidate should always attempt to discover the cause of the haemorrhage and identify any secondary complications by carefully examining both eyes.

Exam questions

Question: *What are the causes of a vitreous haemorrhage?*

Answer: Significant vitreous haemorrhage can complicate proliferative retinopathies when there is rupture of fragile new disc or retinal vessels. The commonest causes of these are diabetes and retinal vein occlusion, others include sickle cell retinopathy, Eales' disease and ROP. Neovascularization with subsequent vessel rupture and vitreous haemorrhage can also occur with trauma, inflammation and intraocular tumours. Trauma, either blunt or penetrating, may cause vitreous haemorrhage directly in an otherwise normal eye. Other less common causes include disciform macular degeneration, blood dyscrasias, retinal or disc angiomas (von Hippel–Lindau syndrome) and the rare Terson's syndrome. Small vitreous haemorrhages can occur with a PVD. The development of a retinal break may rupture a retinal vessel and lead to haemorrhage. This is a cause of the floaters which often herald a detachment.

Question: *What are potential complications of vitreous haemorrhage?*

Answer: Non-clearance or delayed clearance of a vitreous haemorrhage can be included as a complication in their own right but poor clearance is the main cause of all the complications. These include syneresis, inflammation and fibrosis with the risk of traction retinal detachment, haemosiderosis, synchysis scintillans, ochre membrane formation and glaucoma (haemolytic or ghost cell).

Question: *How do the opacities of synchysis scintillans differ from those of asteroid hyalosis?*

Answer: The opacities of synchysis scintillans, also known as cholesterolosis bulbi, consist of cholesterol crystals and are thus more refractile than the calcium soap opacities of asteroid hyalosis. In addition, the former are usually present in degenerate, liquefied vitreous and are not attached to fibrils, such that they tend to settle with rest.

Question: *What is ghost cell glaucoma?*

Answer: This is a complication of a prolonged vitreous haemorrhage or less commonly a prolonged hyphaema. After about 2 weeks the intraocular red blood cells lose their haemoglobin degenerating into ghost cells and Heinz bodies. The ghost cells consist of cell membrane only but since they are very rigid when they eventually reach the anterior chamber they obstruct the trabecular meshwork resulting in a secondary open angle glaucoma. It is an indication for vitrectomy in certain cases may reverse the raised intraocular pressure.

Question: *What is Terson's syndrome?*

Answer: This is the occurrence of a vitreous haemorrhage in a patient who has had a subarachnoid haemorrhage.

Question: *What is von Hippel–Lindau syndrome and how may it affect the eye?*

Answer: This is one of the hereditary phakomatoses, inherited in an autosomal dominant fashion. General features include haemangioblastomas of the cerebellum, medulla, pons or spinal cord; visceral cysts, phaeochromocytoma and/or hypernephroma. Ocular features occur in 50% of cases and include retinal and disc angiomas which may bleed producing a vitreous haemorrhage or leak to cause retinal exudation. Hypertensive retinopathy may occur in the presence of a phaeochromocytoma and papilloedema may occur if there is raised intracranial pressure.

65. Leukocoria

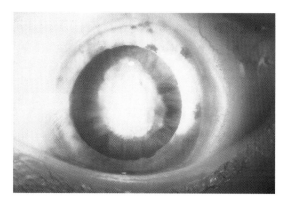

Figure 54 Leukocoria. Due to persistent hyperplastic primary vitreous (courtesy of Stephen Drance MD OC).

Definition

This literally means 'white pupil' and refers to a whitish pupillary reflex. It has also been called an 'amaurotic cat's eye reflex'.

Clinical features

The pupillary reflex, seen best with a direct ophthalmoscope held at a distance from the patient, instead of having the usual orange/red glow is whitish. It is important to determine whether the sign is unilateral or bilateral.
Leukocoria is only a clinical sign, not a condition. Once seen a candidate should examine the patient in more detail and attempt to discover the cause.

Exam questions

Question: *What are the causes of leukocoria?*

Answer: These are numerous but can be classified into more manageable groups:

1. cataract
2. retrolental mass
3. retinal and/or choroidal disease:
   – neoplastic
   – exudative
   – infective
   – other.

Conditions which commonly result in a retrolental mass are persistent hyperplastic primary vitreous, retinopathy of prematurity and Norrie's disease.
Important neoplastic conditions are retinoblastoma and choroidal metastases. Exudative causes include Coat's disease, Eales' disease and familial exudative vitreoretinopathy. Infective causes include toxoplasmosis, toxocariasis and endophthalmitis. Other causes include high myopia, extensive nerve fibre myelination, choroideraemia, retinal dysplasia and many others (but don't say this unless you can remember at least a few others!).

Question: *Why may a patient with retinoblastoma present with leukocoria and is this common?*

Answer: This is a common sign in patients with retinoblastoma, seen in 60–70% of cases and can be due to the presence of a large tumour and/or a total retinal detachment.

Question: *Apart from leukocoria how else can a patient with retinoblastoma present?*

Answer: Ideally all familial and most sporadic cases are identified in the infant at an early stage before any complications occur. A number of patients, however, present relatively late with a squint (strabismus) and amblyopia, secondary glaucoma, chronic uveitis, hyphaema secondary to iris neovascularization, proptosis due to retrobulbar extension, a pseudohypopyon of tumour cells or with evidence of metastatic spread.

Question: *How can patients with anterior PHPV be treated?*

Answer: In selected cases removal of the retrolental mass by closed intraocular microsurgery can prevent future complications and may even restore some vision, although there is a high risk of amblyopia.

Question: *What are the complications of anterior PHPV?*

Answer: The more common complications include cataract, secondary closed angle glaucoma, vitreous haemorrhage and retinal detachment.

66. Diabetic retinopathy

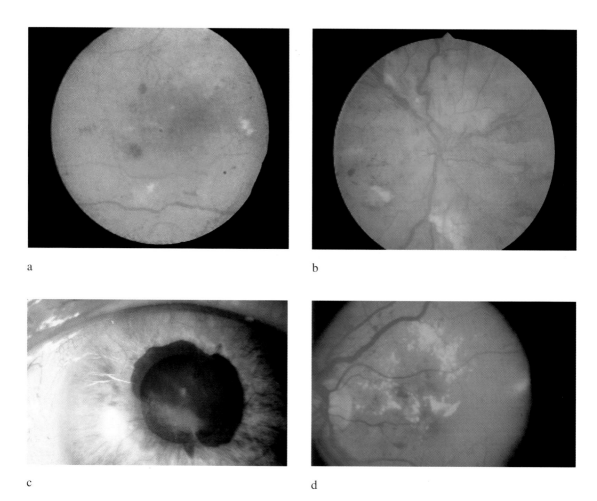

a

b

c

d

Figure 55 a: Haemorrhages and exudates characteristic of diabetic retinopathy (courtesy of Gordon Douglas MD); b: Neovascularization of the optic disc; c: Rubeosis iridis; d: Exudative maculopathy (b–d courtesy of the Department of Medical Illustration, Moorfields Eye Hospital).

Definition

Retinopathy secondary to diabetes mellitus. The retinopathy can be associated with all types of diabetes mellitus:

1. Type I (juvenile onset, 'insulin dependent')
2. Type II (maturity onset, 'non-insulin dependent')
3. Secondary.

Clinical features

Fundus examination

Background diabetic retinopathy
- microaneurysms (in the inner nuclear retinal layer)
- retinal hard exudate; isolated or circinate (in the outer plexiform and inner nuclear retinal layers)

- 'dot' and 'blot' haemorrhages (in the middle retinal layers)
- 'flame' haemorrhages (in the retinal nerve fibre layer).

Diabetic maculopathy
1. *Oedematous*
   - macular oedema (extracellular fluid within Henle's layer)
   - can be subtle and difficult to identify at routine fundoscopy
2. *Exudative*
   - isolated or circinate exudate deposition in the macula region
3. *Ischaemic*
   - central region of retinal non-perfusion (often difficult to identify on routine fundoscopy)
4. *Mixed*
   - features of (1)–(3).

Pre-proliferative diabetic retinopathy
- cotton wool spots
- intraretinal microvascular abnormalities (shunt vessels)
- large 'blot' haemorrhages (in the middle retinal layers)
- venous dilation, loop formation, beading and reduplication
- arterial narrowing
- regions of retinal non-perfusion/ischaemia (often difficult to identify on routine fundoscopy).

Proliferative diabetic retinopathy
- peripheral retinal neovascularization
- optic disc neovascularization
- fibrovascular epiretinal membrane.

Candidates must be very careful not to miss neovascularization.

Advanced posterior segment diabetic eye disease
- vitreous haemorrhage
- tractional retinal detachment (tangential, antero-posterior bridging)
- opaque/ochre membrane of posterior hyaloid face
- synchysis scintillans
- lipaemia retinalis.

Other ocular signs associated with diabetes mellitus
- xanthelasma
- blepharitis
- external hordeolum (stye)
- recurrent corneal erosions (epithelial microcysts)
- ectropion uveae
- iris neovascularization (rubeosis iridis)
- iris depigmentation
- iris neuropathy (with resultant poor pupil dilation)
- neovascular glaucoma
- primary open angle glaucoma
- cataract
- fluctuations in refractive error
- ischaemic optic neuropathy
- diabetic optic nerve papillitis
- third, fourth or sixth cranial nerve palsies.

Exam questions

Question: *When is laser photocoagulation indicated in the management of diabetic retinopathy?*

Answer: There is some controversy concerning the thresholds for laser therapy, although it is accepted that all patients with 'high-risk proliferative disease' or clinically significant macular oedema should be treated with laser photocoagulation. With high-risk proliferative disease pan-retinal photocoagulation is applied to the fundus peripheral to the major vascular arcades with the aim of inhibiting the growth of new vessels. Grid photocoagulation is applied to areas of posterior pole or macular retinal oedema and focal therapy is applied to leaking microaneurysms (e.g. at the centre of a circinate exudate). In general it is felt that patients with pre-proliferative retinopathy do not require laser therapy if they can be followed closely in the clinic.

Question: *What is the value of fluorescein angiography in the assessment of the patient with diabetic retinopathy?*

Answer: Fluorescein angiography adds information to that obtained from clinical examination. In cases of ischaemic retinopathy fluorescein angiography identifies the extent of capillary non-perfusion. When there is significant macular oedema fluorescein angiography helps identify the region to which grid or focal laser photocoagulation should be applied. Fluorescein angiography is also useful in determining the cause of unexplained visual loss (e.g. relatively subtle macular oedema) and identifying sites of subtle neovascularization not seen at fundoscopy.

Question: *Is the degree of glycaemic control important with respect to the progression of diabetic retinopathy?*

Answer: The Diabetes Control and Complications Trial Research Group have reported that intensive insulin based control of blood sugar levels can delay the onset and slow the progression of retinopathy. However, this fact is not an indication for intensive insulin therapy for all patients with Type II diabetes. In addition, there is evidence that too rapid an improvement of chronic poor control may increase the risk of short-term retinopathy progression. In general however, good control is definitely beneficial and it has been shown that the level of glycosolated haemoglobin (which reflects the degree of long-term hyperglycaemia) can be used to predict the incidence and progression of retinopathy.

References:

New Eng J Med 1993; 329: 977–986
Diabetes and Metabolism Reviews 1988; 4: 291–322
JAMA 1988; 260: 2864–2871

Question: *What are the high-risk characteristics of proliferative diabetic retinopathy for severe visual loss?*

Answer: The Diabetic Retinopathy Study Research Group reported that patients at greatest risk of severe visual loss were those with optic disc neovascularization involving more than a quarter to a third of the disc area or those with a vitreous or pre-retinal haemorrhage associated with less extensive disc neovascularization or neovascularization elsewhere with an area of more than half a disc area.

Reference:

Int Ophthalmol Clin 1987; 27: 239–253

Question: *What pathological features may play a role in the pathogenesis of diabetic retinopathy?*

Answer: The two underlying factors of importance in the pathogenesis of diabetic retinopathy are initial increased retinal vascular permeability with eventual vascular closure and ischaemia. Pathological features which may be of importance include loss of vascular pericytes, capillary endothelial cell damage, deposition of glycogen and carbohydrate in basement membrane, increased platelet aggregation and defective oxygen transfer from erythrocytes to the retina.

Question: *What percentage of individuals with diabetes mellitus develop retinopathy?*

Answer: After 5 years about 25% of patients with Type I diabetes have retinopathy. This increases to 60% at 10 years and 80% at 15 years. The prevalence is less for patients with Type II diabetes, although because the condition is more common than Type I more patients with retinopathy and Type II diabetes are seen in practice.

References:

Arch Ophthalmol 1984; 102: 520–526
Ophthalmology 1984; 91: 1–9

Question: *What is the genetic component to the aetiology of diabetes?*

Answer: It has long been known that patients with either type I or II diabetes often have a positive family history for the respective condition. The risk of type I, insulin dependent diabetes in the siblings of affected Caucasian patients is about 6% compared to a population frequency of only 0.4%. Linkage analysis has identified a multitude of genetic loci contributing to the aetiology of type I diabetes including the HLA region of chromosome 6 (6p21). Other loci of probable importance include 11p15 as well as 2q31, 3q21-25, 6q25, 6q27, 10cen, 11q13, 15q and 18q. A genetic component is also involved with the aetiology of type II, non-insulin dependent diabetes. In some patients there is autosomal dominant inheritance with a mutation in the glucokinase gene with a locus on either chromosome 20 or 12. Mutations at the 17q25 locus may play a role in some cases, this being the site of the glucagon receptor gene.

67. Hypertensive retinopathy

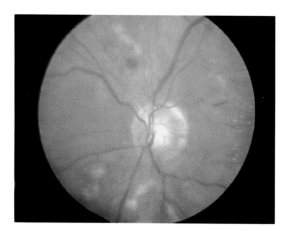

Figure 56 Hypertensive retinopathy. Arteriovenous crossing changes, cotton wool spots and haemorrhages associated with systemic hypertension (courtesy of Gordon Douglas MD).

Definition

A retinopathy secondary to systemic hypertension.

Clinical features

Retinal vessels respond to systemic hypertension by narrowing. The degree to which this can occur depends on the degree of arteriosclerosis and hence vessel wall rigidity. Thus, the classical progressive changes of long-standing hypertension are seen in the eyes of young patients but are modified in the older patient.

The Keith–Wagener–Barker classification of hypertensive retinopathy divides the clinical signs into 4 grades which correlate with the severity and duration of the hypertension. The features of the 4 grades are listed below:

Grade 1

- generalized arteriolar attenuation (i.e. the normal 1.1 : 1 ratio of vein : artery is increased).

Grade 2

- severe Grade 1 changes
- focal arteriolar attenuation (followed by segments of arteriolar dilation)
- arteriovenous crossing changes (e.g. a-v nipping)
- vessel tortuosity
- partial concealment of the venous blood column.

Grade 3

- severe Grade 2 changes
- haemorrhages (mainly flame shaped, some blot)
- retinal exudates (± macular star)
- cotton wool spots (see p. 196).

Grade 4 (accelerated or malignant hypertension)

- severe Grade 3 changes
- disc swelling*.

* Do NOT use the term 'papilloedema' to describe a swollen disc unless the cause is known to be or is thought to be due to raised intracranial pressure. In some cases of Grade 4 hypertensive retinopathy there may be papilloedema since a cerebral tumour or raised intracranial pressure from any cause may result in secondary hypertension (Cushing's reflex).

Exam questions

Question: *What is hypertension?*

Answer: The World Health Organization (WHO) definition of hypertension is a systolic blood pressure of >160 mmHg and a diastolic of >95 mmHg. Patients with a systolic pressure of <140 mmHg and a diastolic of <90 mmHg are defined as normotensive and the rest are considered as borderline hypertensives.

Question: *What are the causes of hypertension?*

Answer: By far the commonest cause is essential hypertension (i.e. the cause is unknown) which accounts for about 95% of cases. Renal disease is the commonest of the other causes; specific conditions including renal artery stenosis, nephritis, polycystic disease, renin secreting tumours, and connective tissue disorders including SLE. Endocrine causes include Cushing's and Conn's syndromes, phaeochromocytoma, acromegaly, pre-eclampsia, oral contraceptive use, hyperparathyroidism and hypothyroidism. Other causes include polycythaemia, coarctation of the aorta and acute porphyria.

Question: *What are the main ocular complications of systemic hypertension?*

Answer: In addition to hypertensive retinopathy, hypertension can be the underlying cause of a retinal vein or artery occlusion, a macroaneurysm, anterior ischaemic optic neuropathy, choroidal infarcts (Elschnig spots and Siegrist streaks) and cranial nerve palsies. Diabetic retinopathy is aggravated by hypertension.

Question: *What are the main systemic complications of hypertension?*

Answer: Hypertension increases a patient's risk of developing left ventricular failure, an acute myocardial infarction, renal failure or a cerebrovascular accident. In addition severe hypertension can cause hypertensive encephalopathy. Patients treated for hypertension are at risk of the side-effects of anti-hypertensive drugs.

Question: *What vascular histopathological changes occur in patients with hypertension?*

Answer: Arterioles throughout the body show hyalinization (i.e. deposition of eosinophilic material below the endothelium). Small and medium sized arteries show medial muscular hypertrophy and fibrosis with intimal proliferation. Large arteries show accelerated arteriosclerosis. Small perforating arteries in the brain show microaneurysms.

Question: *Is visual acuity usually impaired by hypertensive retinopathy?*

Answer: No. The ocular complications of hypertension frequently impair vision but the hypertensive process itself has no effect on vision. Visual acuity is usually normal even in Grade 4 retinopathy unless an exudate or haemorrhage involves the fovea.

Question: *Is the assessment of hypertensive retinopathy useful to the general physician?*

Answer: Yes. The grade of retinopathy correlates well with the systemic effects of the hypertension. Patients with Grade 1 have normal cardiac and renal function, those with Grade 2 have continuously higher blood pressure and may show mildly impaired cardiac or renal function. Patients with Grade 3 invariably show impaired function of these organs and are at high risk of a CVA. Grade 4 also correlates with severe systemic disturbances and many patients have an associated encephalopathy.

Question: *What is the mean life expectancy for a patient with malignant hypertension?*

Answer: About 1 year.

Question: *Is hypertensive retinopathy different from arteriosclerotic retinopathy?*

Answer: Yes. Although arteriosclerotic changes are usually seen in association with hypertensive retinopathy they are also commonly seen in the older normotensive individual. Arteriosclerosis is characterized by thickening of vessel walls and the key features of the retinopathy are arteriovenous crossing changes.

Grade 1
  – broad arteriolar light reflex
  – simple vein concealment
Grade 2
  – Grade 1 changes
  – deflection of veins at a-v crossings (Salus' sign)
Grade 3
  – Grade 2 changes
  – copper-wire arterioles
  – venous dilation distal to a-v crossings (Bonnet's sign)
  – venous tapering either side of a-v crossings (Gunn's sign)
Grade 4
  – severe Grade 3 changes
  – silver-wire arterioles
  – often associated with a branch retinal vein occlusion.

Question: *Is the presence of a macular star exclusive to hypertension?*

Answer: No. A macular star represents exudate deposited radially around the fovea within Henle's layer of the retina. There are, therefore, a number of causes including idiopathic, diabetic retinopathy, retinal periphlebitis, macular vessel obstruction and chronic infections such as syphilis or tuberculosis. A star can also be seen in association with papilloedema or papillitis and after ocular or cerebral trauma.

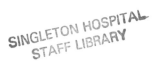

68. Cotton wool spots

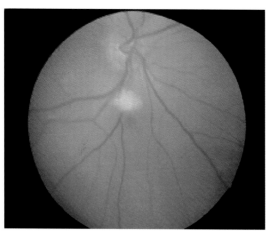

a

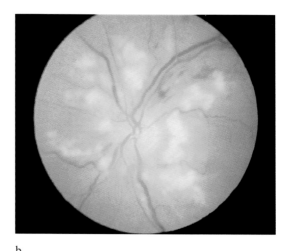

b

Figure 57   a: A relatively large cotton wool spot in a patient with SLE (courtesy of Gordon Douglas MD); b: Multiple cotton wool spots surrounding the optic disc in a patient with AIDS (courtesy of the Department of Medical Illustration, Moorfields Eye Hospital).

Definition

A cotton wool spot is a focal lesion within the nerve fibre layer of the retina due to a hold up of nerve axoplasmic flow (both orthograde and retrograde flow) as a response to ischaemia. Each spot is the result of a micro-infarct in the retinal nerve fibre layer.

Clinical features

Initially each spot appears as a fluffy white patch typically in the retina of the posterior pole where the nerve fibre layer is thickest. Later they shrink and become more circumscribed. They may resorb completely within a few months, leaving a nerve fibre defect.

Exam questions

Question: *What is a soft exudate?*

Answer: The term 'soft exudate' has been used to describe a cotton wool spot. The term is now obsolete since it is incorrect; a cotton wool spot is not an exudate but represents held up axoplasmic flow secondary to focal ischaemia in the nerve fibre layer.

Question: *What are the causes of cotton wool spots?*

Answer: Cotton wool spots are most commonly associated with diseases which cause microvascular ischaemia such as diabetes mellitus, hypertension and collagen vascular disease including SLE and PAN. They are also a common feature of ischaemic retinal vein occlusions. Other causes include anaemia, leukaemia, septicaemia, acquired immune deficiency syndrome (AIDS) and dysproteinaemia.

Question: *What is a cytoid body?*

Answer: A cotton wool spot consists of many cytoid bodies, each being the swollen end or stump of a disrupted axon, a section of which has lost its arteriolar supply. The stumps swell because both orthograde (towards the lateral geniculate body) and retrograde (towards the retinal ganglion cell body) axoplasmic flow persist. Electron microscopy thus shows axonal stumps at the edge of a micro-infarct which are stuffed full of cell organelles, particularly mitochondria.

Question: *How does a cotton wool spot appear on a fluorescein angiogram?*

Answer: Each spot corresponds to an area of hypofluorescence (a filling defect) in the retinal capillary network. These appear in the arterio-venous phase and persist throughout the angiogram. Since they are micro-infarcts they show no extravascular leakage.

Question: *What does the presence of cotton wool spots imply in the eye of a patient with AIDS?*

Answer: It implies the presence of HIV-related microvasculopathy, which is usually asymptomatic. However, the patient is at increased risk of developing CMV retinitis.

69. Retinal macroaneurysm

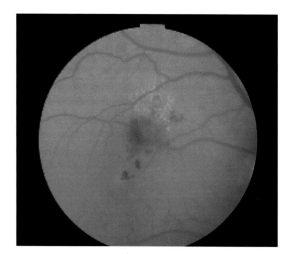

Figure 58 A retinal macroaneurysm with associated exudate and haemorrhage (courtesy of Philip Hykin MD FRCS FRCOphth).

Definition

An acquired aneurysm of a retinal artery which occurs within the first 3 orders of bifurcation.

Clinical features

Macroaneurysms tend to occur in patients with arteriosclerosis who are elderly and hypertensive and are rarely seen in an otherwise normal fundus. They are commonly single but can be multiple and are usually situated at the posterior pole. As their name implies they are large and by definition they occur within the first 3 orders of retinal arterial bifurcation. A macroaneurysm is not always easily identified by ophthalmoscopy, particularly if they bleed or leak and become obscured by haemorrhage or exudate. The latter complications are common (especially in those that present to an ophthalmologist) and most are surrounded by oedema, a ring of exudate or blood. An old aneurysm

may have become thrombosed, the vessel beyond being sclerosed and occluded or a vessel wall plaque (focal yellow material) may develop.

Remember to note any co-existing retinal vascular changes of systemic hypertension or atherosclerosis which may predispose to the development of macroaneurysms. Suggest to an examiner that you would like to measure the patient's blood pressure.

Exam questions

Question: *Are retinal macroaneurysms similar to Leber's miliary aneurysms in aetiology?*

Answer: No. Macroaneurysms have a similar pathology to the Charcot-Bouchard aneurysms of the cerebral circulation. They are acquired and thought to occur secondary to embolization with subsequent damage, weakness and dilation of the arterial wall. Leber's miliary aneurysms in contrast are the result of a developmental vascular malformation.

Question: *How does a retinal macroaneurysm affect vision?*

Answer: An uncomplicated aneurysm usually has no effect on vision. However, haemorrhage (especially if recurrent), macular oedema or an extensive exudative response can reduce vision significantly.

Question: *How does a macroaneurysm appear at fluorescein angiography?*

Answer: The aneurysm itself appears as a hyperfluorescent saccular dilation of the retinal artery which usually shows a degree of leakage. Areas of associated haemorrhage or exudate mask the background choroidal fluorescence. If an aneurysm has become thrombosed the artery beyond the occlusion will not fill. The angiogram invariably shows evidence of arteriosclerotic and/or hypertensive retinopathy.

Question: *How should patients with a retinal macroaneurysm be managed?*

Answer: Systemic hypertension should be treated if indicated. An uncomplicated macroaneurysm can be treated conservatively as can those which haemorrhage. Haemorrhages tend to resolve spontaneously and do not require specific treatment unless large and/or recurrent. Laser photocoagulation of the lesion should be performed if vision is threatened by an exudative response, macular oedema or recurrent haemorrhage.

Question: *Are retinal macroaneurysms a specific complication of essential systemic hypertension?*

Answer: No. Although this is the commonest cause/association they can occur in patients with secondary hypertension and also in patients with no evidence of hypertension.

70. Retinal vein occlusion

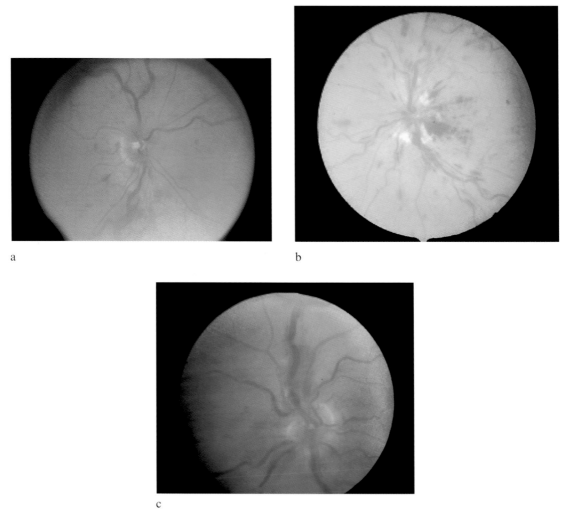

Figure 59 a: A branch retinal vein occlusion (courtesy of Gordon Douglas MD); b: A central retinal vein occlusion (courtesy of the Department of Medical Illustration, Moorfields Eye Hospital); c: The characteristic sausage-like retinal veins of a patient with Waldenström's macroglobulinaemia – a differential diagnosis of a central retinal vein occlusion (courtesy of Peng Khaw PhD MRCP FRCS FRCOphth).

Definition

A common retinal vascular disorder due to occlusion or partial occlusion in the venous part of the retinal circulation.

With a central retinal vein occlusion (CRVO) the site of occlusion is behind the cribiform plate. With a branch retinal vein occlusion (BRVO) the site of occlusion is anterior to the cribiform plate.

Clinical features

A patient with the signs of an acute vein occlusion is unlikely to appear in exams. However, the condition is common and patients may be seen with the signs of a previous occlusion. The signs are highly variable between patients depending on when the occlusion occurred, its cause and its severity. Central vein occlusions affect the whole fundus, branch occlusions only a part of the fundus.

Acute signs

- dilated ($\pm$ tortuous) retinal veins
- flame shaped (superficial intraretinal) haemorrhages
- retinal oedema
- cotton wool spots (if retina is ischaemic)
- macular oedema
- disc swelling.

Chronic signs

- retinal exudates
- venous sheathing
- arterial sheathing (occasionally).

A candidate should examine the patient for clues as to the possible aetiology of the occlusion.

Exam questions

Question: *What are the causes of a retinal vein occlusion?*

Answer: Venous occlusion can occur due to pressure on the vein from outside, vessel wall disease or increased blood viscosity. External pressure is the commonest cause due to either raised intraocular pressure or systemic hypertension. Hypertension results in arterial pressure on a retinal vein where they share a common fibrous adventitial sheath (i.e. just posterior to the lamina cribrosa or at retinal a-v crossings). Diabetes is the commonest cause in the vessel wall disease group, others including conditions which result in retinal periphlebitis such as sarcoidosis, Behçet's disease and Eales' disease. Causes of increased blood viscosity are rare and include chronic leukaemia, polycythaemia and

dysproteinaemias such as Waldenström's macroglobulinaemia and myeloma. Blood hyperviscosity syndromes more commonly cause a bilateral slow-flow (venous stasis) retinopathy characterized by dilated tortuous retinal veins.

Question: *Is the site of a branch retinal vein occlusion related to the aetiology?*

Answer: To some extent this is true. A hemisphere occlusion occurs when the blockage is at the edge of the optic disc. This is more likely if the disc is cupped and there is associated glaucoma. Quadrantic occlusions occur secondary to a-v crossing occlusion and therefore are most common in hypertensive patients. Most of these occur in the upper temporal quadrant where a-v crossings are most common. Peripheral venous occlusions are most common in patients with retinal periphlebitis and are also seen in patients with sickle cell retinopathy. Nasal vein occlusions are often associated with diabetes.

Question: *Why do some patients have persistently reduced visual acuity following a branch retinal vein occlusion?*

Answer: There are two main reasons for this, the commonest being chronic macular oedema. The other is recurrent vitreous haemorrhage secondary to posterior segment neovascularization.

Question: *Is retinal and/or optic nerve head neovascularization a common complication of branch retinal vein occlusion?*

Answer: This occurs in about 25% of the eyes which have undergone a major branch vein occlusion. Neovascularization occurs in the eyes which develop an ischaemic retina with extensive areas of capillary drop-out. It is thought that the ischaemic retina produces a vasoformative substance as in proliferative diabetic retinopathy.

Question: *How can patients with retinal neovascularization secondary to branch retinal vein occlusion be treated?*

Answer: The only specific treatment available is laser photocoagulation to any areas of ischaemic retina. This inhibits the neovascular response and can prevent recurrent vitreous haemorrhage. Some studies have shown, however, that the 10 year visual acuity is no different in patients who have undergone laser treatment from those who have suffered vitreous haemorrhage. Thus some clinicians treat only patients whose other eye is blind so as to avoid total blindness during episodes of vitreous haemorrhage.

Question: *Is retinal neovascularization a common complication of central retinal vein occlusion?*

Answer: No. It is very rare after a central vein occlusion.

Question: *What is the most important complication of central retinal vein occlusion?*

Answer: Rubeosis iridis and associated neovascular glaucoma is the most serious complication of a central retinal vein occlusion. It develops about 3 months after the occlusion when there is an extensive amount of retinal ischaemia as evidenced clinically by cotton wool spots, retinal oedema and dense, dark blot haemorrhages.

Question: *What is 100 day glaucoma?*

Answer: This is another name for the neovascular (or thrombotic) glaucoma which occurs

secondary to an ischaemic central retinal vein occlusion. This classically develops about 3 months (or 100 days) after the occlusion but this is not a hard and fast rule.

Question: *How can neovascular glaucoma be prevented?*

Answer: All patients with an ischaemic central retinal vein occlusion (best demonstrated by fluorescein angiography) should be treated with pan-retinal photocoagulation as soon as possible. This prevents onset of the neovascular response, rubeosis and neovascular glaucoma.

Question: *After a central retinal vein occlusion is disc swelling a bad prognostic sign?*

Answer: Not necessarily. If a central retinal vein occlusion is ischaemic axoplasmic flow is held up in the retina and does not reach the disc. If the occlusion is non-ischaemic the retina is more healthy and axoplasmic flow occurs to the disc where it is then halted resulting in swelling. Disc swelling is thus more likely to be associated with a non-ischaemic occlusion with a better prognosis than an ischaemic type.

71. Retinal emboli

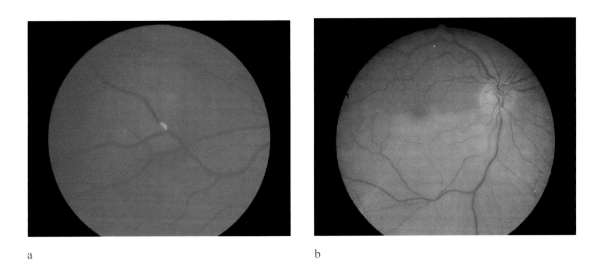

a

b

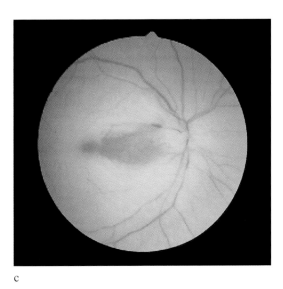

c

Figure 60 Retinal emboli. a: A peripheral calcific embolus (courtesy of the Department of Medical Illustration, Moorfields Eye Hospital); b: A calcific embolus at the optic disc margin associated with an acute branch retinal artery occlusion (courtesy of the Department of Medical Illustration, Moorfields Eye Hospital); c: A central retinal artery occlusion with cilioretinal artery sparing (courtesy of Robert Nozik MD and Carlos Pavesio MD).

Definition

A retinal embolus is a particulate mass circulating in the retinal vasculature which is not a normal component of the circulating fluid.

Types of emboli:

1. Atheromatous:
   – fibrinoplatelet
   – cholesterol
   – calcific
2. Cardiac:
   – thrombus
   – calcific
   – vegetations
   – myxoma
3. Fat
4. Air
5. Neoplastic
6. Talc
7. Amniotic
8. Parasite.

Retinal emboli impacting within a retinal artery can cause branch or central retinal artery occlusion. They originate most commonly from either the heart or the carotid arteries.

Clinical features

Emboli

Fibrinoplatelet
These are usually only visible during an attack of amaurosis fugax and are thus unlikely to be seen during a clinical exam. The emboli are usually numerous, small and white. They tend to pass rapidly through the retinal vessels.

Calcific
These are usually single, relatively large, globular and white. They do not glint with the light of an ophthalmoscope. Since they are large they are often impacted in an arteriole near to the disc. When at the disc margin they are easily missed since they tend to blend in with the colour of disc tissue. Ischaemic retina is often evident distal to the embolus, since they frequently cause complete and permanent arteriolar obstruction.

Cholesterol
These are usually multiple, small, yellow/orange in colour and they tend to glint under the light of an ophthalmoscope. When present, they are often seen at retinal arteriole bifurcations. With time or after ocular massage they may break up and disperse.

Retinal artery occlusion (post-embolic)

Embolization is the commonest cause of both central and branch retinal arterial occlusions. An acute arterial occlusion will not be seen in the exam setting. Signs include:

Central retinal artery occlusion
- reduced visual acuity (usually to no perception of light [NPL])
- afferent pupillary defect
- cotton wool spots (acutely)
- stagnation of the retinal circulation with clumping (cattle trucking) of the blood within arterioles
- cherry-red spot (disappears after about 2 weeks) (see p. 206)
- there may be cilioretinal artery sparing
- retinal atrophy (chronically)
- arteriolar narrowing with irregularity of calibre (chronically)
- optic atrophy and arteriolar attenuation (chronically)
- rubeosis iridis (4% of cases, chronically).

Branch retinal artery occlusion (variable with site)
- sectoral visual field defect
- sectoral retinal ischaemia and secondary changes (as above)
- an embolus may be visible
- lipid deposition in the arterial wall at the site of endothelial cell damage caused by an embolus.

Cilioretinal artery occlusion
- As above affecting the associated region of blood supply.

It is important when an embolus is seen or suspected that the patient's cardiovascular system is examined.

Exam questions

Question: *What is a Hollenhorst plaque?*

Answer: A Hollenhorst plaque is synonymous with a cholesterol embolus. These usually originate from an atheromatous plaque which has undergone ulceration releasing the contents into the circulation. They are small refractile yellowish emboli, frequently found at arteriolar bifurcations, which because of their size rarely produce symptoms.

Question: *Where do calcific retinal emboli originate?*

Answer: These can originate from a calcified aortic valve in the heart, from the ascending aorta or from a calcified atheromatous plaque in the carotid arteries. Thus, the diagnosis of a calcific embolus should be followed by full assessment of the heart and carotid arteries, appropriate treatment and hopefully avoidance of further embolic events, particularly stroke.

Question: *Apart from emboli, what else may be the cause of a retinal artery occlusion?*

Answer: In addition to disease within the lumen (emboli), disease in the wall or outside the wall of the artery may result in occlusion.
Vessel wall diseases which can result in vaso-obliteration fall into two main groups. Firstly localized atheroma and secondly arteritis. Causes of arteritis include giant cell arteritis, SLE, PAN, scleroderma, dermatomyositis and syphilis. Other less common causes of vaso-obliteration include sickle cell disease, pre-eclamptic toxaemia and drug induced retinal artery spasm with ergotamine or quinine.
Increased pressure on the retinal circulation producing occlusion may occur with a high IOP, such as in acute angle closure glaucoma or during retinal detachment surgery. A rise in orbital pressure can also result in arterial occlusion. This may be secondary to a retrobulbar haemorrhage or exophthalmos.

Question: *How should one manage a patient with an acute major retinal artery occlusion?*

Answer: This is an ophthalmic emergency and prompt treatment should be provided immediately. Treatment can improve the visual outcome if started within 48 hours of the occlusion, but earlier treatment is more likely to be successful.
Specific measures include orbital decompression (e.g. for an acute retrobulbar haemorrhage) and lowering a raised IOP (e.g. as with acute glaucoma or during retinal detachment surgery). Non-specific measures are aimed at increasing retinal blood flow and dislodging any emboli. They include, lying the patient flat, applying intermittent, firm digital ocular massage for 15 minutes, administering 500 mg of i/v acetazolamide, inhalation of a 5% CO_2/95% O_2 gas mixture and anterior chamber paracentesis if indicated.
Investigations into the cause of the occlusion should be carried out as soon as is reasonable. In particular it is important to: exclude arteritis (erythrocyte sedimentation rate [ESR], temporal artery biopsy in the elderly), assess the patient for carotid artery stenosis (clinical examination, digital subtraction angiography [DSA] and Doppler sonography) and exclude causes of emboli from the heart (clinical examination, electrocardiogram [ECG], chest X-ray and echocardiogram) especially atrial fibrillation and mitrial stenosis. In addition a biochemical screen including lipids and glucose should be performed and the patients blood pressure measured.

Question: *When may fat emboli be observed on examination of the fundus?*

Answer: These may be seen within retinal blood vessels after the fracture of a long bone or in a patient with pancreatitis.

Question: *What is a cilioretinal artery?*

Answer: These are present in about 20% of individuals and are part of the posterior ciliary circulation. They extend from the optic disc towards the fovea, vary in size and supply a variable area of retina. Since they are separate from the central retinal artery they may be spared in a retinal artery occlusion or they may become occluded in isolation.

72. Cherry-red spot

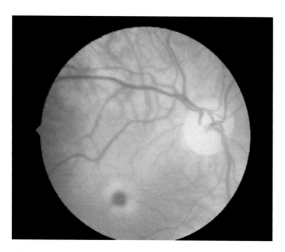

Figure 61 A prominent cherry-red spot (courtesy of Gordon Douglas MD).

Definition

A fundal appearance, where the area of the fovea appears red relative to the surrounding fundus. There are a number of causes:

1. Central retinal artery occlusion (but only if acute, and thus very unlikely to be seen in clinical examinations)
2. Certain lysosomal storage disorders:
   Sphingolipidoses:
   – Tay–Sachs disease
   – Sandhoff's disease
   – Niemann–Pick disease
   Mucolipidoses:
   – generalized gangliosidosis
   – metachromatic leucodystrophy
3. Quinine toxicity (acute, due to retinal oedema)
4. Traumatic retinal oedema
5. Macula retinal hole with surrounding retinal detachment
6. Cherry-red spot myoclonus syndrome.

Clinical features

On ophthalmoscopy the cherry-red spot is usually obvious, the area corresponding to the fovea appearing bright red against a pale fundus. Other signs depend on the cause.

A candidate is more likely to be shown a slide or fundus photograph of this physical sign, rather than a patient.

Exam questions

Question: *What is Tay–Sachs disease?*

Answer: This is also known as infantile amaurotic familial idiocy and GM_2 gangliosidosis type I. It is a familial condition transmitted in an autosomal recessive manner, 70% of patients being Ashkenazi Jews. The disease is due to a deficiency of the enzyme hexosaminidase A, which results in an accumulation of GM_2 ganglioside. The lipid accumulates in retinal ganglion cells and in the large neurones of the grey matter of the brain. Apart from hyperacusis, development is normal for about six months, after which severe progressive neurological changes occur. These include dementia, epilepsy, weakness, spasticity and deafness. A cherry-red spot develops in over 90% of cases, and may be present at two months. Retinal ganglion cell death, secondary to the excessive lipid deposition within them, results in a fading of the cherry-red spot and the development of optic atrophy and blindness. Blindness is usually complete by 18 months, and in most cases death occurs before the age of three years.

Question: *What are Ashkenazi Jews?*

Answer: These are Jewish people of German or East European descent. The name is derived from Ashkenaz, the son of Gomer, a descendant of Noah, who was associated with the ancient Ascanians of Phrygia.

Question: *What is the cause of the cherry-red spot often seen in infants with Tay–Sachs disease?*

Answer: Deposition of GM_2 gangliosidase within retinal ganglion cells gives the normally transparent retina a pale colour, particularly at the posterior pole where the cells are several layers thick. Since ganglion cells are absent at the foveolar and sparse at the fovea, the red colour of the underlying choroidal circulation remains in this region, forming the cherry-red spot. The spot itself is thus the normal appearance, and the pale surround the abnormal fundal appearance.

Question: *What is the cause of the cherry-red spot characteristic of a central retinal artery occlusion?*

Answer: As with Tay–Sachs disease, the retinal ganglion cells are the site of pathology after a central retinal artery occlusion. Ischaemia induces oedema and the oedematous ganglion cells are pale in colour. Again, the cherry-red spot represents the appearance of a normal choroidal circulation at the fovea.

Question: *Apart from a cherry-red spot how else can some of the sphingo- and mucolipidoses affect the eyes?*

Answer: Corneal cloudiness can be a feature of Niemann–Pick disease, generalized gangliosidosis, metachromatic leucodystrophy, and types I, II and III mucolipidoses. Fabry's disease is a cause of verticillata, posterior capsular lens opacities and conjunctival and retinal vessel tortuosity. A brown discolouration of the anterior lens capsule occurs in most cases of Niemann–Pick disease. A pigmentary retinopathy can occur in association with GM_2 gangliosidosis type III, and a maculopathy may complicate metachromatic leucodystrophy or mucolipidosis type I. Farber disease is a rare cause of ocular inflammation and macular pigmentation.

73. Sickle cell retinopathy

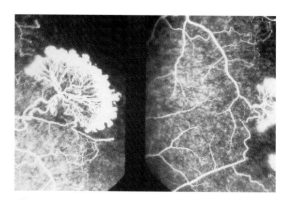

Figure 62 Sickle cell retinopathy. Fluorescein angiography of a sea-fan lesion (courtesy of the Department of Medical Illustration, Moorfields Eye Hospital).

Definition

A retinopathy associated with one of the sickling haemoglobinopathies.

The sickling haemoglobinopathies are a group of disorders predominantly affecting some of the black population, characterized by the presence of one or more abnormal haemoglobins. These are insoluble and form crystals under conditions of low oxygen tension or acidosis. This causes red blood cells to adopt an abnormal (sickle) shape and become less pliable. These deformed cells alter blood flow, impact in small blood vessels and produce hypoxia and eventual ischaemia.

Classifications

Sickle cell haemoglobinopathies
1. Sickle cell trait: HbAS
2. Sickle cell disease/anaemia: HbSS
3. Sickle cell haemoglobin-C disease: HbSC
4. Sickle cell thalassaemia: HbSThal.

Sickle cell retinopathy
1. Proliferative (five progressive stages):
   – peripheral arteriolar occlusions
   – arterio-venous anastomoses
   – neovascularization
   – vitreous haemorrhage
   – retinal detachment
2. Non-proliferative.

Clinical features

The patient will be black. If asked to examine the fundi and the posterior pole appears normal, a candidate should examine the peripheral fundus. This may require the use of an indirect ophthalmoscope (not for MRCP). Sickle cell retinopathy is essentially a condition of the retinal periphery, where oxygen tensions are most likely to be low.

Proliferative

Stage 1
- peripheral arterial occlusions.

Stage 2
- Stage 1 changes
- peripheral arterio-venous anastomoses. These are not new vessels, but represent dilated pre-existent capillary channels
- the retina distal to occlusions and anastomoses is virtually avascular, and perfusion is reduced.

Stage 3
- Stage 2 changes
- neovascular tufts originating from the anastomoses. These have a characteristic 'sea-fan' appearance. Each tuft is usually fed by a single arteriole and drained by a single venule. They are most commonly seen in

the superotemporal quadrant, at the equator or anterior to the equator.

Stage 4
- Stage 3 changes
- vitreous haemorrhage.

Stage 5
- Stage 3 (± Stage 4) changes
- traction retinal detachment (usually, can be rhegmatogenous).

Non-proliferative

Most of these are asymptomatic lesions:

- venous tortuosity
- arteriolar narrowing
- peripheral chorioretinal scars (choriocapillaris infarction), also known as 'black sun-bursts'
- peripheral, superficial retinal haemorrhages (salmon-patch haemorrhages)
- haemosiderin deposits within schisis cavities (refractile dots)
- retinal breaks
- angioid streaks
- vascular occlusions (may be symptomatic).

Exam questions

Question: *What is the biochemical difference between haemoglobin HbS and HbA?*

Answer: In HbS there is substitution of valine for glutamine in the sixth position on the β-chains of the haemoglobin molecule. The HbS molecule is thus Hb $\alpha_2\beta_2^S$ as opposed to Hb $\alpha_2\beta_2$.

Question: *Does sickle cell retinopathy occur with equal incidence in patients with the different types of sickling haemoglobinopathies?*

Answer: No. Ocular complications are the most severe with sickle cell haemoglobin-C disease (HbSC) and sickle cell thalassaemia (HbSThal), even though the systemic features of these anaemias tend to be relatively less severe. Despite the potentially severe systemic features of sickle cell disease, its ocular complications are usually fairly mild; with sickle cell trait they are very rare.

Question: *With what may sickle cell 'sea-fans' be confused?*

Answer: 'Sea-fans' can be confused with other forms of peripheral neovascularization, such as occurs with diabetes, retinal vein occlusion, retinopathy of prematurity, sarcoidosis, Eales' disease, posterior uveitis or familial exudative vitreoretinopathy.

Question: *What are the therapeutic options for proliferative sickle cell retinopathy?*

Answer: Laser photocoagulation to obliterate sea-fans or to areas of capillary non-perfusion can reduce the chance of progression. If this is not available, peripheral retinal cryotherapy can be used as an alternative. The treatment for a prolonged non-clearing vitreous haemorrhage is a vitrectomy, but results tend to be poor. Retinal detachment surgery is sometimes required, but if this is possible the eye is at great risk of anterior segment ischaemia, particularly if scleral buckling is used. To reduce this risk a number of measures can be taken:

- use of local anaesthesia (without adrenaline) if possible
- preoperative partial exchange blood transfusion
- maintenance of a low IOP
- drainage of subretinal fluid whenever possible
- use of segmental scleral buckles rather than an encirclement band.

Question: *What are the non-retinal, ocular manifestations of the sickling haemoglobinopathies?*

Answer: These include lesions of the conjunctiva and iris. The conjunctiva may show dark red vascular segments shaped like commas or corkscrews. Inferior, small-calibre vessels tend to be affected. The iris may undergo ischaemic atrophy, usually between the pupil margin and the collarette. Rubeosis is rarely seen, but if present there is a risk of hyphaema.

NB: If a patient with sickle cell anaemia develops a hyphaema and secondary raised IOP, acetazolamide should be avoided because it induces a metabolic acidosis which (by shifting the oxygen dissociation curve) can increase the risk of sickling and subsequent ocular ischaemia.

74. Eales' disease

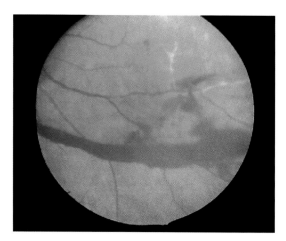

Figure 63 Sheathed vessels, neovascularization and vitreous haemorrhage in the eye of a patient with Eales' disease (courtesy of Gordon Douglas MD).

Definition

A primary idiopathic retinal vasculitis of unknown cause, characterized by obliterative retinal periphlebitis. The diagnosis should only be made after exclusion of other causes of such periphlebitis.

Clinical features

The disease affects young men (15–30 years of age), and mainly the peripheral fundus. Both eyes are affected in over 50% of cases. The condition has four stages.

Stage 1
- sheathing of small peripheral retinal venules with inflammatory exudates
- segmented, dilated, beaded or occluded peripheral retinal venules
- peripheral retinal oedema
- minute peripheral retinal haemorrhages.

Stage 2
- Stage 1 changes extending more posteriorly, behind the equator
- vitreous haze.

Stage 3
- peripheral and equatorial retinal neovascularization.

Stage 4
- proliferative retinopathy (± disc new vessels) associated with retinal and vitreous haemorrhages and/or tractional retinal detachment (in severe cases).

Other clinical signs which may be evident include:

- rubeosis iridis (± neovascular glaucoma)
- cataract.

Exam questions

Question: *What is the aetiology of Eales' disease?*

Answer: The aetiology is unknown and at present it is a clinical diagnosis of exclusion. Some work has suggested that it is a form of T-cell, cell-mediated, vascular hypersensitivity. Histopathological examination has shown the retinal venules to be cuffed with lymphocytes and plasma cells.

Question: *What is the main symptom of Eales' disease?*

Answer: Loss of vision secondary to vitreous haemorrhage. Before a vitreous haemorrhage occurs the condition is relatively symptom free.

Question: *How should patients with Eales' disease be treated?*

Answer: The treatment rationale is similar to that for proliferative diabetic retinopathy. Laser photocoagulation to areas of ischaemic retina and focal photocoagulation to destroy new vessels and/or occlude affected vessels is effective in preventing progression, although it frequently has to be repeated. In advanced cases, a pars plana vitrectomy is required.

Question: *Is there an association between Eales' disease and tuberculosis?*

Answer: There is no definite link between Eales' disease and tuberculosis (TB), although some patients with Eales' disease appear to have an unexplained tuberculin hypersensitivity. TB is also a cause of retinal phlebitis.

Question: *What are known causes of retinal phlebitis?*

Answer: The commonest cause is extension of adjacent chorioretinitis. Other causes include:

- sarcoidosis
- Behçet's disease
- syphilis
- multiple sclerosis
- tuberculosis
- cytomegalic inclusion disease
- necrotizing angiitis.

75. Coats' disease

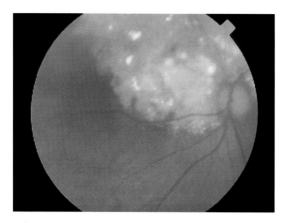

Figure 64 Retinal exudation in a patient with 'adult Coats' disease (courtesy of Philip Hykin MD FRCS FRCOphth).

Definition

This is a congenital anomaly of retinal and optic nerve vasculature, resulting in telangiectasia, aneurysms and massive subretinal exudation.
Also known as Retinal Telangiectasis or Leber's Miliary Aneurysms.

Clinical features

The three main clinical signs are:

- telangiectasia of the paramacular or macular regions
- peripheral retinal aneurysmal dilations
- subretinal exudate

In some cases the only sign is paramacular or macular telangiectasia. This may be associated with macular oedema or deposition of exudate. In other cases the main sign is of massive subretinal exudation due to leakage from peripheral retinal aneurysms affecting both arterioles and venules. The aneurysms have been described as having a light-bulb shape, but may be fusiform or saccular. These are Leber's miliary aneurysms, and they are most commonly seen in the temporal retina.

Exudate is initially deposited in the macular area, often in the form of a macular star. For this reason, a peripheral vascular abnormality should always be sought in patients with an otherwise unexplained macular star.

Subretinal exudation can be of a sufficient degree to produce a retinal detachment and/or leukocoria. Other complications include iridocyclitis, cataract and glaucoma.

Exam questions

Question: *When and in whom does Coats' disease present?*

Answer: Classically, Coats' disease presents in one eye of an otherwise healthy boy of about eight years of age. These cases usually present with Leber's miliary aneurysms, telangiectasia and extensive subretinal exudation. Occasionally patients present in middle age with so-called 'adult Coats' disease'. These cases usually feature paramacular telangiectasia with macular oedema or mild exudation but no aneurysms. The disease probably represents a spectrum of a disease process; the milder the condition, the later the presentation.

Question: *What are the fluorescein angiographic changes which occur with Coats' disease?*

Answer: A fluorescein angiogram shows the telangiectatic vessels as an abnormally coarse net of dilated capillaries. These may involve both superficial and deep retinal vascular networks. Although the disease often appears to be clinically unilateral, an angiogram may show the presence of mild telangiectasia in the other eye.

The peripheral aneurysms affect both arterioles and venules, which show leakage of fluorescein. The angiogram may show evidence of retinal or subretinal exudate and/or haemorrhage.

Question: *How should patients with Coats' disease be managed?*

Answer: In some cases spontaneous regression of the disease occurs, even when quite advanced. Obliteration of peripheral vascular anomalies by laser photocoagulation or cryotherapy should be attempted in patients in whom central vision is threatened or has recently been lost due to retinal or subretinal exudation. Since there is a high incidence of recurrence, these patients should be carefully followed up. In advanced cases retinal detachment surgery can be useful, but the prognosis for such patients is poor.

Question: *What is a macular star?*

Answer: This is a clinical sign which represents the deposition of exudate, in a star shape, within Henle's layer of the retina at the macula.

Question: *What are the causes of a macular star?*

Answer: These include:

- hypertension
- papilloedema
- papillitis
- ocular or cerebral trauma
- macular vessel occlusions
- retinal periphlebitis
- juxtapapillary choroiditis
- chronic infections (e.g. syphilis, TB)
- idiopathic.

76. Roth spots

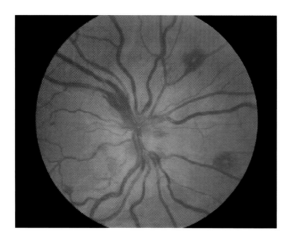

Figure 65 Retinopathy in a patient with anaemia. Two classic Roth spots are clearly visible (courtesy of Peter Shah BSc FRCOphth).

Definition

These are retinal haemorrhages with a pale-coloured or white centre.

Clinical features

Each spot is a superficial retinal haemorrhage with a white or pale-coloured central portion, the composition of which varies with the cause. The haemorrhages are usually roundish in shape, but may be irregular or flame-shaped. They are of variable size, usually being less than one disc diameter.

Exam questions

Question: *What are the causes of Roth spots?*

Answer: Classically, Roth spots are a feature of certain blood disorders, such as anaemia, sub-acute bacterial endocarditis and leukaemia.

They may, however, also be a feature of hypertensive or diabetic retinopathy when a haemorrhage resolves from the centre. A cotton wool spot with surrounding haemorrhage can also be defined as a Roth spot. Of these causes, it is important to remember anaemia and leukaemia since other clinical signs may be subtle or absent.

Question: *What are possible ocular features of leukaemia?*

Answer: Leukaemic infiltration, haemorrhage or a combination of these may affect virtually any part of the eye and orbit. Ocular complications are more likely with acute rather than chronic leukaemia.

Features of leukaemic retinopathy include retinal haemorrhages (including Roth spots), tortuous and dilated retinal veins, cotton wool spots and neovascularization.

Infiltrative optic neuropathy and papilloedema (due to raised intracranial pressure from CNS infiltration) are important sight-threatening complications. Raised intracranial pressure may also be the cause of third, fourth or sixth cranial nerve palsies.

Orbital involvement may be a cause of proptosis, particularly in children. Compression of the lacrimal drainage apparatus in conjunction with abnormal leukocyte function predisposes to dacryocystitis.

Other rare ocular features include lid haemorrhage, conjunctival infiltration, iris involvement with hypopyon or hyphaema and vitreous infiltration.

Question: *What does the white centre of a leukaemic Roth spot consist of?*

Answer: Each white centre consists of a collection of leukaemic white blood cells.

Question: *What are the ocular features of subacute bacterial endocarditis?*

Answer: Roth spots occur in approximately 5%

of cases. Conjunctival splinter haemorrhages have also been described, but these are only very rarely seen. Numerous potential neurological complications may involve the eyes.

Question: *Are Roth spots a feature of Rothmund's syndrome?*

Answer: No. This syndrome is a rare inherited disorder, which predominantly affects females. Systemic features include hypogonadism; skin atrophy, telangiectasia (poikiloderma) pigmentation and sclerosis; disturbed hair and nail growth and bony defects, including a saddle-nose. Ocular involvement, with the rapidly progressive development of cataracts, only occurs in about 15%. The eyes are otherwise not involved.

77. Age-related (senile) macular degeneration (ARMD, SMD)

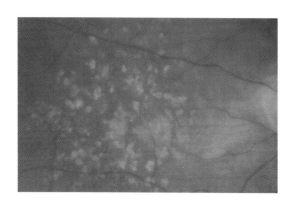
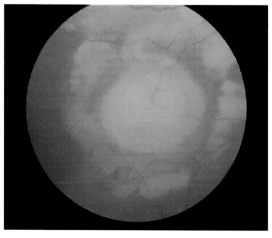

a   b

Figure 66 Age-related macular degeneration. a: Macular drusen (courtesy of Gordon Douglas MD); b: A large disciform scar (courtesy of the Department of Medical Illustration, Moorfields Eye Hospital).

Definition

An age-related degenerative condition of the macula, which is the leading cause of blindness in the western world.

Classification

1. Age-related changes (ARC):
   - drusen (colloid bodies)
   - RPE atrophy/hypertrophy
2. Non-exudative, atrophic or dry ARMD (choroidal sclerosis)
3. Exudative or wet ARMD:
   - RPE detachment
   - subretinal neovascular membrane (SRNVM).

Clinical features

The patient is usually over 60 years of age, and although the disease is often highly asymmetrical it is essentially bilateral.

Age-related changes (ARC)

A term applying to the presence of retinal drusen and/or areas of RPE atrophy and hypertrophy. The patient is rarely under 45 and commonly over 60 years of age.

Retinal drusen
- bright yellowish-white, slightly raised circular lesions at the posterior pole
- with time, secondary calcification makes each lesion whiter
- the lesions are either small and discrete or large and fluffy in size and nature
- present deep in the retina (on Bruch's membrane).

RPE atrophy and hypertrophy
- the RPE at the macula, and particularly perifoveally, has a mottled appearance
- drusen lesions, especially if large, may be surrounded with hypertrophied RPE.

Non-exudative ARMD

- areolar, geographical, atrophic or dry ARMD
- large areas of well-circumscribed RPE and choriocapillaris atrophy (with secondary neurosensory retinal atrophy)
- prominent large choroidal vessels
- ARC.

Exudative ARMD

RPE detachment

- sharply circumscribed dome-shaped elevations of variable size, usually orange in colour
- associated RPE atrophy
- ARC.

Subretinal neovascular membrane (SRNVM)

- choroidal neovascularization. Early membranes may be invisible at ophthalmoscopy, but later develop a greyish colour and produce an elevation of the retina
- exudative detachment of RPE or neurosensory retina
- sub-RPE, subretinal or vitreous haemorrhage
- disciform scarring (chronic change)
- ARC.

Exam questions

Question: *What is the pathology of retinal drusen?*

Answer: Each lesion is a collection of a hyaline material situated between the inner collagenous part of Bruch's membrane and the basement membrane of the RPE. The lesions may represent a reduction in RPE phagocytosis or discharge of RPE phagosomes, and thus may consist of old photoreceptor outer segments. Associated pathology includes atrophy and depigmentation of the RPE over each drusen lesion, irregularities in the thickness of Bruch's membrane with the risk of splitting and subsequent RPE detachment, or choroidal neovascularization.

Question: *What are the causes of retinal drusen?*

Answer: The commonest cause is as an age-related change (ARC), but drusen may also be seen in association with a number of vascular, inflammatory or neoplastic conditions which result in choroidal and/or retinal degeneration. Drusen are thus seen overlying some choroidal malignant melanomas, and are common in early phthisis. A rare cause is a primary retinal dystrophy – autosomal dominant familial drusen. Drusen may also be seen in association with other retinal dystrophies, such as fundus flavimaculatus.

Question: *What are the fluorescein angiographic features of retinal drusen?*

Answer: The classical early feature is of multiple small hyperfluorescent spots or 'RPE window defects'. These occur because of the associated atrophy of the RPE overlying the drusen, which allows a localized apparent increase in background choroidal fluorescence. The appearance is similar for some 20 minutes after fluorescein injection because of staining of the lesions by the fluorescein, which increases as the choroidal fluorescence diminishes.

Question: *How should patients with non-exudative ARMD be managed?*

Answer: At present there is no specific therapy available but retinal rotational procedures may prove useful in some patients. Patients with relatively mild disease should be asked to report back to an ophthalmologist if they develop central visual distortion, which may be due to the development of a subretinal neovascular membrane. To aid detection of distortion, patients should be provided with (and instructed on the use of) an Amsler grid. Patients with more extensive visual loss should be managed with low visual aids (LVA) if required, and should be registered blind or partially-sighted if desired and indicated.

Question: *What are the fluorescein angiographic features of an RPE detachment?*

Answer: The early appearance is of a uniformly hyperfluorescent area which gradually increases in intensity. The area later develops well-circumscribed margins, marking the extent of the detachment as the fluorescein pools in the sub-RPE space.

Question: *What are the possible outcomes of an RPE detachment?*

Answer: Some undergo spontaneous resolution and some others progress to detachment of the neurosensory retina. Up to 66%, however, become complicated by subretinal neovascularization and the risk of exudative maculopathy, particularly if the RPE detachment is associated with an RPE rip.

Question: *What are subretinal neovascular membranes (SRNVMs)?*

Answer: These are membranes of fibrovascular tissue which sprout from the choriocapillaris through defects in Bruch's membrane into the subretinal space.

Question: *With what may a SRNVM be associated?*

Answer: A SRNVM may occur after any cause or RPE, Bruch's membrane and/or choriocapillaris disruption. The commonest association is with ARMD, but there are numerous others including:

- high myopia (Fuchs' spot)
- angioid streaks
- presumed ocular histoplasmosis syndrome
- chorioretinitis
- excessive laser photocoagulation
- choroidal naevus, haemangioma or melanoma
- traumatic choroidal rupture
- retinal dystrophy (Best's vitelliform and cone dystrophies)
- rubella retinopathy
- serpiginous choroidopathy
- retinitis pigmentosa.

Question: *What are the fluorescein angiographic features of a SRNVM?*

Answer: The classical first sign occurs very early as the new vessels of the membrane fill in a lacy or bicycle wheel pattern. After 20–30 seconds the vessels fluoresce maximally, and after one to two minutes they start to leak into the subretinal space. Leakage is followed by staining of the fibrous elements of the membrane, which thus hyperfluoresce.

Question: *What are the possible outcomes of a SRNVM?*

Answer: The main problem with SRNVMs is that they are prone to haemorrhage. This may result in a haemorrhagic detachment of the RPE or neurosensory retina. If blood breaks through the retina, a vitreous haemorrhage occurs. Organization of subretinal haemorrhages results in the most likely outcome of a SRNVM, namely a disciform scar. Some membranes do not bleed but leak profusely, resulting in exudative retinal detachment. Whatever the specific outcome, the prognosis for vision is poor.

Question: *Is laser photocoagulation of a SRNVM an appropriate form of management?*

Answer: Laser photocoagulation can be beneficial, but only in certain patients. The criteria adopted for selection of suitable patients vary from centre to centre, but most consider therapy appropriate if:

- VA is 6/18 or better
- SRNVM is outside the foveal avascular zone
- eyes have other evidence of ARMD (e.g. drusen)
- there is recent onset of symptoms.

Photocoagulation is only beneficial if the membrane is totally obliterated, and it is thus important to perform a fluorescein angiogram no more than 72 hours before treatment so as to identify the extent of any membrane. Unfortunately the long-term recurrence rate is high. Experimental forms of therapy include surgical membranectomy, radiotherapy and administration of interferon.

78.   Angioid streaks

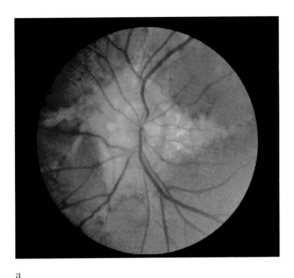

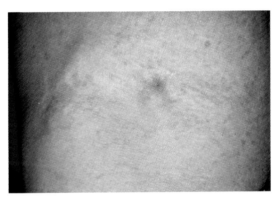

a   b

Figure 67   a: Angioid streaks in association with optic nerve head drusen (courtesy of Gordon Douglas MD); b: The 'plucked chicken' skin appearance of a patient with pseudoxanthoma elasticum who also had angioid streaks (courtesy of the Department of Medical Illustration, Moorfields Eye Hospital).

Definition

Streaks usually visible at fundoscopy due to cracks in the collagenous and elastic portions of Bruch's membrane associated with secondary changes to the RPE and choriocapillaris.

Clinical features

The streaks

- red/brown streaks
- irregular contour with serrated edges
- usually darker and wider than retinal blood vessels
- positioned deep to the retinal vessels
- usually present in a radial fashion (based on the disc)
- run an irregular course to end abruptly posterior to the equator
- almost always bilateral.

The patient

- usually middle-aged
- more commonly male
- look for signs of associated systemic disease (e.g. pseudoxanthoma elasticum, Paget's disease, Marfan's syndrome, sickle cell anaemia).

Exam questions

Question: *What other fundal signs may be seen in patients with angioid streaks?*

Answer: Associated fundal signs which may be present include:

- peau d'orange (stippled pigmentary retinal mottling)
- salmon spots (small, round yellow-white spots)

- peripapillary chorioretinal atrophy
- optic nerve head drusen
- crystalline bodies (multiple small subretinal crystals).

Question: *What are the fluorescein angiographic features of angioid streaks?*

Answer: Each streak appears as a line of hyperfluorescence due to the associated overlying RPE window defect.

Question: *Do angioid streaks affect vision?*

Answer: Sometimes. Central vision may be reduced in one of three ways:

- by a streak crossing the fovea
- by development of a SRNVM
- by choroidal rupture with an associated subretinal haemorrhage.

Question: *What are the systemic associations of angioid streaks?*

Answer: In 50% of cases no systemic association can be identified. In the other 50% of cases, most are associated with conditions affecting skin, bone or blood. These include:

- pseudoxanthoma elasticum (Grönblad–Strandberg syndrome)
- Paget's disease
- sickle cell anaemia
- Ehlers–Danlos syndrome
- senile elastosis of skin
- thrombocytopenic purpura
- familial hyperphosphataemia
- Marfan's syndrome
- acromegaly
- lead poisoning.

Question: *What are the ocular features of Ehlers–Danlos syndrome?*

Answer: In addition to an association with angioid streaks, other features include blue sclera, ectopia lentis, microcornea, keratoconus and an increased risk of rhegmatogenous retinal detachment.

79. Central serous choroidoretinopathy (CSCR)

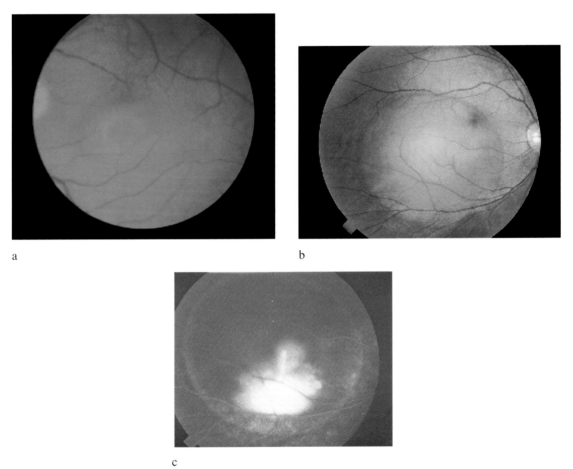

a

b

c

Figure 68 a: Subtle macular elevation in a patient with central serous choroidoretinopathy (courtesy of the Department of Medical Illustration, Moorfields Eye Hospital); b: A less subtle example of a central serous choroidoretinopathy and; c: the associated fluorescein angiogram (courtesy of Robert Nozik MD and Carlos Pavesio MD).

Definition

A small serous neurosensory retinal detachment at the macula due to a localized breakdown of the outer blood–retinal barrier (RPE level).

Also known as:

- Central Serous Retinopathy (CSR).

Clinical features

Visual defects

- usually unilateral
- mildly reduced VA (6/6–6/18)
- improved VA with a +1.00D lens (acquired hypermetropia)

- positive paracentral or central scotoma
- red desaturation
- abnormal photo-stress test.

Fundoscopy

- shallow roundish elevation of the neurosensory retina at the posterior pole, usually at or near the fovea
- absent foveolar reflex
- detached retina is transparent and of normal thickness
- surrounding glistening reflex
- shadows of overlying retinal vessels on underlying RPE
- small yellowish precipitates on undersurface of detached retina (chronic cases).

Remember to look for an optic disc pit, which is an uncommon associated finding.

Exam questions

Question: *In what type of patient is central serous choroidoretinopathy (CSCR) most common?*

Answer: The classical patient is a young (20–45 years) male myope of dynamic personality type A. Not all patients with CSCR, however, fit these criteria.

Question: *What symptoms may a patient with central serous choroidoretinopathy (CSCR) report?*

Answer: Occasionally the condition is extrafoveal and asymptomatic. Most patients, however, complain of a relatively sudden reduction in vision with a mild reduction in visual acuity and a positive relative scotoma (i.e. something obstructing central vision, cf. a hole). Other symptoms include:

- visual distortion (micropsia, metamorphopsia)
- generalized darkening/dimming
- decreased recovery from glare
- symptoms of (relative) hypermetropia.

Question: *What are the fluorescein angiographic features of central serous choroidoretinopathy (CSCR)?*

Answer: The angiographic features occur due to local breakdown of the blood–retinal barrier and subsequent leakage of fluorescein into the subretinal space. One of two specific patterns may be evident, of which the ink-blot type is the more commonly seen. Here a small hyperfluorescent spot at the site of the defect appears early and this gradually increases in size like an ink-blot until by the late venous phase the whole subretinal space of the lesion is filled. The smoke-stack type is less common, occurring when there is an associated small RPE detachment. Here fluorescein collects early in the angiogram beneath the RPE detachment, producing a tiny hyperfluorescent spot. During the late venous phase the dye streams into the subretinal space and then ascends vertically to the upper limit of the detachment like the smoke from a chimney. It then spreads laterally to umbrella outwards and eventually fill the entire detachment.

Question: *What is the visual prognosis for patients with central serous choroidoretinopathy (CSCR)?*

Answer: Generally good, up to 90% undergoing spontaneous resolution within six months. Symptoms such as metamorphopsia or micropsia may persist for a longer period and in some patients the visual acuity and distortions, although improving, never return to normal. Up to 40% of patients suffer recurrence, and in these and in persistent cases there is a risk of local RPE degeneration or (rarely) cystoid macular oedema (CMO). The prognosis is unrelated to severity of the condition or the age of the patient.

Question: *How should patients with central serous choroidoretinopathy (CSCR) be managed, and are any drugs such as steroids useful?*

Answer: In most cases reassurance is all that is required, some patients finding a + 1.00D addition helpful. In cases that fail to undergo spontaneous resolution within six months, laser photocoagulation should be considered for selected patients, particularly when:

- recurrent episodes have caused visual impairment
- vision in an affected fellow eye is impaired
- there is associated CMO or retinal lipid deposition
- the subretinal fluid appears turbid
- the patient requires 'perfect' vision for work.

Steroids are of no value, and there is no evidence that drugs such as acetazolamide help resolution.

80. Epiretinal membrane

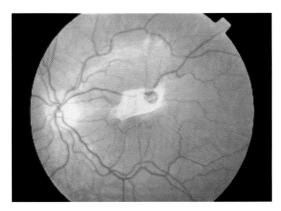

Figure 69 A Grade 2 epiretinal membrane exerting retinal traction (courtesy of the Department of Medical Illustration, Moorfields Eye Hospital).

Definition

Membrane formation at the vitreoretinal interface which can cause a maculopathy.

Also known as:

- Simple Membrane
- Pre-Retinal Fibrosis
- Vitreoretinal Interface Maculopathy
- Cellophane Maculopathy
- Surface Wrinkling
- Macular Pucker (when all retinal layers are involved).

Clinical features

Grade 1

Early:
- translucent membrane seen only as a sheen (irregularity of the light reflex)
- best visualized with red-free light

Late:
- grey-coloured membrane
- mild retinal striae

- traction on the temporal vessels produces tortuosity and pulls them towards the median raphe
- traction on vessels of the papillomacular bundle stretches and straightens them.

Grade 2

- dense membrane
- partially obscured retinal vessels
- marked vessel distortion
- marked retinal striae
- macular oedema (severe cases).

Exam questions

Question: *What is metamorphopsia?*

Answer: Metamorphopsia is the symptom of altered image size, and is common in early macular disease. A decrease in image size (or micropsia) occurs if foveal cones are spread apart, and an increase in image size (or macropsia) occurs if they are compressed.

Question: *What are the causes of an epiretinal membrane?*

Answer: Most cases are idiopathic, occurring in eyes which are normal apart from the presence of a posterior vitreous detachment. Other causes include:

- vitreoretinal surgery (7% of cases)
- retinal vascular disorders (e.g. diabetic retinopathy or retinal vein occlusion)
- posterior ocular inflammation
- trauma
- excessive retinal laser photocoagulation
- retinitis pigmentosa.

Question: *Why does an epiretinal membrane reduce visual acuity?*

Answer: This is usually due to a combination of factors such as:

- physical covering of the retina
- macular distortion
- low traction retinal detachment of the macula
- vascular leakage/retinal oedema/CMO
- obstructed axoplasmic flow.

Question: *What do epiretinal membranes consist of?*

Answer: These membranes consist of cells and secreted extracellular material. Early simple membranes contain mainly glial cells, but the more complex membranes contain glial cells, fibroblast-like cells, RPE cells and inflammatory cells, including activated T-lymphocytes. The extracellular material consists mainly of collagen (types I and III), glycosaminoglycans and glycoproteins such as fibronectin.

Question: *When is surgical membrane peeling with vitrectomy indicated?*

Answer: Indications vary from centre to centre, but results are best if the patients visual acuity is better than 6/18 and there is only a short history of visual disturbance, particularly if this is of distortion rather than visual loss. Full visual recovery is rare, and since the procedure is often technically difficult, it should not be undertaken by an inexperienced surgeon.

81. Cystoid macular oedema (CMO)

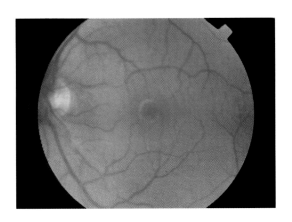 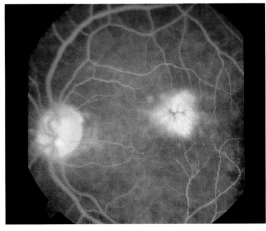

a b

Figure 70 a: Post-operative pseudopakic cystoid macular oedema; b: The classical appearance of cystoid macular oedema at fluorescein angiography (both courtesy of Rajni Jain MB BS and Philip Hykin MD FRCS FRCOphth).

Definition

An accumulation of extracellular fluid in Henle's (outer plexiform) layer and the inner nuclear layer of the retina, based about the fovea, due to leakage from macular capillaries.

Clinical features

Visual defects

- reduced central vision (positive central scotoma, metamorphopsia, micropsia)
- reduced visual acuity
- abnormal photo-stress test.

Fundoscopy

- absent foveal depression
- retinal thickening
- multiple fluid-filled microcysts in neurosensory retina
- large intraretinal cysts (chronic cases, may herald lamellar hole formation).

Exam questions

Question: *What are the causes of cystoid macular oedema (CMO)?*

Answer: There are many causes, including:

- diabetic retinopathy
- retinal vein occlusion (BRVO, non-ischaemic CRVO)
- inflammatory eye disease (especially pars planitis)
- retinal vascular lesions (macroaneurysm, telangiectasia)
- topical adrenaline (in aphakic patients)
- drugs (e.g. chloroquine)
- Irvine–Gass syndrome
- retinitis pigmentosa
- epiretinal membrane formation
- inherited
- central serous choroidoretinopathy.

Question: *What is Irvine–Gass syndrome?*

Answer: This is the occurrence of CMO in the post-operative cataract extraction eye, the incidence being considerably higher following intracapsular extraction as opposed to extracapsular extraction. The incidence is higher in eyes in which vitreous loss occurred at the time of surgery. It may be due in part to excessive light stimulation of the fovea during surgery. In most cases, spontaneous resolution occurs within six months. The incidence can be reduced by prescribing oral indomethacin in the post-operative period. In some cases, persistent CMO has resolved following pars plana vitrectomy.

Question: *What are the fluorescein angiographic features of CMO?*

Answer: Leakage of fluorescein into Henle's layer of the retina produces a distinctive angiographic appearance. Parafoveal focal leakage begins during the early arteriovenous phase. By the end of the arteriovenous phase the areas of leaked fluorescein coalesce and, due to the radial arrangement of nerve fibres around the fovea, this produces a characteristic 'flower-petal' pattern of hyperfluorescence. This persists into the later phases of the angiogram. Fluorescein angiography is sensitive in detecting CMO that is not evident at fundoscopy.

Question: *Is CMO common following a branch retinal vein occlusion?*

Answer: Yes. CMO occurs in 50–60% of cases with a temporal vein occlusion, although it is rare following a nasal occlusion, and chronic CMO is the commonest cause of persistently poor central vision following an occlusion. Focal laser photocoagulation to intraretinal microvascular abnormalities and aneurysms (but not shunts) should be considered in cases that continue to deteriorate after six months.

Question: *How can CMO associated with retinitis pigmentosa be managed?*

Answer: CMO may occur in up to 70% of eyes with retinitis pigmentosa, and in many of these cases it appears to have relatively little effect on visual acuity. In cases where VA is reduced there is evidence that low-dose acetazolamide may be useful.

82. Macular hole

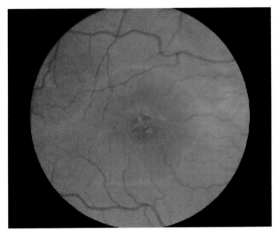

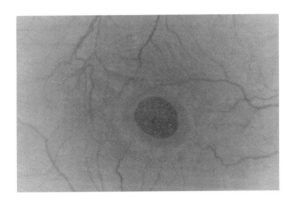

a   b

Figure 71   a: A Stage 3 macular hole; b: A Stage 4 macular hole (courtesy of the Department of Medical Illustration, Moorfields Eye Hospital).

Definition

A full thickness retinal hole at the fovea.

Clinical features

Visual defects

- reduced central vision
- reduced VA.

Fundoscopy

- round or oval, punched out, full-thickness foveal lesion
- usually $\frac{1}{4}$ disc diameter
- yellow pigment in base (probably xanthophyll in macrophages)
- surrounding grey halo of oedema
- Watzke sign.

Fluorescein angiography

- area of hyperfluorescence (an RPE window defect).

Exam questions

Question: *Why is the foveal region particularly susceptible to retinal hole formation?*

Answer: The retina at the fovea is thin, avascular, and has little supporting tissue. It is thought that this makes it weaker and more susceptible to damage.

Question: *What are the causes of macular holes?*

Answer: It is currently thought that prefoveal vitreous traction on weakened foveal retina is the cause of true macular hole formation. The commonest aetiology is due to an age-related atrophy of the retina (spontaneous idiopathic/ senile macular holes), together with prefoveal vitreous cortex shrinkage. These are more common in women and those over 60 years, and are bilateral in 10% of cases. Other causes or aggravating factors include:

- high myopia
- trauma (e.g. following commotio retinae)
- solar retinopathy
- direct vitreous traction with incomplete posterior vitreous detachment in association with a retinal detachment
- severe chorioretinitis following severe CMO.

Question: *Are patients with spontaneous idio-pathic/senile macular holes at increased risk of retinal detachment?*

Answer: No.

Question: *What is the differential diagnosis of a macular hole?*

Answer: Pseudo-macular holes, macular cysts and lamellar holes can be confused with true macular holes.

A pseudo-macular hole is produced by a defect in an epiretinal membrane overlying the fovea. Lamellar holes usually occur following rupture of macular cysts due to chronic CMO.

Pseudo and lamellar holes do not produce RPE window defects at fluorescein angiography be-cause the RPE remains unaffected.

Question: *Can vitrectomy prevent progression of an impending macular hole?*

Answer: There is increasing evidence that in certain cases vitrectomy may be of benefit. Gass has classified macular holes into four stages, based on the effect of prefoveal vitreous cortex shrinkage and foveal traction:

1. Stage 1:
   a) Partial foveolar detachment
   b) Full-thickness foveolar detachment
2. Stage 2: Dehiscence in inner limiting membrane
3. Stage 3: Full-thickness macular hole with overlying operculum (i.e. a localized pre-foveal PVD)
4. Stage 4: Full-thickness macular hole with complete vitreous separation (PVD).

Since spontaneous resolution of Stage 1 holes can occur, vitrectomy is not indicated unless the hole is either at Stage 2, 3 or 4. Patients have to accept that post-operative, face-down posturing is required for 1–3 weeks.

83. Bull's eye maculopathy

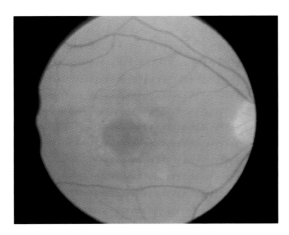

Figure 72 Bull's eye maculopathy. Chloroquine maculopathy (courtesy of Gordon Douglas MD).

Definition

A characteristic macular lesion with the ringed appearance of a dartboard, usually secondary to chloroquine (or high-dose hydroxychloroquine) toxicity, which results in RPE degeneration and loss of photoreceptors.

Clinical features

Visual defects

- reduced visual acuity
- reduced colour vision
- impaired peripheral and central vision (field loss).

Fundoscopy

A central area of hyperpigmentation at the fovea is surrounded by a zone of depigmentation, which is itself further surrounded by an annulus of hyperpigmentation.

Exam questions

Question: *Who is at risk of developing a bull's eye maculopathy?*

Answer: Patients receiving long-term, high-dose chloroquine (used in the treatment of rheumatoid arthritis, SLE and malaria) are at risk. The incidence is proportional to the cumulative dose, and is rare unless a total dose of 300 g has been exceeded. Patients taking hydroxychloroquine are also at risk, but to a lesser degree. In addition, clofazimine (used to treat atypical mycobacterial infections in patients with AIDS) can produce a bull's eye maculopathy.

Question: *What abnormalities may be detected in patients with chloroquine toxicity before they develop a bull's eye maculopathy?*

Answer: Before there is a detectable maculopathy at fundoscopy, a red target scotoma may be evident between 5° and 10° from fixation. The electro-oculogram (EOG) may be subnormal at this stage. With continuing drug treatment these changes become more severe and less reversible, non-specific pigment stippling of the RPE occurs and the foveolar reflex is lost. In addition to retinal changes corneal deposition of chloroquine may occur, this being unrelated to the dose of drug and reversible upon withdrawal. Another ocular side-effect of chloroquine is a transient difficulty with accommodation when the drug is first taken – it is of little significance.

Question: *How should patients on long-term chloroquine therapy be monitored?*

Answer: Ideally, a baseline eye examination should be carried out before the patient commences long-term, high-dose therapy. This should consist of:

- visual acuity testing
- colour vision testing

- assessment of visual fields
- ophthalmoscopy
- fundus photography.

Follow-up should be arranged after nine months and continued six monthly, the aim being to detect the reversible premaculopathy, particularly by looking carefully for a red target scotoma between 5° and 10° from fixation.

Question: *What conditions can mimic a bull's eye maculopathy?*

Answer: In addition to the maculopathy of chloroquine and hydroxychloroquine toxicity, a similar fundal appearance may be seen in patients with one of the bull's eye macular syndromes:

- cone dystrophy
- Stargardt's disease
- Batten's disease
- benign concentric annular macular dystrophy.

Question: *What drugs can produce a toxic maculopathy?*

Answer:

1. chloroquine
2. hydroxychloroquine
3. quinine
4. chlorpromazine
5. thioridazine
6. tamoxifen.

84. Stickler's syndrome

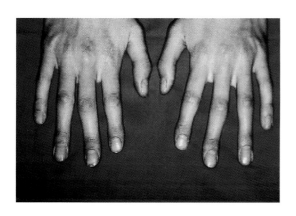
a

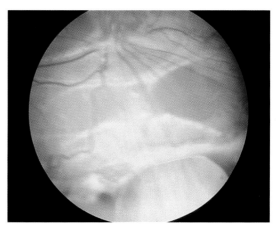
b

Figure 73 a: The typical hands of a patient with Stickler's syndrome (Marfanoid); b: Vitreoretinal degeneration of Stickler's syndrome (note the retinal vessel dragging at the disc and a dislocated lens) (courtesy of the Department of Medical Illustration, Moorfields Eye Hospital).

Definition

A hereditary progressive arthro-ophthalmopathy with both specific and certain marfanoid features, which is classified as one of the connective tissue dysplasias.

Clinical features

Vitreoretinal degeneration

- vitreous veils (condensations)
- vitreous lacunae
- posterior vitreoretinal adhesions
- perivascular pigment deposition
- retinal vessel dragging at the optic disc
- peripheral retinal degeneration (lattice-like)
- retinal breaks (including giant) and detachment.

Other ocular features

- cataract (posterior subcapsular)
- myopia
- glaucoma.

Maxillofacial and skeletal

- mid-facial flattening
- extended philtrum
- Pierre–Robin features:
  - cleft lip and palate
  - micrognathia (small mandible)
  - glossoptosis
- Marfanoid habitus
- joint hyperextensibility
- arthropathy.

Exam questions

Question: *How is Stickler's syndrome inherited?*

Answer: In an autosomal dominant manner.

Question: *What are the genetic abnormalities associated with Stickler's syndrome?*

Answer: Two genotypes corresponding with the phenotype of Stickler's syndrome have been described. Type I is due to a mutation in gene encoding Type 2 procollagen at the locus 12q13. Type II is due to an abnormality at 1p21, although the exact function of the abnormal gene(s) remains unknown.

Question: *What type of glaucoma is most common in patients with Stickler's syndrome?*

Answer: Secondary open angle glaucoma.

Question: *What diagnoses would you think of when examining a child with a vitreoretinal degeneration?*

Answer: One would have to consider:

- juvenile retinoschisis (XLR)
- Stickler's syndrome (AD)
- Goldmann–Favre syndrome (AR)
- Wagner's disease (AD).

Question: *What is Wagner's disease?*

Answer: This is an autosomal dominantly inherited vitreoretinal degeneration indistinguishable from Stickler's syndrome except that there are no systemic features.

Question: *Is Stickler's syndrome more or less common than Marfan's syndrome?*

Answer: More.

85. Retinitis pigmentosa

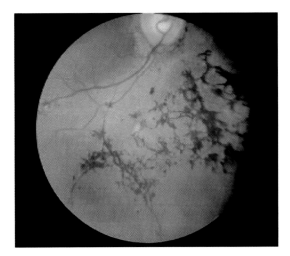

Figure 74 The classical bone-spicule pigmentation of typical retinitis pigmentosa (courtesy of the Department of Medical Illustration, Moorfields Eye Hospital).

Definition

A group of diseases characterized by bilateral night blindness, constricted visual fields and, typically, a pigmentary retinopathy.

(There is preferential degeneration of the rod photoreceptor system, the cone system only being affected late in the disease.)

Classification

Typical retinitis pigmentosa
- autosomal recessive (51%)
- autosomal dominant (26%)
- X-linked recessive (23%).

Atypical retinitis pigmentosa
- retinitis pigmentosa sine pigmento
- retinitis punctata albescens (fundus albipunctatus or progressive albipunctate dystrophy)

- sector retinitis pigmentosa
- pericentric retinitis pigmentosa.

Secondary retinitis pigmentosa/systemic associations
- abetalipoproteinaemia (Bassen–Kornweig syndrome)
- phytanic acid storage disease (Refsum's syndrome)
- Friedreich's ataxia
- Laurence–Moon–Bardet–Biedl syndrome
- Usher's syndrome
- Cockayne's syndrome
- Kearns–Sayre syndrome
- mucopolysaccharidosis (Hurler's, Hunter's and Sanfilippo's syndromes).

Pseudo-retinitis pigmentosa
(Can be unilateral)
- trauma
- posterior ocular inflammation (syphilis, rubella)
- drug toxicity (quinine, phenothiazines)
- post ophthalmic artery occlusion
- spontaneous retinal reattachment
- calcium oxalate retinopathy.

Clinical features (typical RP)

Visual defects

- night blindness
- reduced dark adaptation
- visual field defects (ring scotoma, 2–3°–tunnel vision)
- photophobia.

Fundoscopy

Classic triad:
- retinal pigmentary changes (bone-spicule pigmentation)
- arteriolar attenuation
- waxy disc pallor.

Other posterior segment features

- CMO ($\pm$ lamellar hole formation)
- RPE atrophy and hypertrophy
- retinal microaneurysms
- retinal telangiectasia $\pm$ exudation
- retinal venous sheathing
- tessellate fundus/choroidal atrophy
- vitreous changes (PVD, vitreous deposits)
- optic nerve head drusen
- epiretinal membrane.

Female carriers of the X-linked type may show a golden metallic tapetal reflex temporal to the macula.

Anterior segment

- myopia
- keratoconus (rare)
- cataract (posterior subcapsular)
- open angle glaucoma.

Exam questions

Question: *What is the visual prognosis of typical retinitis pigmentosa?*

Answer: In 75% of cases there is a gradual deterioration in vision with age. These are usually the X-linked and autosomal recessive cases. By the age of 50 years, 50% of affected patients have a visual acuity of 6/60 or below and significantly constricted visual fields.
In the other 25%, the visual acuity remains good (often better than 6/18) even if there is progressive, severe loss in visual field and loss of an electro-retinogram (ERG) response. These are mainly the patients with the autosomal dominant form.

Question: *What are the electrodiagnostic test features of typical retinitis pigmentosa?*

Answer: The EOG is lost early in the disease, and the ERG amplitude falls with disease progression and loss of photoreceptors. The ERG amplitude is usually subnormal before obvious fundal changes occur. The scotopic ERG is affected more and earlier than the photopic ERG, indicating a predominant loss of rods. Dark adaptation tests demonstrate a rise in both rod and cone thresholds.

Question: *How should one manage patients with retinitis pigmentosa?*

Answer: It is important when diagnosing retinitis pigmentosa to exclude pseudo-retinitis pigmentosa and associated systemic disorders, in particular those which are treatable.
Once diagnosed patients should be offered:

- genetic counselling
- referral to self-help groups
- management of associated features, including cataract, glaucoma, keratoconus and CMO
- advice on avoiding excessive illumination
- low vision aids
- partial sight registration.

Question: *What is Refsum's syndrome, and why is it important for clinicians to recognize it?*

Answer: This is an autosomal recessive storage disease characterized by accumulation of phytanic acid because of a deficiency of the enzyme phytanic acid hydroxylase. Clinical features include:

- hypertrophic peripheral neuropathy (loss of deep tendon reflexes and superficial sensation to pain, touch or temperature)
- cerebellar ataxia
- deafness
- cardiomyopathy
- ichthyosis
- atypical retinitis pigmentosa.

The presenting feature is invariably night blindness and/or the associated pigmentary retinopathy in a patient of young or middle age. It is important that the diagnosis is not missed because the condition is treatable by eliminating phytates from the patient's diet. Phytates are present in dairy products, ruminant fats and green vegetables.

Question: *What are the clinical features of Laurence–Moon–Bardet–Biedl syndrome?*

Answer: This autosomal recessive disorder is characterized by:

- deafness
- polydactyly
- mental retardation
- obesity
- hypogonadism
- atypical retinitis pigmentosa.

86. Cone dystrophy

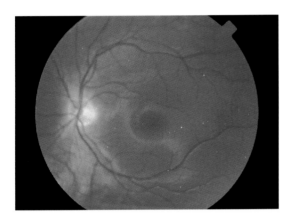

Figure 75 The abnormal macular reflex associated with cone dystrophy (courtesy of Philip Hykin MD FRCS FRCOphth).

Definition

An inherited retinal dystrophy characterized by degeneration of the cone photoreceptor system. (Rod photoreceptor system degeneration only occurs late in the disease – cf. retinitis pigmentosa.)

Classification

1. Type I – less severe, later onset
2. Type II – more severe, earlier onset.

Clinical features

Visual defects

- reduced central vision
- reduced vision in good illumination (cf. night blindness)
- reduced colour vision
- photophobia
- nystagmus.

Fundoscopy

- bull's eye-like macular lesion (a ring of depigmentation centred on the fovea)
- temporal disc pallor (waxy pallor in severe cases)
- attenuated retinal arterioles
- peripheral pigmentary retinopathy (mild).

Exam questions

Question: *How is cone dystrophy inherited?*

Answer: Most familial cases are inherited by an autosomal dominant or X-linked mode, but autosomal recessive cases have been reported.

Question: *At what age do most patients with cone dystrophy present?*

Answer: Onset of Type I cone dystrophy is usually between the ages of 10 and 30 years. Type II tends to present earlier than Type I.

Question: *What are the electrodiagnostic test features of cone dystrophy?*

Answer: The photopic ERG is subnormal in the presence of a normal scotopic ERG.

Question: *What is the differential diagnosis of cone dystrophy?*

Answer:
The differential diagnosis includes:

- bull's eye maculopathy (chloroquine toxicity)
- benign annular macular dystrophy
- Batten's disease (ceroid-lipofuscinosis)
- retinitis pigmentosa.

Question: *Are patients with cone dystrophy easy to examine at ophthalmoscopy?*

Answer: In some cases ophthalmoscopy is difficult because these patients often have an aversion to bright light. Such patients often complain of photophobia and a reduced visual acuity in conditions of good illumination.

87. Stargardt's disease

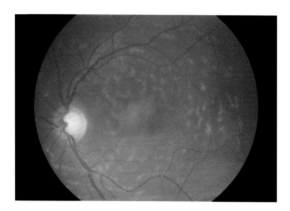

Figure 76 The classical fundus appearance of Stargardt's disease (courtesy of the Department of Medical Illustration, Moorfields Eye Hospital).

Definition

An inherited, bilateral disorder of the macula, classified as one of the 'flecked retina' syndromes.

Also known as:

– Stargardt's Macular Dystrophy

Classification

1. Central
2. Central and pericentral
3. Central and peripheral.

Clinical features

Visual defects

- bilateral, symmetrical
- reduced central vision
- reduced colour vision
- unrelated to fundus appearance
- (normal night vision).

Fundoscopy

Central
- ovoid, atrophic foveal lesion (1.5 disc diameters) (beaten-bronze or snail-slime appearance).

Central and pericentral
- foveal lesion (as above)
- yellow-white, linear, round and fishtail-shaped 'fleck' lesions at the posterior pole (present late in the disease)
- pigmentary retinopathy.

Central and peripheral
- foveal lesion (as above)
- pigmentary retinopathy
- vessel narrowing
- disc pallor.

Exam questions

Question: *What is the mode of inheritance for Stargardt's disease, and when does it present?*

Answer: Autosomal recessive, presentation with loss of central vision occurring between 10 and 20 years of age. (Autosomal dominant cases are rare but have been reported.)

Question: *What is the treatment of Stargardt's disease?*

Answer: There is no specific treatment, but patients should be offered genetic counselling and low vision aids if appropriate.

Question: *What are the yellowish flecks characteristic of Stargardt's disease?*

Answer: These are collections of engorged RPE cells full of lipofuscin. Late in the disease the flecks are associated with focal areas of retinal degeneration and RPE atrophy.

Question: *What is fundus flavimaculatus?*

Answer: This is a variant of Stargardt's disease which has a slightly different fundal appearance and tends to present later. Unlike Stargardt's disease, the yellowish fleck lesions are seen early and are more prominent and widespread. A maculopathy (often of the beaten-bronze type) occurs in 50% of cases, and is usually a late feature. Most current literature use the terms Stargardt's and fundus flavimaculatus interchangeably.

Question: *What is the differential diagnosis of Stargardt's disease or fundus flavimaculatus?*

Answer: The main condition that should be considered is familial dominant drusen. Other conditions characterized by yellowish fundal flecks are very rare, such as fundus albipunctatus, primary oxalosis and the flecked retina of Kandori syndrome.

88. Best's vitelliform macular dystrophy

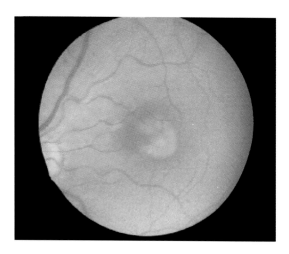

Figure 77 Best's vitelliform macular dystrophy.
A vitelliform lesion of the macula with the
appearance of a fried egg (sunnyside-up) (courtesy of
Gordon Douglas MD).

Definition

An inherited bilateral disorder of the macula
which usually presents in childhood and initially is associated with a near normal visual
acuity.

Also known as:

– Best's disease
– Best's macular dystrophy
– Vitelliruptive macular degeneration
– Vitelliform degeneration.

Stages

1. Previtelliform
2. Vitelliform
3. Pseudohypopyon
4. Vitelliruptive
5. End stage.

Clinical features

The clinical signs are highly variable, and
patients do not always progress though all the
classical stages described below. The lesions
rarely occur eccentrically.

Previtelliform

- asymptomatic
- normal fundus
- reduced EOG.

Vitelliform

- patient usually under 10 years of age
- normal or slightly reduced VA
- 'fried-egg yoke' lesion of the macula
  (a 0.5–3 disc diameter cyst of lipofuscin
  sited between the sensory retina and RPE).

Pseudohypopyon

- the superior half of the vitelliform lesion is
  absorbed, revealing RPE atrophy
- reduced colour vision.

Vitelliruptive

- patient usually under 15 years of age
- 'scrambled-egg' lesion of the macula
  reduced VA.

End stage

- severely reduced VA
- macular scar – atrophic, fibrous (hypertrophic) or fibrovascular (disciform).

Exam questions

Question: *What is the mode of inheritance for Best's vitelliform dystrophy?*

Answer: Autosomal dominant, although there is variable penetrance and expressivity.

Question: *What are the electrodiagnostic test features of Best's vitelliform dystrophy?*

Answer: The light–dark ratio of the EOG is reduced in all cases and at all stages, and is also reduced in carriers of the condition, even if their fundi appear clinically normal. Dark adaptation is mildly affected, but the ERG remains unaffected.

Question: *What are the pathological changes seen in Best's vitelliform dystrophy?*

Answer: The condition is thought to start with an abnormal accumulation of cone outer segment material in the RPE cells of the fovea. The RPE cells accumulate in elevations, and become diffusely engorged with lipofuscin. In established cases, macrophages also become engorged with both lipofuscin and pigment and are found in the subretinal space. Eventually the condition is associated with photoreceptor outer segment, RPE and choriocapillaris atrophy.

Question: *Is colour vision affected by Best's vitelliform dystrophy?*

Answer: Yes. There is usually a deutan–tritan defect, although this is only of a moderate degree.

Question: *What is adult pseudovitelliform macular degeneration?*

Answer: This is an acquired macular degeneration, which has some similarities in clinical appearance with Best's vitelliform dystrophy. The lesions are smaller, although they tend to affect vision at an earlier stage than in Best's disease. Presentation is later in life, usually in the fifth decade, and the EOG is unaffected throughout the course of the disease.

89. Choroideremia

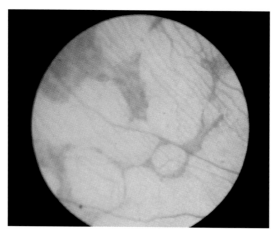
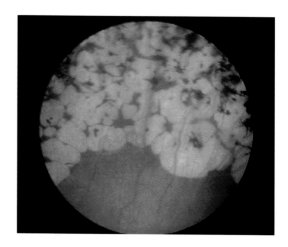

a   b

Figure 78 a: Choroidal atrophy characteristic of choroideraemia (courtesy of Gordon Douglas MD); b: Gyrate atrophy (courtesy of Peng Khaw PhD MRCP FRCS FRCOphth).

Definition

An inherited bilateral disorder of the choroid and RPE, associated with night blindness and a characteristic fundal appearance.

Clinical features

Early

- onset between 5 and 10 years of age
- reduced night vision
- granular pigmentary changes
- a normal (or moderately reduced) scotopic ERG.

Established

- moderate night blindness
- annular scotoma
- 'salt and pepper' fundus (pigmentation and depigmentation)

- RPE and choroidal atrophy with exposure of the larger choroidal vessels, spreading centrally and peripherally from the equatorial region.

End stage

- reduced visual acuity (CF by 30–40 years)
- severe night blindness
- grossly constricted visual fields
- total choroidal atrophy with exposure of the sclera in the equatorial region
- the retinal vessels and the optic disc retain a normal appearance until very late in the progression.

Exam questions

Question: *What is the mode of inheritance for choroideraemia?*

Answer: X-linked recessive.

Question: *Are female carriers of choroideraemia affected?*

Answer: The carrier state is asymptomatic, but the fundus shows mid-peripheral pigmentary changes which are similar to those of early choroideraemia although they do not progress. Areas of hyperpigmentation are small (<0.1 disc diameters) with an irregular squarish appearance. The areas of depigmentation are larger (<0.5 disc diameters), may be under or adjacent to the pigment spots, and appear either pale or bright yellow.

Question: *What conditions are characterized by choroidal degeneration?*

Answer: The commonest condition associated with atrophy of the choroid is degenerative myopia. Rarer causes include:

- choroideraemia
- central areolar sclerosis
- generalized choroidal atrophy
- gyrate atrophy.

Question: *Why is it important not to miss the diagnosis of gyrate atrophy in a patient with a choroidal degeneration?*

Answer: This rare autosomal recessive condition is due to a deficiency of ornithine keto-acid aminotransferase and raised levels of ornithine. It is important not to misdiagnose, because high doses of vitamin B_6 and proline can normalize levels of ornithine and slow disease progression if given early enough.

Question: *What are the ocular complications of gyrate atrophy?*

Answer:

- myopia (first decade)
- night blindness (second decade)
- posterior subcapsular cataract (third decade)
- pigmentary maculopathy with loss of central vision (fourth decade)
- blindness (fifth decade).

90. Myopia

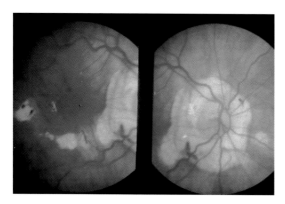

Figure 79 A myopic optic nerve head with characteristic peripapillary atrophy (courtesy of the Department of Medical Illustration, Moorfields Eye Hospital).

Definition

An optical condition in which parallel rays of light from an object are brought to focus in front of the retina. The refractive error is correctable with a concave (negative) lens.

Classification

Mechanism
1. Axial myopia – the globe is too long relative to its dioptric power
2. Refractive myopia – the dioptric power of the globe is too high relative to its length.

Type
1. Physiological myopia (common) – can be predominantly axial or refractive
2. Pathological myopia
   - Degenerative myopia – myopia associated with numerous ocular signs (see below)
   - Index myopia – lenticular (myopia due to pathologically increased lens power (e.g. nuclear sclerotic cataract), or cor-neal (myopia due to pathologically increased corneal power (e.g. kerato-conus).

Clinical features

Physiological myopia

Apart from the refractive error (usually $< -6.00D$) there may be no signs because the condition is only due to a mismatch between the refractive power of the globe and its length, both factors of which lie within their normal distribution curves.

Pathological myopia

Degenerative myopia

Fundus
1. *Optic disc*:
   - myopic crescent, usually temporal but can encircle disc
     - white = exposed sclera
     - pigmented = exposed choroid
   - pallor
   - apparent enlargement (optical magnification)
   - T-sign (visible bifurcation of central retinal vessels)
2. *Sclera/choroid*:
   - posterior pole staphyloma
3. *Choroid/RPE*:
   - pallor
   - tessellation atrophy
   - lacquer cracks in Bruch's membrane (yellow-white lines)
   - subretinal neovascularization
   - Foster–Fuchs' spot (foveal hyperpigmentation following resorption of haemorrhage from a SRNVM)
4. *Vessels*:
   - straightening of retinal vessels

Vitreous:
1. Syneresis and synchysis
2. Opacities.

Cornea:
Increased corneal diameter.

Other features:
Increased risk of:

- Peripheral retinal degeneration
- Peripheral retinal holes
- Posterior vitreous detachment
- Macular hole
- Rhegmatogenous retinal detachment
- Posterior subcapsular cataract
- Nuclear sclerotic cataract
- Primary open angle glaucoma
- Steroid-induced glaucoma.

Exam questions

Question: *What are the causes of refractive myopia?*

Answer: An increased refractive power of the lens may occur with:

- nuclear sclerotic cataract
- uncontrolled diabetes mellitus
- certain systemic drugs – carbonic anhydrase inhibitors, phenothiazines, hydralazine, chlorthalidone
- topical miotics (e.g. pilocarpine) – these give rise to a fluctuating myopia due to contraction of the ciliary muscle, which produces accommodation
- pregnancy.

An increased refractive power of the cornea may occur with:

- keratoconus
- following corneal surgery.

Question: *What is the basic underlying pathology of degenerative myopia?*

Answer: The primary known pathological change is that of scleral thinning and weakness. This is associated with secondary axial lengthening of the globe and chorioretinal degeneration. The actual cause of scleral degeneration remains a mystery.

Question: *Is myopia a common cause of blind registration?*

Answer: Yes. It is the seventh commonest cause of legal blindness in the UK, and is of particular importance because many of those affected are young adults.

Question: *In which groups of patients is degenerative myopia more common?*

Answer: Women tend to be affected more than men, and the highest incidence occurs among the Chinese, Japanese, Arabs and Jews. Hereditary factors play a role in many cases, a strong family history often being evident.

Question: *What is the principle behind the surgical procedure of radial keratotomy?*

Answer: This is a method of reducing the radius of curvature of the axial cornea by weakening the peripheral cornea with a series of 8–16 radial incisions. These incisions, of about 4 mm in length, extend through most of the corneal thickness from near to the limbus to the edge of the central optical zone. A normal intraocular pressure pushes the weakened peripheral cornea anteriorly, flattening the axial cornea and thus reducing its dioptric power. Radial keratotomy is able to correct moderate degrees of myopia (-2.00 to -4.00), but is not suitable for correcting high myopia.

91. Albinism

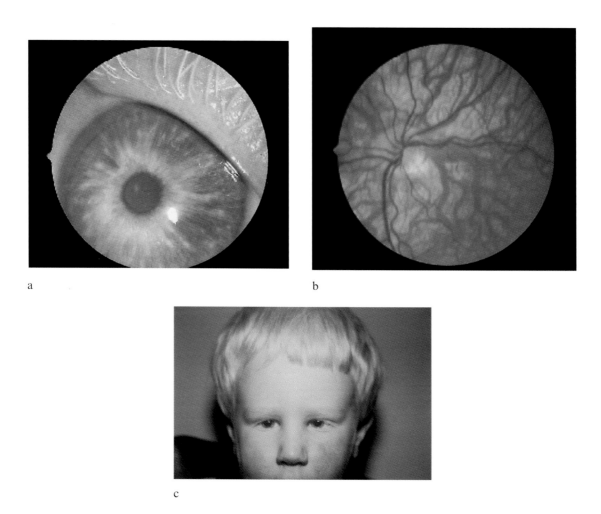

Figure 80 a: An albino iris; b: An albino fundus (courtesy of Gordon Douglas MD); c: The classic hair and skin of a patient with albinism (courtesy of Peng Khaw PhD MRCP FRCS FRCOphth).

Definition
(From an ophthalmic view-point only)

A group of inherited disorders characterized by a lack, or reduction in the degree of ocular melanin pigmentation.

Classification

Oculocutaneous albinism
Affects skin, hair and eyes, and is due to an abnormality of melanocytes throughout the body.

Types
1. Tyrosinase-negative (complete, generalized) (Hermansky–Pudlak syndrome)
2. Tyrosinase-positive (incomplete)
3. Chédiak–Higashi syndrome
4. Yellow mutant albinism
5. Menke's kinky hair syndrome
6. Cystinosis
7. Oculocerebrohypopigmentation (Cross syndrome).

Ocular albinism:
Affects eyes only, and is due to an abnormality of the optic cup-derived melanocytes.

Clinical features

Tyrosine-negative oculocutaneous albinism

- pale/pink skin
- skin sun damage
- white hair
- white eyelashes (pseudopoliosis)
- reduced vision (VA <6/60)
- tendency to high myopia
- tendency to strabismus (squint)
- photophobia
- nystagmus
- light blue-grey irides
- complete iris transillumination
- prominent fundal red-reflex (whole eye appears pink)
- non-pigmented fundus (visible choroidal vasculature)
- absent foveal reflex (macular hypoplasia/aplasia).

Tyrosinase-positive oculocutaneous albinism

- similar signs to above, but less severe (improvement with age)
- reduced vision, nystagmus, refractive errors
- partial iris transillumination.

Ocular albinism

The ocular signs of tyrosinase-negative oculocutaneous albinism in the absence of skin and hair changes.

- Type 1: severe hypopigmentation, normal colour vision
- Type 2: mild/moderate hypopigmentation, normal colour vision
- Type 3: severe hypopigmentation, abnormal colour vision.

Exam questions

Question: *What is the mode of inheritance for albinism?*

Answer: The various forms of oculocutaneous albinism are inherited in an autosomal recessive manner, but ocular albinism differs being inherited in an X-linked manner. Rare forms of ocular albinism and partial oculocutaneous albinism have been reported to have an autosomal dominant mode of inheritance.

Question: *What test can be used to differentiate between tyrosinase-negative and tyrosinase-positive oculocutaneous albinism?*

Answer: Hair bulb incubation in a solution of tyrosine can differentiate between these subgroups of albinism, providing the hair is taken from a patient over the age of four years. The hair bulb from a patient with tyrosinase-positive albinism will produce pigmentation, whereas that from a tyrosinase-negative albino will not.

Question: *Why is albinism of interest to neurologists and neuro-ophthalmologists?*

Answer: There are three main reasons why albinism is of interest to these specialists:

1. As a cause of nystagmus
2. As a cause of strabismus (squint)
3. Because patients with tyrosinase-negative oculocutaneous albinism have an abnormal arrangement of neurones in the optic chiasm and hence lateral geniculate body (LGB). In these patients, 90% of neurones decussate at the chiasm. This arrangement gives rise to atypical visual field defects following lesions to the optic chiasm, tract or radiation. In addition, the visual evoked potential to monocular stimulation is abnormally small. The LGB is abnormal in having only three layers rather than the normal six.

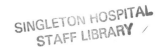

Question: *Why do patients with albinism develop nystagmus?*

Answer: The nystagmus of albinism is of the sensory deprivation type, which occurs secondary to macular hypoplasia and the associated poor visual acuity. The nystagmus thus arises due to an afferent defect in the control of fixation, and can be considered to be searching in nature. The nystagmus is usually pendular and horizontal. In mild cases, it can be reduced in amplitude by convergence. Prolonged exposure to bright light tends to aggravate the nystagmus.

Question: *What are the features of the Hermansky–Pudlak and Chédiak–Higashi syndromes?*

Answer: Hermansky–Pudlak syndrome is classified as a subgroup of tyrosinase-negative oculocutaneous albinism. It shares the features of this form of albinism in association with a haemorrhagic diathesis and the features of Batten's disease (ceroid-lipofuscin storage disease). The hair of such patients is not always white, and may be dark brunette.

Chédiak–Higashi syndrome is a fatal disease of childhood with the features of mild albinism (although total lack of RPE pigmentation), altered immunity and susceptibility to recurrent infections. Neutrophils from these patients show large inclusion bodies.

92. Iris melanoma

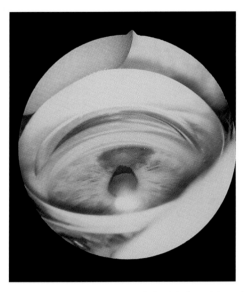

Figure 81   A melanoma of the iris involving the angle (courtesy of Gordon Douglas MD).

Definition

A malignant tumour of iris melanocytes.

Classification:
1. *By pigmentation*:
   - pigmented
   - amelanotic (tapioca melanoma)
2. *By form*:
   - nodular
   - diffuse (superficial spreading)
3. *By cell type*:
   - spindle A
   - spindle B
   - epithelioid
   - mixed.

Clinical features

Patient

Usually 40–50 years of age.

Tumour

- usually a solitary pigmented nodule (may be non-pigmented and/or diffuse – iris heterochromia)
- usually sited in peripheral iris
- inferior iris more commonly affected.

Associated ocular features

- ectropion uveae
- pupil distortion
- iris neovascularization
- focal lens opacification
- secondary glaucoma
- secondary uveitis.

Exam questions

Question: *What lesions may be confused with an iris melanoma?*

Answer: The differential diagnosis includes:

- iris naevus (<3 mm in diameter, <1 mm thick)
- iris freckle (<1 mm in diameter, <1 mm thick)
- iris cyst (congenital, traumatic, surgical)
- ICE syndrome (Cogan–Reese iris naevus type)
- inflammatory granuloma
- juvenile xanthogranuloma
- leiomyoma
- metastasis.

Question: *Are patients with neurofibromatosis predisposed to development of iris melanomas?*

Answer: No. These patients have an increased prevalence of iris naevi called Lisch nodules. (Remember that Lisch nodules are melanocytic lesions, NOT neurofibromas.)

Question: *How should a patient with an iris melanoma be managed?*

Answer: Iris melanomas are usually slow-growing and benign in nature, and observation of pigmented iris lesions is thus frequently sufficient. Active surgical management is indicated if there is evidence of growth, if the lesion is greater than 3 mm in diameter or thicker than 1 mm, or if there are secondary complications such as glaucoma or uveitis. Excision can often be achieved with a broad iridectomy. An irido-cyclectomy or iridotrabeculectomy may be required if there is angle invasion or involvement of more than five clock hours of peripheral iris. Incomplete excision increases the risk of metastasis, and it is thus important to excise the tumour with adequate margins. If a biopsy of an aggressively behaving tumour (often of the diffuse type) or an excision-biopsy of any melanoma reveals the histology to be epithelioid, then an enucleation rather than excision is advised. Fortunately this is rare.

Question: *What is the prognosis for life in patients with iris melanoma?*

Answer: Excellent. Most iris melanomas are slow-growing, benign in nature and composed of spindle A cells. Metastasis, which doesn't occur with spindle A tumours, occurs in less than 5% of all cases. Following surgical excision, the five year survival rate is almost 100%.

Question: *What is juvenile xanthogranuloma, and how may it involve the eye?*

Answer: This is a skin disorder of childhood characterized by yellow-orange coloured, vascular tumours. These are benign, sited in the dermis and are composed of macrophages and abnormal vessels. Involvement of the iris can give rise to spontaneous hyphaema and/or secondary glaucoma. The tumours usually resolve, and may have disappeared by the age of five years. Topical steroid or low-dose radiotherapy to the iris can hasten resolution.

93. Choroidal melanoma

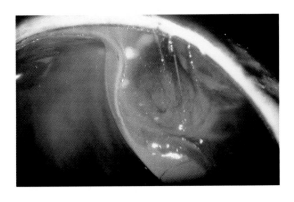
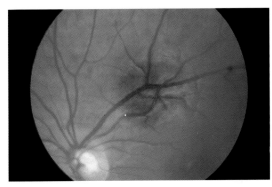

a   b

Figure 82   a: A pathological specimen showing a choroidal melanoma and an associated retinal detachment (courtesy of Gordon Douglas MD); b: A choroidal naevus, unchanged in clinical appearance over a 10 year period (courtesy of the Department of Medical Illustration, Moorfields Eye Hospital).

Definition

A malignant tumour of choroidal melanocytes.

Classification

1. *By pigmentation*:
   - pigmented
   - amelanotic
2. *By form*:
   - localized
   - diffuse
3. *By cell type*:
   - spindle A
   - spindle B
   - epithelioid
4. *By histology*:
   - simple
   - fascicular
   - mixed
   - necrotic.

Clinical features

These are highly variable, and many of the features listed below are not always evident.

Patient

Usually white, and 40–60 years of age.

Vision

- reduced VA (macular involvement)
- visual field defect
- photopsia.

Tumour

- elevated (usually >3 mm) oval-shaped fundal mass (pigmented, brown or mottled; amelanotic, yellow-orange) overlying orange (lipofuscin) pigmentation in the RPE
- overlying drusen (yellow-white)
- large vessels
- negative to transillumination.

Other ocular features

- pre-existing choroidal melanoma
- serous retinal detachment
- choroidal neovascularization
- choroidal folds

- haemorrhage (vitreous, subretinal or intra-retinal)
- retinal exudates (yellow) and cystoid changes
- secondary glaucoma
- cataract
- ocular inflammation
- masquerade uveitis (tumour necrosis).

Exam questions

Question: *How can a choroidal melanoma present?*

Answer: In some patients the tumour is asymp-tomatic and is detected at routine fundoscopy. Symptoms or signs are dependent on the site, size and state of the tumour and include:

- reduced visual acuity (with macular in-volvement)
- visual field defect
- serous retinal detachment
- uveitis (true or masquerade)
- secondary glaucoma
- trans-scleral spread
- metastasis (e.g. enlarged liver).

Question: *What lesions may be confused with a choroidal melanoma?*

Answer: The differential diagnosis includes:

- choroidal naevus
- retinal detachment
- retinoschisis
- choroidal haemorrhage/detachment
- choroidal metastasis (e.g. breast, lung or gut carcinoma)
- lymphoid deposits
- pigment epithelial hyperplasia
- choroidal haemangioma
- disciform degeneration (with subretinal haemorrhage)
- melanocytoma
- astrocytoma
- congenital ciliary body cyst
- posterior uveitis.

Question: *What features of a choroidal mela-noma indicate a poor prognosis?*

Answer: A poor prognosis is more likely with:

- metastatic tumour
- large tumours

- diffuse tumours
- highly pigmented tumours
- anterior tumours
- tumours near optic disc (includes Knapp–Ronne variant)
- overlying lipofuscin deposition in the absence of drusen
- presence of subretinal fluid
- rupture of Bruch's membrane
- extraocular spread
- tumours of epithelioid cell type
- tumour necrosis
- absence of choroidal neovascularization
- increasing age of patient (especially if >65 years)
- damage to tumour during surgery.

Question: *What are the histological features of the various tumour cell types and variants of choroidal melanoma, and how do these relate to prognosis?*

Answer: A spindle A cell is a slender spindle-shaped cell with a flattened nucleus, no nucleo-lus and a prominent basophilic nuclear line which is caused by an infolding of the nuclear membrane.

A spindle B cell is a larger spindle-shaped cell with a round or oval nucleus, a prominent nucleolus and poorly differentiated cytoplasmic borders. These cells thus appear to merge with each other into a syncytium.

An epithelioid cell is a large oval or round cell with a large, round, eccentrically positioned nucleus, a prominent nucleolus, an eosinophilic cytoplasm and a well-demarcated cell mem-brane. Epithelioid cells vary in size, shape and degree of pigmentation. When epithelioid cells are found in a tumour, mitotic figures are plentiful.

Histology of a choroidal melanoma may be simple, that is composed of one cell type only with the cells present in a random fashion. Of these, spindle B tumours are the commonest (35%). Simple spindle A tumours (5%) and epithelioid tumours (5%) are less common. Spindle A tumours have a 95% five year survival rate, spindle B 85% and epithelioid 30%.

A fascicular pattern (5%) in which spindle cells (either A or B) are arranged in palisades is purely a descriptive term, and does not influ-ence prognosis.

Mixed tumours (45%) consist of spindle and epithelioid cells, and have an average five year survival rate of 50%, depending on the proportion of the particular cell types.

Tumours which show signs of necrosis (5%) have a 50% five year survival rate.

Metastatic tumour is associated with a negligible five year survival rate, most patients dying within a year of diagnosis.

Question: *What treatment modalities are available in the management of choroidal melanoma?*

Answer: The management of choroidal melanomas is controversial and differs from centre to centre. However, all agree that management is tailored both to the tumour and the patient. It is important that the ophthalmologist does not omit a general examination and investigation for metastases. The therapeutic options include:

- observation
- enucleation
- laser photocoagulation ($+/-$ photosensitizing agent)
- irradiation using a local scleral plaque – ^{60}Co, ^{106}Ru, ^{125}I, ^{222}Ra, ^{189}Au
- irradiation using a charged particle beam – proton, helium nuclei
- local resection
- cryotherapy
- exenteration
- palliation.

In general, observation, laser photocoagulation or local scleral plaque radiotherapy is suitable for small tumours. Medium-sized tumours are best treated with charged particle beam irradiation, local scleral plaque radiotherapy or local resection unless central, when only laser photocoagulation is appropriate. Large tumours will invariably have metastasized, but if treatment is indicated, only charged particle beam irradiation, enucleation or exenteration are appropriate. Enucleation or exenteration should only be considered if the eye has no useful visual potential or if there is intractable pain from glaucoma, or for cosmesis.

94. Third cranial nerve palsy

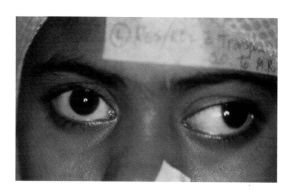

Figure 83 A left third cranial nerve palsy (primary position) (courtesy of Jane Gardiner MD).

Definition

A third cranial nerve palsy is due to interruption of the oculomotor nerve at some point during its course, resulting in failure of some or all of the third nerve functions. It may be congenital (very rare) or acquired.
A lesion may interrupt the nerve:

- in the brainstem
- at the edge of the tentorium cerebelli
- at the junction of the posterior communicating artery and the internal carotid artery
- in the cavernous sinus
- in the orbit.

Clinical features

General survey

If the ptosis is incomplete, there may be a compensatory face-turn away from the side of the palsy. Look for signs of diabetes, hypertension, vasculitis, ischaemia or demyelinating disease.
If there is a fascicular lesion, there may be hemiparesis, hemitremor or ataxia.

Ocular signs

Eyelids
Ptosis (bilateral if there is a nuclear lesion).
It is unnecessary to examine for myasthenic fatigue if the pupil is involved, since the pupil is unaffected in myasthenia gravis.

Ocular movements
Examination is variable but may show:

1. A complete limitation of all ocular movements except in the temporal direction (abduction)
2. Partial limitation of the actions of the supplied muscles, if the palsy is incomplete
3. Limited up-gaze only (with ptosis and a normal pupil) if the lesion is of the superior division alone
4. An inability to look nasally (adduction) and inferiorly (with a dilated pupil) if the lesion is of the inferior division.

Examine for the cavernous sinus syndrome, checking for fourth, fifth and sixth cranial nerve involvement.
To examine for a coexisting fourth nerve palsy, ask the patient to look down and nasally. The eye will only intort if the fourth nerve is intact (focus on a limbal blood vessel with the slit-lamp to help confirm this).

Pupil
The pupil may be involved (dilated with no direct reaction to light), spared or partially involved (partially dilated with some direct response to light).
The pupil and pupil reactions may be abnormal with aberrant regeneration of the third nerve and may vary with eye position (see p. 254).

Optic disc
Remember that the palsy may be due to an intracranial aneurysm, a brainstem lesion, meningitis, encephalitis, toxic polyneuritis or

an intracranial tumour, and thus the optic disc may be swollen or pale.

Additional points

1. Check for the bruit of a caroticocavernous fistula
2. Don't forget possible aberrant regeneration (see p. 254).

Exam questions

Question: *What factors may help decide clinically whether a third nerve palsy is compressive or ischaemic?*

Answer: In an ischaemic palsy the pupil is involved in just 5% of cases, there is never any aberrant regeneration, associated signs are infrequent and presentation is usually in late adulthood.
In a compressive lesion, 95% of cases have pupillary involvement, there may be aberrant regeneration and it may present at any age. Other signs may be present, and pain is more common than when ischaemia is the cause.

Question: *Which patients with a third nerve palsy should receive urgent investigation?*

Answer: Those with pupil involvement, other neurological abnormalities, or who are younger than 50 years of age (unless there is a known ischaemic risk factor and there are no other signs); those with a palsy of greater than three months duration with no resolution or when the palsy is a partial third with evolving signs, and those with aberrant regeneration.

Question: *What are the signs of a unilateral nuclear third nerve palsy?*

Answer: An ipsilateral third nerve palsy with contralateral superior rectus weakness and ptosis.

Question: *What is the prognosis for a 'diabetic' pupil-sparing third nerve palsy?*

Answer: Good. Almost all recover 100% of function within six months.

Question: *What is the commonest cause of an isolated third nerve palsy with pupillary involvement?*

Answer: A posterior communicating artery aneurysm at the junction of the posterior communicating artery and the internal carotid artery which enlarges (usually due to haemorrhage) and compresses the third nerve. The event is usually painful.

Question: *What are the differences between Benedikt's syndrome, Weber's syndrome and Nothnagel's syndrome?*

Answer: Benedikt's syndrome is due to a lesion in the red nucleus, resulting in an ipsilateral third nerve palsy with contralateral tremor; Weber's syndrome is due to a lesion of the third nerve in the region of the cerebral peduncle, resulting in an ipsilateral third nerve palsy with contralateral hemiparesis. Nothnagel's syndrome is an ipsilateral third nerve palsy with cerebellar ataxia, and occurs with a lesion in the superior cerebellar peduncle.
(NB: Claude's syndrome is a combination of Benedikt's and Nothnagel's syndrome.)

95. Aberrant regeneration of the third cranial nerve

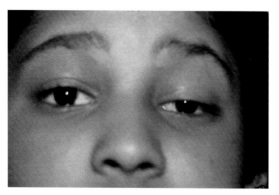

a

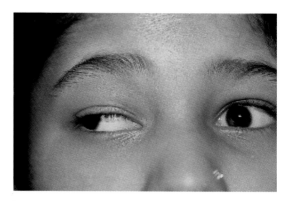

b

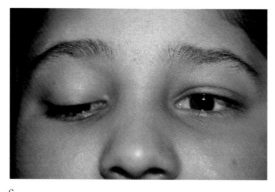

c

Figure 84 Left aberrant regeneration of the third nerve, showing; a: the primary position of gaze; b: right gaze and; c: downgaze. Note the classic lid-gaze dyskinesis (courtesy of the Department of Orthoptics, Moorfields Eye Hospital).

Definition

Aberrant regeneration consists of a constellation of clinical findings presumed to be due to a 'miswiring' following a break in the axon cylinders in the third nerve, and misdirection of the sprouting axons.

Clinical features

One of the following may be elicited:

1. Lid-gaze dyskinesis – lid elevation on adduction (inverse Duane's syndrome) or downgaze (pseudo-von Graefe's sign) with a partial third nerve palsy

2. Pupil-gaze dyskinesis – pupillary constriction on downgaze or on adduction/convergence (pseudo-Argyll Robertson pupil).

Exam questions

Question: *What is the commonest cause of aberrant regeneration?*

Answer: A lesion in the cavernous sinus which initially caused an acute oculomotor palsy.

Question: *Is ischaemia a common cause of aberrant regeneration?*

Answer: No, ischaemia is never a cause of aberrant regeneration and so, if present, the patient requires early investigation for a compressive lesion such as an intracavernous aneurysm, meningioma or neuroma.

Question: *Apart from aberrant regeneration of the third nerve, what other abnormalities may be present in the cavernous sinus syndrome?*

Answer: Third, fourth, fifth, sixth cranial nerve palsies and a small or large pupil, depending on the relative involvement of the third and oculosympathetic nerves (the pupillary fibres are often spared).

Question: *Does a clinically detectable third nerve palsy always precede aberrant regeneration?*

Answer: No, misdirection may be the first clinically detectable abnormality, usually subsequent to an intracavernous lesion such as meningioma or aneurysm. This is referred to as primary aberrant regeneration.

Question: *What is the inverse Duane's syndrome?*

Answer: As part of aberrant regeneration of the third nerve some of the axons originally supplying the medial rectus end up innervating the levator, resulting in lid retraction on adduction.

96. Fourth cranial nerve palsy

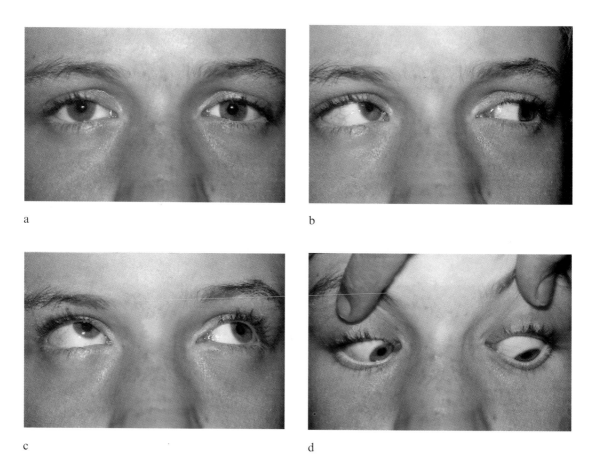

a

b

c

d

Figure 85 A right fourth cranial nerve palsy. a: Primary position; b: Left gaze. Note that the hypertropia is worse on left gaze; c: The patient attempts to look up and to the left; d: The patient attempts to look down and to the left. Note that there is underaction of the right eye (courtesy of the Department of Orthoptics, Moorfields Eye Hospital).

Definition

A fourth cranial nerve palsy is due to an interruption of the trochlear nerve (which supplies the superior oblique muscle) at some point during its course, resulting in failure of some or all of the fourth nerve functions. It may be congenital or acquired.

Remember that the fourth cranial nerve is the only cranial nerve that exits at the dorsal aspect of the brainstem and that it has the longest intracranial course. A lesion may interrupt the nerve:

- in the midbrain
- in the subarachnoid space

- in the cavernous sinus
- in the orbit.

Clinical features

General survey

The characteristic head position is of head tilt to the opposite shoulder, chin depression, and a face turn away from the side of the lesion.

Ocular signs

Ocular movements
There is deficient inferior movement of the eye when the patient attempts to look down and in.

The Parks–Bielschowsky three-step test
1. Step 1: Which eye is higher (hypertropic)? The involved eye is hypertropic on looking straight ahead
2. Step 2: Is the hypertropia worse on left or right gaze? The hypertropia increases on looking away from the side of the lesion
3. Step 3: Is the hypertropia worse on head tilt to the left or right? The hypertropia increases on tilting the head to the ipsilateral shoulder.

Pupils
If palsy is due to a fascicular lesion, there may be a contralateral Horner's syndrome since the sympathetic pathway descends through the midbrain adjacent to the trochlear fascicles.

Additional points

1. Remember to look for signs of diabetes, hypertension, trauma or demyelinating disease.
2. There may be signs of the cavernous sinus syndrome.

Exam questions

Question: *What are the causes of an acquired fourth nerve palsy?*

Answer: The more common causes include ischaemia, haemorrhage, trauma and demyelinating disease. Rare causes include postneurosurgical trauma, meningitis, orbital inflammation or tumours and intracranial tumours (meningioma, pinealoma).

Question: *How can a congenital and an acquired fourth nerve lesion be distinguished?*

Answer: By measuring the vertical fusion range, which is large in congenital palsies (>10 prism dioptres); by checking old photographs, which may reveal a long-standing head tilt indicative of a congenital aetiology; and by examining for cyclotropia, which is often absent in congenital cases.

Question: *How can the presence of a bilateral fourth cranial nerve palsy be confirmed?*

Answer: The patient will exhibit hypertropia of the right eye on looking to the left and hypertropia of the left eye on looking to the right. A V-esotropia will be present. More than 10° of extorsion confirms the diagnosis. In addition there may be evidence of previous trauma, since the commonest cause of a bilateral palsy is severe head trauma with contusion of the anterior medullary velum at the point where the fourth nerve fascicles cross.

Question: *What treatment options are available for a non-resolving fourth nerve palsy?*

Answer: Treatment options include patching the affected eye or incorporating prisms in glasses (if the deviation is small). Again if the deviation is small, botulinum toxin may be used to the contralateral inferior rectus. Surgical treatment may be offered when the lesion is long-standing and stable. Choice of surgery depends on the amount of deviation.

Question: *What conditions may mimic a fourth nerve palsy?*

Answer: Myasthenia gravis, thyroid eye disease, orbital inflammatory disease, skew deviation, atypical Brown's syndrome and vertical hypertropia.

97. Sixth cranial nerve palsy

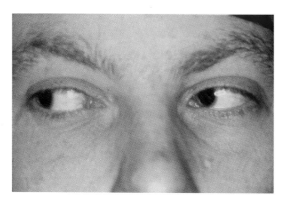
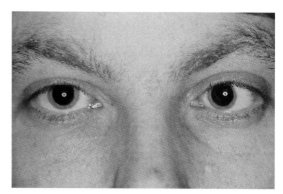

a   b

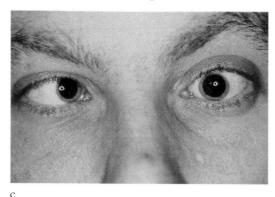

c

Figure 86 A sixth cranial nerve palsy. a: Right gaze; b: Primary position. Note the esotropia, which was greatest for distance; c: Left gaze. Note the absent abduction of the left eye. Note that the pupil has been dilated so that the fundus can be examined (courtesy of the Department of Orthoptics, Moorfields Eye Hospital).

Definition

A sixth cranial nerve palsy is due to an interruption of the abducens nerve (which supplies the lateral rectus muscle) at some point during its course, resulting in failure of some or all of the sixth nerve functions. It may be congenital or acquired.

A lesion may interrupt the nerve:

- in the brainstem (lower pons)
- in the subarachnoid space (between pons and Dorello's canal)
- at the apex of the petrous bone (Dorello's canal)
- in the cavernous sinus
- in the orbit.

Clinical features

General survey

The characteristic abnormal head posture is of a face turn towards the side of the lesion.
If there is a pontine lesion there may be a contralateral hemiplegia due to involvement of

the pyramidal tract and/or an ipsilateral seventh cranial nerve palsy.

Ocular signs

Ocular movements
There is an esotropia (convergent squint) and reduced abduction of the eye on the affected side.

If there is a pontine lesion there may be an ipsilateral horizontal conjugate gaze palsy due to involvement of the paramedian pontine reticular formation (PPRF), or an ipsilateral internuclear ophthalmoplegia due to the lesion involving the medial longitudinal fasciculus (MLF).

Pupils
An ipsilateral Horner's syndrome can occur with brainstem lesions that affect the sixth nerve and the oculosympathetic central neurone or cavernous sinus lesions that affect the sixth nerve and the carotid oculosympathetic plexus.

Optic disc
There may be papilloedema in patients with pseudotumour cerebri and an associated sixth nerve palsy.

Additional points

Remember to look for signs of diabetes, hypertension, trauma or demyelinating disease. There may be signs of the cavernous sinus syndrome.

Exam questions

Question: *What are the Millard–Gubler, Raymond and Foville syndromes?*

Answer: These are all brainstem lesion syndromes affecting lateral gaze. The Millard–Gubler syndrome consists of a sixth nerve palsy, an ipsilateral seventh nerve palsy and contralateral hemiparesis. Raymond's syndrome consists of a sixth nerve palsy with contralateral hemiparesis, and Foville's syndrome comprises a horizontal gaze palsy, an ipsilateral Horner's syndrome and ipsilateral fifth, seventh and eighth nerve palsies.

Question: *What is a 'non-localizing' sixth nerve palsy?*

Answer: This occurs in association with raised intracranial pressure (ICP) due to inferior displacement of the brainstem and consequent stretching of the nerve in the subarachnoid space between the pons and Dorello's canal.

Question: *What is the commonest causes of an isolated sixth nerve palsy in the elderly, and how are such patients managed?*

Answer: An ischaemic mononeuropathy is the commonest cause, and this may be associated with hypertension or diabetes. Management should be aimed at the cause, and with respect to the eye should simply be supportive for six months since recovery frequently occurs. Conservative measures include occlusion or the use of a prism to avoid diplopia. If there has been no improvement and the palsy is stable at six months, surgery can be considered. Primary surgery should be maximum recession of the ipsilateral medial rectus muscle. If this proves insufficient other procedures which should be considered include:

- recession of the contralateral medial rectus
- resection of the paretic lateral rectus (for a mechanical advantage)
- transposition of part of the ipsilateral superior and inferior recti to respective folds of the paretic lateral rectus muscle insertion.

Question: *What is Gradenigo's syndrome?*

Answer: Gradenigo's syndrome is periostitis of the petrous apex usually secondary to otitis media causing a sixth nerve palsy, an ipsilateral seventh nerve palsy, ipsilateral facial pain (fifth nerve distribution) and ipsilateral hearing loss.

Question: *What is the differential diagnosis of a sixth nerve palsy?*

Answer:

- thyroid eye disease
- trauma (medial orbital wall fracture with restrictive myopathy)
- type A Duane's syndrome
- myasthenia gravis
- near reflex spasm
- fusional breakdown of a congenital esophoria.

98. Brown's syndrome

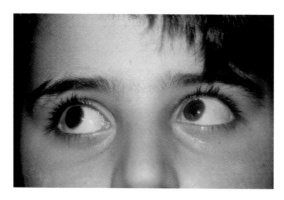

a

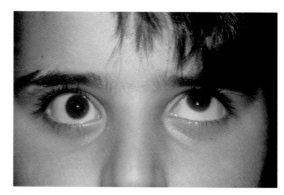

b

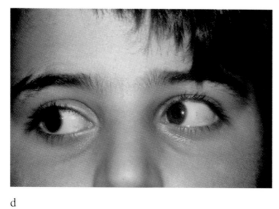

d

e

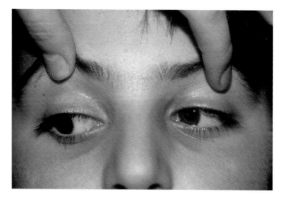

g

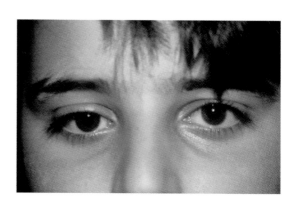

h

Figure 87 Nine positions of gaze (a–i) for a child with a right-sided Brown's syndrome. Note the inability to elevate the right eye in adduction (courtesy of the Department of Orthoptics, Moorfields Eye Hospital).

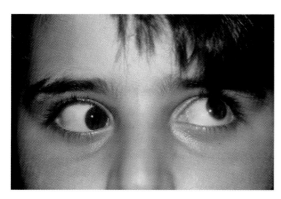

c

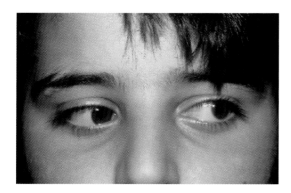

f

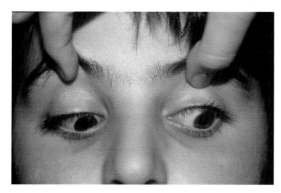

i

Definition

Brown's (superior oblique tendon sheath) syndrome is an ocular motility disorder featuring a limitation of passive as well as active elevation in adduction. It may be constant or intermittent in nature, and either congenital or acquired.

Clinical features

General features

There may be an abnormal head posture, with the chin up and a face turn to the opposite side (to place the affected eye in abduction).

Ocular signs

There is an inability to elevate the eye in adduction, and elevation improves in the primary position or in abduction. There is little or no overaction of the ipsilateral superior oblique. Discomfort may be felt in the region of the trochlea on attempted elevation in adduction, and it may be associated with an audible and palpable 'click'. There may be widening of the palpebral aperture on adduction (associated with the restriction in elevation).

Investigation of choice

Positive traction test.

Exam questions

Question: *What are the causes of an acquired Brown's syndrome?*

Answer: Surgery (e.g. following tucking of the superior oblique), orbital trauma or inflammatory disease.

Question: *What are the indications for surgical treatment?*

Answer: Indications for surgery in an adult include hypotropia in the primary position with significant diplopia. In children, surgery should be considered if there is concern about loss of binocularity or a significant anomalous head posture.

Question: *What are the surgical treatments available?*

Answer: Tenotomy or tenectomy can be used to correct a Brown's syndrome. However, patients (and/or parents) should be warned that such procedures do not always improve head posture or ocular movements.

Question: *Do all patients with a congenital Brown's syndrome need to be treated?*

Answer: No, mild cases should always be observed.

Question: *Is there any medical treatment available for Brown's syndrome?*

Answer: Locally injected or systemic steroids may be used in acquired cases, particularly if there is evidence of an inflammatory aetiology.

99. Duane's syndrome

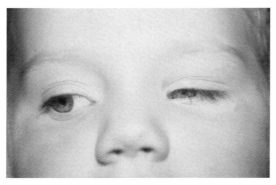

a

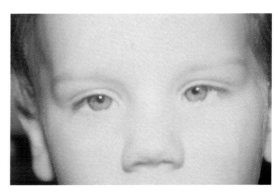

b

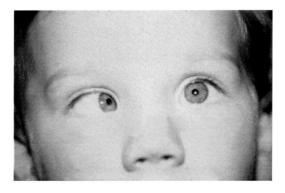

c

Figure 88 a: Type A, 1 or typical left Duane's syndrome (right gaze). Note narrowing of the left palpebral fissure on adduction (which is slightly reduced); b: Primary position. Note the left esotropia; c: Left gaze. Note reduced abduction and widening of palpebral fissure of the left eye (courtesy of the Department of Orthoptics, Moorfields Eye Hospital).

Definition

A congenital anomaly of unknown aetiology characterized by abnormal eye movements, which may be due to paradoxical innervation of extraocular muscles.

Also known as:

– Duane's Retraction Syndrome

Clinical features

Type A or 1: (Most common type)

- reduced/absent abduction of affected eye
- narrowing of palpebral fissure on adduction of affected eye (+ widening on abduction)
- globe retraction on adduction of affected eye

- face turn towards the affected side
- poor convergence.

Type B or 2:

- reduced adduction
- normal abduction.

Type C or 3:

- reduced abduction
- grossly reduced or absent adduction
- face turn away from the affected side.

Exam questions

Question: *What can Type A Duane's syndrome in a child be confused with?*

Answer: The differential diagnosis includes:

- a simple infantile congenital esotropia
- a congenital sixth cranial nerve palsy
- Möbius syndrome
- an acquired type of Duane's syndrome following excessive lateral rectus resection, orbital trauma or localized orbital inflammation.

Question: *What are the possible aetiologies that have been proposed in order to explain Type A Duane's syndrome?*

Answer: One theory proposes that there is abnormal innervation of the horizontal recti with co-contraction of the medial and lateral recti, explaining the globe retraction and palpebral fissure narrowing on adduction. Evidence for this has come from electro-

myography (EMG), which has shown low lateral rectus firing with attempted abduction and high lateral rectus firing with attempted adduction.

Other theories have proposed mechanical abnormalities of the horizontal recti or dysplasia of the sixth cranial nerve nucleus and/or brainstem.

Question: *Is Duane's syndrome ever bilateral?*

Answer: Yes, about 15% of cases are bilateral.

Question: *What ocular and non-ocular abnormalities can Duane's syndrome be associated with?*

Answer: Duane's syndrome usually occurs in isolation, but may be seen in association with:

- microphthalmos
- colobomata
- a persistent pupillary membrane
- iris heterochromia
- cataract
- A- or V-pattern eye movements
- skeletal abnormalities
- facial abnormalities
- neural abnormalities.

Question: *How should a child with Type A congenital Duane's syndrome be managed?*

Answer: The management is essentially conservative, with regular orthoptic assessment. Most patients' eyes are straight in the primary position and they do not develop amblyopia. If amblyopia is present it is usually anisometropic (not strabismic), and thus responds to spectacle correction. Surgical correction is indicated for the few patients whose eyes are not straight in the primary position or who develop a significant abnormal compensatory head posture.

100. Ankylosing spondylitis

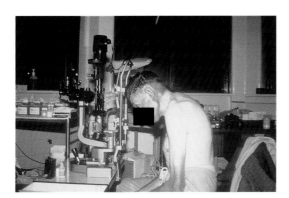

Figure 89 Kyphosis in a patient with ankylosing spondylitis. It is often difficult to examine the eyes of a patient such as this on a conventional slit-lamp (courtesy of Peng Khaw PhD MRCP FRCS FRCOphth).

Definition

A seronegative spondylarthropathy characterized by the involvement of the sacroiliac joints.

Clinical features

It is important to note articular as well as extra-articular complications. The condition is most common in males between 20 and 40 years of age.

Articular features

These include loss of lumbar lordosis, spasm of muscles (reduced full lumbar flexion) and a resultant exaggerated thoracic kyphosis (a 'question mark' posture) with compensatory neck hyperextension and fixed flexion of hips. Peripheral joint involvement may affect the hips, shoulders, knees or ankles. An additional feature is reduced chest expansion (<5 cm).

Extra-articular features

Ocular
The major ocular feature is anterior uveitis – cells and flare in the anterior chamber, keratic precipitates (white cells on the corneal endothelium), posterior synechiae (adhesions of the iris to the lens) resulting in a small sluggish pupil, and injection of the perilimbal blood vessels. Additional features include occasional cataract, altered ocular pressure (ask to check intraocular pressures and look for glaucomatous cupping) and cystoid macular oedema.

Pulmonary
Fibrosis occurs in the upper lung fields, which gives rise to inspiratory crackles and poor chest expansion.

Cardiovascular
Cardiac features include aortic incompetence (early diastolic murmur, collapsing pulse), cardiomegaly and conduction defects diagnosed by ECG.

General
Weight loss, fatigue and low-grade fever may occur.

Other
- osteoporosis
- bone fractures
- amyloidosis
- IgA nephropathy.

Exam questions

Question: *What is the genetic association of ankylosing spondylitis?*

Answer: Approximately 10% of HLA-B27 positive individuals develop ankylosing spondylitis following an unknown environmental event.

Over 90% of those with ankylosing spondylitis are HLA-B27 positive. Identical twins, homozygous for HLA-B27, may be discordant for ankylosing spondylitis. The reason for the link is not clear, but it may be that the HLA-B27 acts as a receptor site for an infective agent, a marker for an immune response gene. The infective agent remains poorly defined. Numerous Gram −ve organisms have been thought to precipitate the disease, for example klebsiella, chlamydia, yersina and salmonella.

Question: *What are the extra-articular manifestations of ankylosing spondylitis?*

Answer: They include general features such as fatigue, weight loss and low grade fever. Cord compression secondary to fractures may occur. Uveitis develops in up to 40% of patients. Patients with severe disease may have chronic fibrotic changes in the upper lung fields, and the cardiovascular system may be involved resulting in aortic incompetence, cardiomegaly and conduction defects. Osteoporosis may occur, and is usually early in onset. Rarely, amyloidosis and an IgA nephropathy can occur.

Question: *What radiological abnormalities are found in the spine and sacroiliac joints?*

Answer: Early changes in the lumbar spine are the squaring of the superior and inferior margins of the vertebral bodies secondary to inflammation of the annulus fibrosus. Late changes result in calcification of the intervertebral ligaments, causing a 'bamboo spine'. The sacroiliac joints are irregular, with sclerosis of the articular margins.

Question: *Describe the typical course of eye involvement in ankylosing spondylitis.*

Answer: The anterior uveitis is typically non-granulomatous, and occurs in recurrent acute bouts at variable intervals. It is frequently bilateral, although often only one eye will be involved at each episode. The attacks may be severe, with hypopyon formation. Recurrent attacks may result in extensive posterior synechiae formation, resulting in iris bombe, cataract, glaucoma and band keratopathy.

Question: *Describe the approaches to the treatment of ankylosing spondylitis?*

Answer: General management points include patient education and genetic counselling (those that are B27-positive pass on the gene to 50% of their children, who then have a one in three chance of developing the disease, i.e. one in six overall). Specific treatments include pain relief with NSAIDs (e.g. indomethacin) and intra-articular steroids for persistent local disease. Exercise should be encouraged (e.g. swimming) and physiotherapy given. Surgical treatment is occasionally indicated, most frequently to replace hips.

(See also Reiter's syndrome, p. 270.)

101. Acquired immune deficiency syndrome (AIDS)

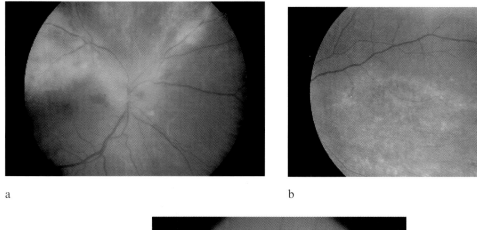

a   b

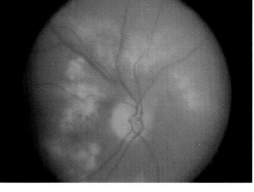

c

Figure 90 a: Cytomegalovirus (CMV) retinitis in a patient with AIDS, characterized by retinal necrosis, a granular border and patchy retinal haemorrhage (courtesy of Gary N. Holland MD); b: Treated CMV retinitis in a patient with AIDS, with early border reactivation (courtesy of Gary N. Holland MD); c: Cotton wool spots in a patient with AIDS who subsequently developed haemorrhagic CMV retinitis (courtesy of Peng Khaw PhD MRCP FRCS FRCOphth).

Definition

A syndrome suffered by an HIV (human immunodeficiency virus) positive individual who has exhibited AIDS indicator diseases (or by an HIV-positive individual with a CD4+ T lymphocyte count of less than 200/ml).

The eye may be affected by secondary infections, autoimmunity, neoplasia or drug toxicity.

Clinical features

75% of HIV-positive individuals develop ocular complications, which include the following:

Eyelids/orbit

- Kaposi's sarcoma (a red/violaceous palpable skin papule, nodule or plaque)

- molluscum contagiosum (waxy umbilicated skin lesions with/without follicular conjunctivitis)
- herpes zoster ophthalmicus (rash in V1 distribution)
- blepharitis (crusting, Meibomium gland dysfunction, telangiectasia)
- long eyelashes
- proptosis (may be due to a number of possible infective or neoplastic causes).

Conjunctiva/episclera

- microvasculopathy
- keratoconjunctivitis sicca (see p. 127)
- Kaposi's sarcoma
- Reiter's syndrome (see p. 270)
- herpes zoster conjunctivitis or episcleritis.

Cornea

- herpes zoster keratitis
- herpes simplex keratitis
- fungal (including microsporidial) keratitis
- bacterial keratitis
- non-specific keratitis (with dry eye)
- non-infectious peripheral corneal ulceration.

Uvea

- iridocyclitis (infective, iatrogenic due to drug toxicity, malignant, idiopathic).
- immune-recovery uveitis.

Retina/choroid

- HIV microvasculopathy – cotton wool spots near large vessels ($\pm$ small superficial haemorrhages, microaneurysms)
- cytomegalovirus (CMV) retinitis – white, opaque, granular areas of retinitis at lesion edge, with or without irregular feathered edges and associated haemorrhage. When severe, the condition has been called 'pizza retinopathy'. There may be areas of necrosis, secondary cystoid macula oedema and papillitis, and exudative and rhegmatogenous retinal detachments
- Roth spots
- acute retinal necrosis (ARN) – this may be related to herpes varicella-zoster infection

- progressive outer retinal necrosis syndrome (PORN)
- toxoplasmosis retinochoroiditis (see p. 157)
- syphilitic retinitis
- herpes simplex retinitis
- fungal chorioretinitis (e.g. cryptococcus or histoplasmosis)
- pneumocystis carinii choroiditis.

(NB: opportunistic infections involving the posterior segment in patients with AIDS are not usually accompanied by much vitreous inflammation due to the low number of CD4+ helper T lymphocytes.)

Neuro-ophthalmic

- optic neuritis, which may be secondary to CMV, cryptococcus, HIV, syphilis, PML
- posterior visual pathway lesions secondary to lymphoma, toxoplasmosis, cryptococcus, mycobacterium, PML
- cranial nerve palsies
- other motility disturbances (skew-deviation, gaze palsies, Parinaud's syndrome).

Exam questions

Question: *What laboratory tests are used to diagnose HIV?*

Answer: ELISA testing to detect antibody to HIV is the best screening test. It is sensitive, but not specific. If an HIV test is positive it should be repeated, and one should consider doing a Western blot test which is more specific (tests for GP120/41/21). If the ELISA test is negative one should consider a repeat test in three to six months, since there may be an interval between exposure and seroconversion. It is important to remember that patient counselling should be carried out before any test is performed.

Question: *What is the treatment for CMV retinopathy?*

Answer: Specific medical treatments include the use of the antivirals ganciclovir, forscarnet and cidofovir. The drugs may be given systemically or locally as intravitreous injections or slow-release implants. They are all equally effective in halting the progress of CMV retinitis when given in standard intravenous regimens. Intravenously, the drugs are given as an initial high-dose induction followed by maintenance doses to prevent recurrence. Following response to treatment, the areas of retinitis stop enlarging, the haemorrhage clears and the retinal opacification resolves, leaving atrophic, non-functioning retinal scars.

Question: *What are the major advantages and disadvantages of treating CMV retinitis in patients with AIDS?*

Answer: Successful treatment of CMV retinitis may preserve vision and in addition may prolong life by preventing or reducing systemic infection with CMV. The main side-effect of gancyclovir is myelosuppression. If this occurs, it may be given intravitreally, using slow-release implants or in combination with granulocyte stimulating factor. Forscarnet's main side-effect is renal toxicity, but it may offer a survival advantage in patients with normal renal function. Cidofovir can cause renal failure, hypotony and/or uveitis.

Question: *What are the ocular signs of so-called 'HIV-retinopathy'?*

Answer: The HIV virus itself causes a microvasculopathy giving rise to cotton wool spots near large vessels that may be associated with small superficial blot haemorrhages. It is nearly always asymptomatic. The differential diagnosis includes early CMV and diabetic or hypertensive retinopathy. The cotton wool spots typically disappear within two months in HIV retinopathy. Other posterior segment changes include microaneurysm formation and ischaemic optic neuropathy. A conjunctival microvasculopathy occurs with dilated capillaries, microaneurysms and sluggish flow.

102. Reiter's syndrome

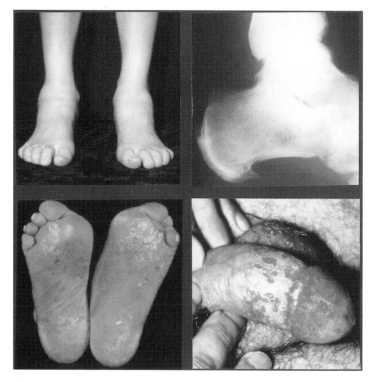

Figure 91   Top left – acute arthritis of ankles; top right – radiograph showing calcaneal spur; bottom-left – keratoderma blennorrhagica; bottom right – circinate balanitis (courtesy of Jack Kanski MD MS FRCOphth).

Definition

A syndrome of unknown aetiology character-ized by the triad of recurrent conjunctivitis, urethritis and a seronegative arthritis.

Clinical features

General survey

The patient is usually a young male (M : F; 20 : 1).

Systemic features

- non-specific urethritis
- asymmetrical seronegative arthritis
- keratoderma blennorrhagica (palms, soles or penis)
- circinate balinitis
- painless oral ulcers
- fingernail dystrophy and subungal keratosis
- plantar fasciitis, os calcis periostitis
- aortic incompetence (rare).

Ocular features

- conjunctivitis
- non-granulomatous acute anterior uveitis

- keratitis
- retinitis (rare)
- optic neuritis (rare).

Exam questions

Question: *Is there an HLA association with Reiter's syndrome?*

Answer: At least 70% of patients with Reiter's syndrome are HLA-B27 positive.

Question: *How do patients with Reiter's syndrome first present?*

Answer: The commonest mode of presentation is with a non-specific (non-gonococcal) urethritis, usually occurring two weeks following sexual intercourse. In some cases there is evidence of chronic prostatitis or vesiculitis. Less commonly, the syndrome develops following an episode of dysentery (salmonella, shigella, campylobacter or yersinia) or a fever. Acute arthritis may be the presenting symptom but this usually occurs two to three weeks after the onset of urethritis, dysentery or fever. The arthritis is asymmetrical, seronegative, and usually affects the knee joint. Later, the sacroiliac joints may be involved, and this is associated with an increased risk of developing anterior uveitis.

Question: *What are the features of Reiter's syndrome conjunctivitis?*

Answer: The conjunctivitis is usually mild and mucopurulent and associated with a mild papillary reaction rather than the development of follicles. It usually follows development of urethritis, precedes any joint involvement and is self-limiting.

Question: *How do the oral ulcers associated with Reiter's syndrome differ from those associated with Behçet's syndrome?*

Answer: The oral ulcers of Reiter's syndrome are painless, whereas those of Behçet's syndrome are painful.

Question: *Is anything known about the aetiology of Reiter's syndrome?*

Answer: Essentially the aetiology is unknown. However, it has been proposed that it may be an immune complex deposition disease secondary to an unusual host response triggered by exposure to chlamydia.

103. Neurofibromatosis

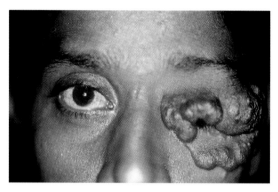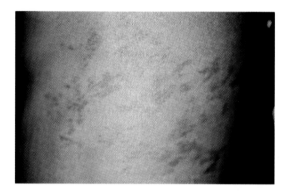

a   b

Figure 92 Neurofibromatosis. a: Left eyelid neurofibromas; b: Café-au-lait spots (both courtesy of Jane Gardiner MD)

Definition

The name given to two disorders classified as phakomatoses. Type I is characterized by neurofibromas, café-au-lait spots and gliomas. Type II is characterized by bilateral acoustic neuromas.

Clinical features

General survey

- multiple neurofibromas (more than two) – sessile pedunculated skin lesions
- café-au-lait spots (more than 6 spots, >15 mm diameter in an adult)
- axillary freckling
- kyphoscoliosis
- pseudoarthrosis (tibia)
- pressure effects on nerves (acoustic neuroma, signs of cord compression)
- signs of associated phaeochromocytoma (raised blood pressure, signs of cardiac failure, hypertensive retinopathy).

Ocular signs

Eyelids
- café-au-lait spots
- neurofibromas.
- plexiform neuromas ('bag of worms')

Anterior segment
- prominent corneal nerves (associated with MEA Type II)
- iris nodules (Lisch)
- congenital glaucoma
- hamartomas in the trabecular meshwork.

Posterior segment
- hamartomas in the uvea, retina or optic nerve head.

Neuro-ophthalmic
- optic nerve glioma (pale/swollen or glaucomatous like disc).

Orbit
- proptosis (due to a plexiform neuroma, neurolemmoma or optic nerve glioma)

- pulsating exophthalmos (due to absence of the greater wing of sphenoid).

Exam questions

Question: *What are the abnormalities of Type 2 neurofibromatosis?*

Answer: Type 2 neurofibromatosis is characterized by bilateral acoustic neuromas that tend to present in the second or third decade. Schwannomas may also be present, and other tumours include neurofibromas, meningiomas and gliomas. Early posterior subcapsular cataract and combined hamartomas may be present in the eye.

Question: *What is the genetic abnormality in Type 1 neurofibromatosis?*

Answer: There is an abnormality in the NF-1 gene on chromosome 17, which is a tumour suppressor gene.

Question: *Describe the histology of an optic nerve glioma?*

Answer: They are mostly low-grade pilocytic astrocytomas, which can invade through the pia and arachnoid. There is controversy as to whether they are true neoplasms or hamartomas.

Question: *What is the treatment for an optic nerve glioma?*

Answer: The treatment of optic nerve gliomas is controversial. The prognosis of optic nerve as opposed to chiasmal glioma is reasonably good, and some would advocate treating an optic nerve glioma only if it was causing significant proptosis. Treatment options include complete excision and radiotherapy, of which excision is the only clearly advantageous option.

Question: *What comprises the MEA II syndrome?*

Answer: This is Sipple syndrome, the features of which are phaeochromocytoma, medullary carcinoma of the thyroid, parathyroid hyperplasia, prominent corneal nerves, gliomas and meningiomas.

104. Systemic lupus erythematosis (SLE)

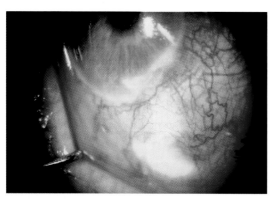

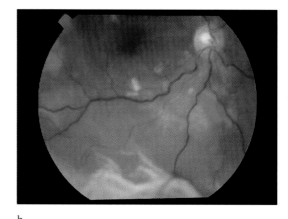

a   b

Figure 93   a: Scleritis in a patient with systemic lupus erythematosis (SLE) (courtesy of Robert Nozik MD and Carlos Pavesio MD); b: Retinochoroidopathy with an exudative retinal detachment in a patient with SLE (courtesy of the Department of Medical Illustration, Moorfields Eye Hospital).

Definition

Systemic lupus erythematosis (SLE) is a chronic multisystem inflammatory disease with a variable clinical presentation. It is characterized by the presence of many autoantibodies, of which antibodies to double-stranded DNA are most specific.

Clinical features

General survey

The patient is often young and female.

Skin/oral

- red, papular butterfly facial rash
- alopecia
- rash in sun-exposed areas (photosensitivity)
- vasculitic rash
- subcutaneous nodules
- Raynaud's phenomenon
- nail fold infarcts
- oral ulcers.

Cardiovascular

- pericarditis (friction rub)
- myocarditis (± cardiac failure)
- endocarditis (Libmann–Sachs murmurs).

Renal

- nephritic syndrome
- glomerulonephritis
- renal failure.

Pulmonary

- pleurisy
- pleural effusions.

Reticuloendothelial

- splenomegaly
- lymphadenopathy
- parotid swelling.

Musculoskeletal

- arthritis (usually non-deforming, migratory and symmetrical).

Neurological

- peripheral neuropathy
- psychosis.

Ocular features

Anterior segment
- episcleritis
- scleritis (either diffuse or nodular)
- conjunctivitis (rare, but may occur with secondary fibrosis)
- keratitis (punctate or with peripheral ulceration)
- keratoconjunctivitis sicca (dry eye, poor tear film, corneal punctate epithelial erosions, interpalpebral Rose Bengal staining)
- anterior uveitis.

Posterior segment
- cotton wool spots
- retinal haemorrhages
- retinal oedema
- optic disc oedema
- hard exudates (relatively rare)
- vasculitis (relatively rare)
- vascular occlusions (relatively rare)
- hydroxychloroquine/chloroquine maculopathy
- secondary hypertensive retinopathy
- retinochoroidopathy.

Neuro-ophthalmic
- intranuclear ophthalmoplegia
- nystagmus
- cranial nerve palsies
- homonymous hemianopia
- papilloedema.

Exam questions

Question: *What drugs may cause an SLE-like syndrome?*

Answer: Hydralazine, procainamide, quinidine, phenytoin and isoniazid.

Question: *What groups in the population are most commonly affected by SLE?*

Answer: There is a female preponderance (10:1), and it is more common in Afro-Caribbeans.

Question: *What abnormalities may be found in laboratory investigations?*

Answer: Presence of antinuclear antibodies anti-dsDNA (in 90%), anti-ssDNA (in 60%), and anti-DNA histone (in 50%, and in 95% with cases of drug-induced SLE). Other auto-antibodies that may be present include anti-nRNP and anti-cardiolipin antibodies. In addition, there may be low levels of serum complement c3 and c4. Anaemia, neutropaenia, lymphopaenia and thrombocytopaenia are relatively common findings, and the ESR is raised in active disease.

Question: *What drug treatments are commonly used in the management of SLE?*

Answer: With severe SLE, corticosteroids form the mainstay of therapy. Intravenous pulsed steroid therapy with the addition of other immunosuppressive agents (such as azathioprine or cyclophosphamide) may be required in severe disease. In mild disease with predominately cutaneous features, hydroxychloroquine may be useful.

Question: *Do patients with SLE retinopathy require treatment?*

Answer: There are several reports showing that the presence of retinal lesions correlates with the systemic course of the disease. Therefore if a patient with SLE develops retinopathy, a thorough search for systemic disease activity should be performed and, if positive, aggressive therapy should be instigated. If the retinopathy is secondary to hypertension, antihypertensive therapy should be started and specific renal investigations carried out by a physician.

105. Sturge–Weber syndrome

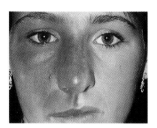

Figure 94 Sturge–Weber syndrome. Hemifacial port-wine stain in a patient with unilateral glaucoma (courtesy of the Department of Medical Illustration, Moorfields Eye Hospital).

Definition

Sturge–Weber syndrome is a sporadic phakomatosis characterized by cutaneous and leptomeningeal angiomatosis with possible ocular involvement.

Clinical features

General survey

- port-wine stain in the distribution of the first or second divisions of the trigeminal nerve
- hemiplegia contralateral to the port-wine stain (evidence for an intracranial capillary haemangioma).

Ocular features

Ocular involvement occurs in one third of cases.

Eyelids
- cavernous haemangioma.

Anterior segment
- congenital glaucoma (buphthalmos, enlarged corneal diameter, striae, cupped disc).

Posterior segment
- cavernous haemangioma of the choroid ('bright red' fundus compared to the fellow eye).

Neuro-ophthalmic
- pale disc
- homonymous hemianopia (rare).

Exam questions

Question: *What is a port-wine stain?*

Answer: It is a collection of telangiectatic vessels forming a haemangioma. They contain deoxygenated blood, which gives them their dark appearance.

Question: *What is the cause of glaucoma in Sturge–Weber patients?*

Answer: It is said to be caused by raised episcleral venous pressure, but it is probable that these patients have an abnormal drainage angle as well.

Question: *What problems (apart from glaucoma) may develop for Sturge–Weber patients later in life?*

Answer: The child may develop epilepsy if cerebral irritation from an intracranial capillary haemangioma occurs.

Question: *What abnormality may be shown on a skull X-ray in a patient with Sturge–Weber?*

Answer: Subcortical 'tramline' calcification, typically in the parieto-occipital area, may be evident.

Question: *What is the management of a child with suspected glaucoma?*

Answer: Once the diagnosis has been confirmed, the patient should be referred to a paediatric glaucoma specialist for assessment for possible surgery (trabeculectomy or goniotomy).

106. Polyarteritis nodosa

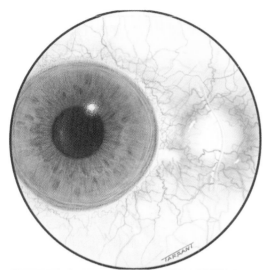

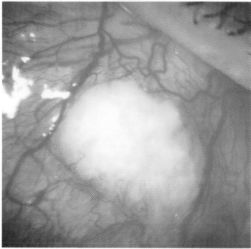

Figure 95 Necrotizing scleritis with inflammation. Top: early avascular patch; bottom: more advanced avascularity (courtesy of Jack Kanski MD MS FRCOphth).

Definition

Polyarteritis nodosa is a multisystem disorder characterized by vasculitis affecting small and medium-sized arteries, with resultant fibrinoid necrosis and occlusion.

Clinical features

General survey

- most common in middle-aged males
- often presents with fever, malaise and weight loss.

Ocular features

- scleritis
- peripheral corneal ulceration
- retinal arteritis (± occlusions)
- hypertensive retinopathy
- AION
- choroidal infarcts
- transient focal retinal detachments.

Skin

- nailfold infarcts
- tender subcutaneous nodules.

Renal

- nephritic syndrome
- nephrotic syndrome
- renal failure.

Cardiovascular

- hypertension (50% of cases)
- pericarditis
- ischaemic heart disease.

Pulmonary

- pulmonary infiltrate leading to asthma

Neurological

- painful mononeuritis multiplex
- polyneuropathy.

Gastrointestinal

- abdominal pain (secondary to infarcts).

Musculoskeletal

- non-deforming, migratory arthritis
- myalgia.

Exam questions

Question: *How can polyarteritis nodosa (PAN) be diagnosed?*

Answer: The diagnosis is based on the clinical picture, and on the presence of leucocytosis (eosinophils predominating) and raised alkaline phosphatase. A renal biopsy may show fibrinoid necrosis, and angiography may show small aneurysms. There are no specific immune markers.

Question: *What is the treatment of PAN?*

Answer: Corticosteroid therapy forms the mainstay of treatment, with the addition of azathioprine or cyclophosphamide if the disease is severe.

Question: *What is the prognosis for PAN?*

Answer: The five-year survival rate is 40–60%, with renal failure being the commonest cause of death.

Question: *What other vasculitides may affect the eye?*

Answer: Vasculitis secondary to SLE, scleroderma, polymyositis, Wegener's granulomatosis, giant cell arteritis, Behçet's disease, Takayasu's disease and rheumatoid arthritis may all have ophthalmic features.

Question: *What is Cogan's syndrome?*

Answer: Cogan's syndrome consists of interstitial keratitis, vestibulo-auditory impairment and an associated systemic disease in most cases. The systemic condition is often a vasculitis such as PAN. Patients are seronegative for syphilis.

107. Wegener's granulomatosis

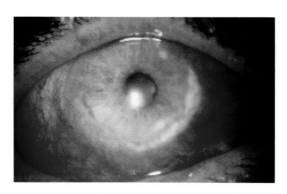

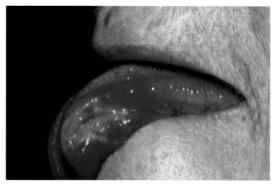

a   b

Figure 96   a: Peripheral ulcerative keratitis in a patient with Wegener's granulomatosis (courtesy of Robert Nozik MD and Carlos Pavesio MD); b: Mouth ulcers associated with Wegener's granulomatosis (courtesy of Peng Khaw PhD MRCP FRCS FRCOphth).

Definition

Wegener's granulomatosis is a systemic disease of unknown aetiology characterized by granulomatous inflammation and necrotizing vasculitis, typically affecting the respiratory tract and kidneys.

Clinical features

General survey

- saddle nose (in established cases, due to nasal septal perforation and loss of supporting structures)
- fever, weight loss, wasting.

Skin

- papules
- purpuric rash.

Pulmonary

- haemoptysis
- breathlessness
- nodal infiltrates which migrate
- cavitational lesions
- atelectasis.

Renal

- renal impairment/failure (hypertension, peripheral/pulmonary oedema, lemon yellow tinge to skin, pericarditis, left ventricular failure [LVF]).

Cardiovascular

- pericarditis
- cardiomyopathy.

Neurological

- mononeuritis multiplex
- cranial nerve palsies.

Ocular features

Ocular involvement occurs in 30–50% of cases.

Orbit
- orbital inflammation (may cause proptosis or nasolacrimal duct obstruction which is often contiguous with sinus inflammation).

Anterior segment
- non-specific conjunctivitis with subconjunctival haemorrhage
- episcleritis
- scleritis (10%)
- peripheral ulcerative keratitis (looks like a Mooren's ulcer).

Posterior segment (rare)
- retinopathy (narrow arteries, tortuous veins, cotton wool spots, cystoid macular oedema, chorioretinitis and choroidal thickening with infarcts)
- anterior ischaemic optic neuropathy (AION)
- central retinal artery occlusion (CRAO).

Neuro-ophthalmic
- cranial nerve palsies.

Exam questions

Question: *What serological abnormalities may occur in Wegener's granulomatosis?*

Answer: Non-specific findings include a normochromic normocytic anaemia, leucocytosis, a raised ESR and C-reactive protein (CRP) and positive rheumatoid factor. A more specific abnormality is a raised level of ANCA (antineutrophil cytoplasmic antibody) mainly of the C-ANCA and occasionally P-ANCA subtypes. The level of ANCA is a sensitive index of generalized disease, correlates with disease activity and can be useful in monitoring the effect of treatment.

Question: *Apart from blood tests, what other investigations may be useful in assessing patients with possible Wegener's granulomatosis?*

Answer: Chest X-rays may show migrating nodal infiltrates, cavities and evanescent areas of atelectasis.
Urinalysis may reveal the presence of red cell casts or cells.
Biopsy of inflamed tissue (e.g. nasal mucosa, sinus, lung) enables histopathological diagnosis, identifying necrotizing granulomas.

Question: *What are the typical histopathological features of Wegener's granulomatosis?*

Answer: Necrotizing granulomatous inflammation and vasculitis.

Question: *What treatment is most commonly used in the management of Wegener's granulomatosis?*

Answer: Prednisolone, usually in combination with cyclophosphamide.

Question: *How may a Mooren's ulcer and peripheral corneal ulceration in Wegener's granulomatosis be differentiated?*

Answer: Both give a peripheral ulcer that progresses centrally and circumferentially, but the sclera is never involved with a Mooren's ulcer.

108. Polymyositis/dermatomyositis

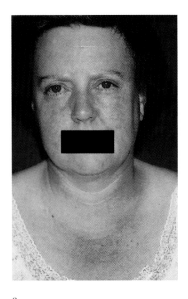

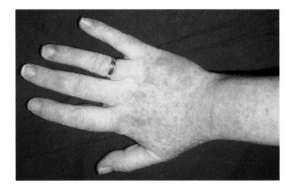

a   b

Figure 97   a: A lady with dermatomyositis, showing the typical purplish-red heliotrope erythema on the eyelids, upper cheeks, forehead and upper chest, and b: the right hand of the same lady with dermatomyositis showing the dusky erythema around the base of the nails, the dorsal aspects of the distal ends of the fingers and the dorsal aspect of the hand (both courtesy of Graeme Stables MRCP).

Definition

Polymyositis is a myopathy characterized by an inflammatory cell infiltration and muscle necrosis. When accompanied by characteristic skin lesions, it is called dermatomyositis.

Clinical features

General survey

The patient is more commonly female.

Ocular features

Eyelids
- purple heliotrope rash
- periorbital/subcutaneous oedema
- ptosis.

Orbital
- ophthalmoplegia (ocular myopathic diplopia).

(NB: The candidate should check for the presence of fatiguability when assessing ptosis or ophthalmoplegia since there may be coexisting myasthenia gravis.)

Anterior segment

- sicca syndrome
- episcleritis
- scleritis
- iritis.

Posterior segment

- retinopathy with cotton wool spots.

Skin

- purple heliotrope rash (back of hand and/ or around the eyes)
- telangiectasia
- nail-fold infarcts
- Raynaud's phenomenon.

Neurological

- symmetrical proximal muscle weakness wasting and tenderness (ask the patient to get up from a chair or to stand up from a squatting position and note difficulty due to girdle weakness)
- diminished or normal reflexes
- dysphagia (pharyngeal weakness)
- dysphonia (laryngeal weakness).

Cardiovascular

- cardiomyopathy.

Pulmonary

- pulmonary fibrosis.

Exam questions

Question: *What is the treatment of polymyositis?*

Answer: Initial treatment is with systemic corticosteroids (prednisolone 60 + mg/day);

higher doses may be necessary in acute forms or if the bulbar/respiratory muscles are involved. The dose is adjusted to the clinical and laboratory findings (ESR, creatine phosphokinase [CPK]). Steroid sparing drugs may be required in severe cases.

Question: *What are the causes of a proximal myopathy?*

Answer: Proximal myopathy can be a feature of chronic corticosteroid therapy, Cushing's disease/syndrome, polymyalgia rheumatica, carcinomatous neuropathy, diabetic amyotrophy, muscular dystrophies, dystrophia myotonica, alcoholism, thyrotoxicosis and osteomalacia.

Question: *How can polymyositis be differentiated from polymyalgia rheumatica?*

Answer: Both disorders give rise to a proximal myopathy and malaise. However, polymyalgia occurs in the elderly, significant weakness and muscle wasting is uncommon, the ESR is usually high and there may be coexisting temporal arteritis. In contrast, polymyositis occurs in a younger age group, the ESR is only moderately elevated, wasting and weakness may be marked, dysphagia is relatively common and a heliotrope rash may be present (dermatomyositis).

Question: *Is ophthalmoplegia a common feature of polymyositis or dermatomyositis?*

Answer: No, it is not common. If it is present, coexisting myasthenia must be excluded.

Question: *What investigations may reveal abnormalities in patients with polymyositis or dermatomyositis?*

Answer: Raised levels of muscle enzymes (e.g. creatinine phosphokinase [CPK]), electromyogram (EMG) abnormalities and characteristic muscle biopsy findings are present in polymyositis. In addition, there may be a raised ESR and the patient may be RhF and/or anti-nuclear antibody (ANA) positive. Other investigations may be necessary to exclude carcinoma, myasthenia or coexisting autoimmune diseases.

109. Behçet's disease

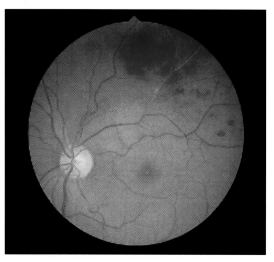 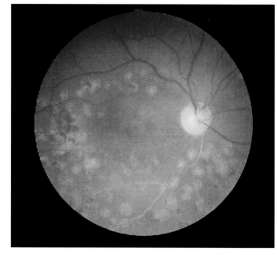

a   b

Figure 98   The fundi of a 36 year old Egyptian male patient with Behçet's disease, showing; a: a recent left superior-temporal branch retinal vein occlusion and; b: an old right inferior-temporal branch retinal vein occlusion (post-sector pan-retinal laser photocoagulation treatment) (courtesy of Philip Hykin MD FRCS FRCOphth).

Definition

Behçet's disease is a systemic vasculitic disease which commonly causes uveitis, oral and genital ulcers and skin lesions.

Clinical features

General survey

The patient is more commonly Japanese or of Mediterranean origin.

Ocular features

These are more common in males and HLA-B5 positive individuals.

Anterior segment
- conjunctivitis
- episcleritis
- scleritis (unusual)
- keratitis
- acute recurrent iridocyclitis often with a hypopyon (common).

Posterior segment
- vitritis
- vasculitis (resulting in diffuse leakage, retinal oedema, CMO, exudation, retinal infarction)
- periphlebitis (may cause retinal venous occlusions and possible secondary retinal neovascularization)
- retinitis.

Neuro-opthalmic

- optic neuritis
- cranial nerve palsies
- transient ischaemic attacks (TIAs).

Skin/oral

- painful mouth ulceration (most consistent feature)
- genital ulceration
- erythema nodosum
- thrombophlebitis.

Neurological

- meningo-encephalitis
- cranial nerve palsies
- TIAs
- confusion.

Other

- occlusion of major vessels
- non-deforming arthritis
- colitis
- epidydimitis
- arthritis.

Exam questions

Question: *What population groups are most commonly affected by Behçet's disease?*

Answer: Behçet's disease most commonly affects people of Mediterranean, Middle Eastern or Japanese origin. It also affects males more commonly than females.

Question: *What is the HLA association of Behçet's disease?*

Answer: There is an association with HLA-B5 and HLA-B51 (a split antigen of HLA-B5) in the Mediterranean and Japanese patient groups.

Question: *What are the treatment options for the ocular manifestations of Behçet's disease?*

Answer: Treatment of anterior uveitis alone is with topical steroids and mydriatics. Initial treatment of sight-threatening retinal vasculitis is with systemic steroids, but it often requires additional immunosuppression with chlorambucil, cyclosporin or azathioprine.

Question: *What diseases can give rise to oral/genital ulcers and uveitis?*

Answer: Reiter's syndrome, Behçet's disease, syphilis, Crohn's disease, ulcerative colitis and herpes simplex may all give rise to uveitis in combination with either oral or genital ulceration.

Question: *What are the differences between the mouth ulcers of Reiter's syndrome and those of Behçet's disease?*

Answer: In Reiter's syndrome the ulcers are painless, the predominant ocular complication is conjunctivitis and long-term marked ocular disability is rare. In Behçet's disease the ulcers are typically painful, the predominant ocular complication is uveitis and significant ocular morbidity is common.

110. Psoriasis

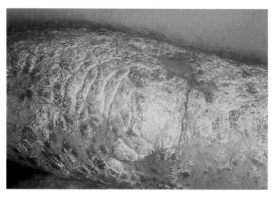
a

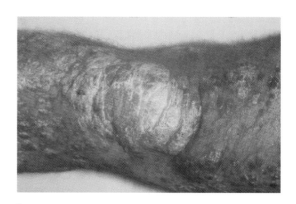
b

Figure 99 Psoriasis: classical large plaque psoriasis affecting the common sites of a: the elbow and b: the knee. Note the thick adherent silvery scale (both courtesy of Graeme Stables MRCP).

Definition

Psoriasis is a common proliferative papulosquamous inflammatory skin disease that often affects extensor surfaces and may have non-dermatological manifestations.

Clinical features

Skin

- erythematous well-defined plaques with a scaly surface (typically on extensor surfaces)
- occasional sterile pustulosis and fissuring
- exhibits Koebner phenomenon (physical insult results in associated linear fissure formation)
- nail pitting (more common when arthropathy present)
- onycholysis.

Musculoskeletal

- asymmetrical arthropathy.

Ocular features

- blepharoconjunctivitis (in up to 20%)
- dry eye (rare)
- iridocyclitis
- keratitis (occasional raised marginal infiltrates).

Exam questions

Question: *What treatments are available for the skin lesions of psoriasis?*

Answer: First line treatments include dithranol and coal tar. Second line treatments are exposure to ultraviolet light (UVB, PUVA [with psoralens]) and topical steroids. Rarely, the use of etretinate (retinoids), methotrexate or cyclosporin may be necessary.

Question: *What forms of arthritis are associated with psoriasis?*

Answer: 5–10% of patients with psoriasis have arthritis. The majority of these (about 70%) have an asymmetrical monoarthropathy, usually affecting the joint of a hand, foot or a sacro-iliac joint. Other forms of arthritis that occur are an asymmetrical arthropathy of the distal interpharyngeal joints, arthritis mutilans or ankylosing spondylitis.

Question: *What ocular problems may occur in a patient with psoriasis?*

Answer: Ocular manifestations are blepharo-conjunctivitis (in up to 20%), dry eye (rare), iridocyclitis, keratitis (occasional raised marginal infiltrates), and side-effects from treatment of the skin lesions. Retinoids can cause blepharo-conjunctivitis, keratitis, optic neuritis and papilloedema (due to benign intracranial hypertension). Psoralen derivatives and PUVA can cause lid erythema and/or keratitis.

Question: *What abnormality occurs in the epidermal cells of skin affected by psoriasis?*

Answer: The epidermal cell cycle time is markedly reduced from over 200 hours to less than 48 hours.

Question: *What factors may trigger psoriasis?*

Answer: Stress, infection, trauma, chloroquine and use of systemic β-blockers have all been identified as triggers for psoriasis, but in many cases no specific cause is identified.

Question: *Is psoriasis associated with any HLA type?*

Answer: There is an increased incidence of HLA-B17 and HLA-B27 in patients with psoriatic arthritis.

111. Giant cell arteritis (GCA)

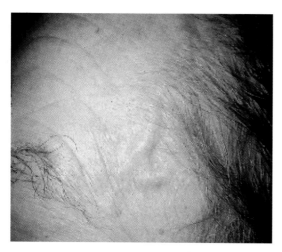

Figure 100 Giant cell arteritis. Temporal arteritis (courtesy of Duncan Anderson MD).

Definition

Giant cell arteritis (GCA) is a systemic vasculitis of unknown aetiology involving medium-sized arteries in the carotid circulation which sometimes affects the aorta and its primary branches.
Also frequently referred to as Temporal Arteritis.

Clinical features

In an exam setting the patient is most likely to have the ocular sequelae of giant cell arteritis, and the candidate may be asked to try to elucidate the cause of these. The candidate should ask about symptoms of acute temporal arteritis that may have been evident in the past. A history of appropriate treatment may also be helpful.

General survey

The patient is usually over 60 years and more commonly female than male.

Symptoms/signs of acute GCA

- headache (often located to temporal or occipital areas)
- tenderness over the temples
- jaw claudication
- non-specific symptoms (fatigue, weight loss and anorexia)
- symptoms of polymyalgia rheumatica (see p. 283).

Ocular features

These occur in about 50% of patients with GCA:

- anterior ischaemic optic neuropathy (often marked visual loss with a Marcus Gunn pupil and loss of colour vision)
- central or branch retinal artery occlusions
- cranial nerve palsies (mainly sixth and third cranial nerve palsies)
- cortical blindness
- scleritis (rare; occurs due to ciliary artery involvement)
- anterior segment ischaemia (rare, since only medium-sized arteries are usually involved).

Cardiovascular

- myocardial infarction
- aortitis.

Musculoskeletal

- myalgia
- arthralgia.

Other

- bowel infarction
- cerebral infarction.

Exam questions

Question: *If giant cell arteritis is suspected, how should the patient be managed?*

Answer: The condition should be considered a medical emergency. Blood should be drawn immediately to obtain an ESR. If the ESR is abnormally high or the clinical picture is consistent with GCA, the patient should have a temporal artery biopsy and a course of high-dose corticosteroid. Providing the temporal artery biopsy is obtained within 48 hours of commencing steroid therapy, the characteristic histological features will still be evident. However, absence of a positive biopsy does not exclude the disease. Once a diagnosis has been made the dose of steroid can slowly be tapered to a maintenance dose, governed by symptoms and the ESR. Some patients have to be maintained on a dose of at least 5 mg/day for life. Referral to a physician is recommended.

Question: *What are the histopathological features characteristic of giant cell arteritis seen in a temporal artery biopsy?*

Answer: The main feature is thickening of the arterial wall with an associated granulomatous inflammation consisting of infiltration by macrophages, lymphocytes and giant multinucleated cells directed against muscle cells of the arterial media and the internal elastic lamina, which is eventually destroyed. The classic granulomatous phase is preceded by an acute necrotizing phase associated with fibrin exudation into the vessel wall. The latter induces a subsequent proliferation of fibroblasts and phase of muscle cell regeneration, both of which, together with the granulomatous inflammation, can result in complete occlusion of the arterial lumen.

Question: *If a patient develops a unilateral ischaemic optic neuropathy secondary to GCA, is the fellow eye at risk?*

Answer: Yes. Without treatment the risk of fellow eye involvement is 75%. Treatment reduces the risk significantly, although not totally. Even more importantly, without treatment the patient is at risk of life-threatening complications such as myocardial or cerebral infarction.

Question: *Is the ESR always raised in patients with GCA?*

Answer: No. In the majority of cases it is significantly higher than normal, but if within the normal range and clinical suspicion of GCA is high one should not exclude it as a diagnosis and a temporal artery biopsy should be performed. Furthermore, in treated cases symptoms of GCA may recur without an associated rise in the ESR.

Question: *Is GCA associated with anaemia?*

Answer: Yes. In about half the cases the condition is associated with a normocytic hypochromic anaemia.

112. Rheumatoid arthritis

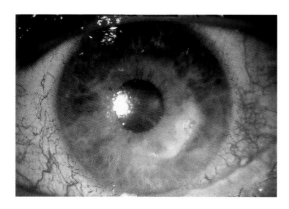
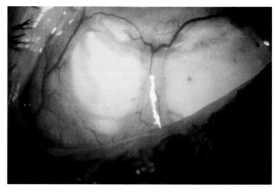

a   b

Figure 101 a: A peripheral corneal melt in a patient with rheumatoid arthritis (courtesy of the Department of Medical Illustration, Moorfields Eye Hospital); b: Necrotizing scleritis in another patient with rheumatoid arthritis (courtesy of Robert Nozik MD and Carlos Pavesio MD).

Definition

Rheumatoid arthritis is a common systemic disease of unknown aetiology, with the dominant clinical features of persistent, peripheral, symmetrical synovitis and polyarthritis. These cause pain, swelling and eventual destruction of joints.

Clinical features

Musculoskeletal

- symmetrical deforming arthropathy
- swelling of the proximal interphalangeal (PIP) and metacarpophalangeal (MCP) joints
- ulnar deviation of fingers
- wasting of the small muscles of the hand
- 'swan-neck' deformity of fingers (hyperextension of PIP joint and fixed flexion of the distal interphalangeal [DIP] and MCP joints)
- Boutonniere deformity (flexion of the PIP joints and extension contracture of the DIP joints)
- Z-shaped thumb deformity
- carpal tunnel syndrome (median nerve distribution sensory loss over the palmar aspect of the first $3\frac{1}{2}$ fingers, wasting of the thenar eminence and abduction, opposition and flexion of the thumb)
- hip, knee and/or ankle arthritis
- atlanto-axial subluxation (risk of spinal cord compression).

Ocular features

Anterior segment
- pale conjunctiva
  (if anaemia severe; poor clinical sign)
- keratoconjunctivitis sicca
- episcleritis
- scleritis
  (often severe and resistant to therapy)
- keratitis
- peripheral corneal melting/perforation
  (often associated with scleritis)

- corneal verticillata (whorl pattern, secondary to therapy with chloroquine or indomethacin)
- iritis (rare)
- cataract (steroid- or chloroquine-induced).

Posterior segment
- 'bull's eye' maculopathy (chloroquine toxicity)
- optic neuropathy (penicillamine toxicity).

Skin/oral

- palmar erythema
- nail-fold splinter haemorrhages and infarcts
- Raynaud's phenomenon
- elbow nodules
- skin ulceration
- oral thrush (secondary to steroid therapy)
- stomatitis (secondary to gold therapy).

Pulmonary

- pleural effusion
- fibrosing alveolitis
- pulmonary nodules.

Cardiovascular

- pericarditis
- myocarditis
- cardiac valve lesions (rare).

Gastrointestinal

- enlarged spleen (Felty's syndrome)
- hepatosplenomegaly (secondary to amyloidosis).

Renal

- amyloidosis.

Neurological

- peripheral neuropathy
- mononeuritis multiplex (primary or secondary to gold or penicillamine therapy or amyloidosis)
- myasthenia (secondary to penicillamine).

Exam questions

Question: *What is the most significant ocular complication of rheumatoid arthritis, and what is its treatment?*

Answer: Scleritis and peripheral corneal ulceration. The treatment options include the use of NSAIDs for one week if the scleritis is non-necrotizing. If there is a poor response to NSAIDs or there is necrotizing scleritis, then systemic steroids should be used (60–100 mg for one week followed by a slowly reducing dosage). If there is poor response to steroids or an associated systemic vasculitis such as PAN (see p. 278) or Wegener's granulomatosis (see p. 280), then immunosuppressants should be added. Surgery may be used to treat perforations or threatened perforations, but these are classically difficult complications to deal with and invariably require aggressive post-operative immunosuppression.

Question: *What abnormalities may be found on investigating patients with active rheumatoid arthritis?*

Answer: Patients are rheumatoid factor (RhF) positive in 80% of cases and ANA positive in 30% of cases. The ESR and CRP are raised in proportion to the activity of the disease process. Anaemia may be present, and is usually the normochromic and normocytic anaemia of chronic disease. Joint X-rays often show erosions, cysts, porosis and loss of joint spaces.

Question: *What systemic treatment options are available for the management of rheumatoid arthritis?*

Answer: Initial management is with NSAIDs, and involves educating the patient about joint protection and physiotherapy. Intra-articular steroids can be used in particularly troublesome joints. If the disease is progressive or NSAIDs fail to control the pain, then immunosuppressive treatment with penicillamine, gold, azathioprine, or hydroxychloroquine should be considered. Joint replacement may eventually be required.

Question: *What are the pathological features of anterior scleritis associated with rheumatoid arthritis?*

Answer: Scleritis may be diffuse, nodular and necrotizing, either with inflammation or without (scleromalacia perforans). All other forms of scleritis show scleral oedema and inflammation, but with the nodular scleritis of rheumatoid arthritis there is usually a granulomatous reaction surrounding necrotic scleral collagen.

Question: *Apart from rheumatoid arthritis, what other systemic diseases are associated with scleritis?*

Answer: Scleritis may be a feature of various other connective tissue disorders such as PAN, Wegener's granulomatosis, SLE and ankylosing spondylitis. Scleritis may also complicate a number of systemic infections, including herpes zoster, syphilis, TB, other bacterial infections and Lyme disease. Other associations include gout, sarcoidosis and relapsing polychondritis, and following ocular surgery.

Question: *Apart from scleritis, what are the possible ocular features of gout?*

Answer: Gout may be associated with conjunctivitis, episcleritis and band keratopathy. Rarely, urate deposits can be seen within the cornea, sclera, lens, tarsus and/or extraocular muscle tendons.

Section C
Appendices

An exam candidate may be asked to discuss ophthalmic conditions in relation to disorders of the various body systems. An approach to such a discussion may be by (1) isolating various disorders and considering how they affect the eye, or (2) considering the anatomy of the eye and isolating ocular conditions which relate to the system in question. The following appendices are not supposed to be comprehensive, but aim to help the candidate determine how to approach these subjects.

1. The eye and skin or mucous membrane disorders

Apart from involvement of eyelid skin there are many associations between dermatological and ophthalmological conditions.

Dermatitis

Endogenous

1. *Seborrhoeic*:
   - blepharitis
2. *Atopic*:
   - conjunctivitis
   - keratitis
   - keratoconus
   - dry eyes
   - cataracts.

Exogenous

1. Irritant – associated chemical or physical ocular injury
2. Allergic – conjunctivitis (drugs, cosmetics)
3. Contact – conjunctivitis (drugs, cosmetics).

Rosacea

(See p. 149)

Systemic features

- seborrhoeic
- dermatitis rhinophyma.

Ocular features

- blepharitis
- chalazia
- conjunctivitis
- keratitis.

Psoriasis

(See p. 286)

Systemic features

- proliferative papulosquamous inflammatory skin disease
- nail disease
- arthropathy.

Ocular features

- blepharoconjunctivitis
- uveitis
- keratoconjunctivitis sicca
- keratitis.

Bullous/cicatrizing skin disease

Systemic features

- pemphigoid
- pemphigus
- erythema multiforme (Stevens–Johnson syndrome)
- dermatitis herpetiformis
- epidermolysis bullosa
- toxic epidermal necrolysis.

Ocular features

- cicatricial eyelid disease (see pp. 94, 97)
- conjunctival cicatrization (see p. 132)
- cataract (rare association with pemphigus).

Inflammatory disorders with skin and ocular manifestations

Systemic features

- VKH (vitiligo, poliosis, alopecia)
- Behçet's disease (erythema nodosum, thrombophlebitis)
- Reiter's syndrome (keratoderma blennorrhagica, circinate balinitis, fingernail dystrophy)
- sarcoidosis (erythema nodosum, lupus pernio)
- SLE (butterfly rash, photosensitivity, discoid rash)
- scleroderma (leathery tense skin)
- dermatomyositis (heliotrope rash)
- PAN (purpuric rash, nail-fold infarcts)
- temporal arteritis (inflammation over temporal arteries ± ulceration)
- Wegener's granulomatosis (papules, purplish rash).

Ocular features

- inflammatory eye disease (see pages 107, 270, 274, 278, 280, 284, 288).

Infective skin disease associated with possible ocular disease

Systemic and ocular features

Bacterial
1. *Local*:
   - staphylococcal, streptococcal infections
2. *Systemic*:
   - syphilis (chancre, maculopapular rash, condylomata lata, multiple ocular features)
   - leprosy (lepromas, madarosis, prominent corneal nerves, keratitis, uveitis)
   - tuberculosis (multiple systemic, dermatological and ocular features; e.g. lupus vulgaris, phlyctenular conjunctivitis, scleritis, granulomatous panuveitis, chorioretinal granuloma, exudative retinal detachment, cranial nerve palsies [TB meningitis], optic neuropathy secondary to ethambutol therapy)
   - Lyme disease (erythema chronicum migrans, scleritis, vitritis)

3. *Viral*:
   - herpes zoster (shingles, ocular muscle palsies, Bell's palsy, keratoconjunctivitis, uveitis, scleritis, glaucoma, retinal vasculitis and necrosis)
   - herpes simplex (keratoconjunctivitis, uveitis, glaucoma, chorioretinitis, congenital cataract)
   - measles (conjunctivitis, Koplik's spots, corneal erosions, uveitis, optic neuritis)
   - rubella (conjunctivitis, congenital eye disease)
   - mumps (keratoconjunctivitis, episcleritis, scleritis, dacryoadenitis, optic neuritis)
4. *Parasitic*:
   - onchocerciasis (nodules, lichenification, depigmentation, papular rash, microfilarial ocular infestation, conjunctivitis, keratitis, glaucoma, uveitis, cataract, chorioretinitis).

Metabolic disorders with skin and ocular manifestations

- diabetes mellitus (see p. 190)
- Addison's (pigmentation of the eyelid, conjunctiva and uvea).

Neoplastic disease with skin and ocular manifestations

- dermatomyositis (extraocular muscle palsies)
- secondary skin metastasis (ocular secondaries)
- Kaposi's sarcoma (AIDS).

Hereditary/developmental disease with skin and ocular manifestations

- Sturge–Weber syndrome (facial port-wine stain, choroidal haemangioma, dilated episcleral veins, glaucoma)
- neurofibromatosis (neurofibromas, café-au-lait spots, prominent corneal nerves, iris nodules, glaucoma, ocular hamartomas, retinitis pigmentosa, optic nerve glioma)

- tuberous sclerosis (ash-leaf and shagreen skin patches, retinal and optic nerve head tumours)
- Wyburn–Mason syndrome (oculocutaneous telangiectasia, pulsatile proptosis, retinal a-v aneurysm)
- pseudoxanthoma elasticum (hyperelastic skin, angioid streaks)
- juvenile xanthogranuloma (hyphaema, glaucoma, iris and skin tumours)
- naevus of Ota (pigmented eyelid, conjunctival, scleral and choroidal lesions, glaucoma)
- xeroderma pigmentosa (malignant skin lesions, symblepharon, keratitis)
- epidermolysis bullosa (lid bullae, blepharitis, keratitis)
- incontinentia pigmenti (strabismus, nystagmus, blue sclera, chorioretinitis)
- ichthyosis (skin ichthyosis, ectropion, conjunctivitis, dry eye, keratitis, cataract)
- cutaneous albinism (unpigmented skin, iris and fundus, white hair and eyelashes, strabismus, nystagmus, macular hypoplasia)
- Ehlers–Danlos syndrome (keratoconus, microcornea, blue sclera, lens ectopia, angioid streaks, retinal detachment).

2. The eye and haematological disorders

Anaemia and the eye

Aetiology

1. *Decreased production*:
   - iron deficient
   - B_{12}/folate deficient
   - thalassaemia
   - anaemia of chronic disease
   - lead poisoning
   - marrow aplasia
2. *Increased destruction*:
   - autoimmune
   - mechanical
   - haemoglobinopathies
   - enzymatic
3. *Increased loss*:
   - haemorrhage.

Systemic features

These depend on the rate of onset.

- lethargy
- dyspnoea
- angina
- heart failure
- confusion.

Ocular features

1. *General*:
   - conjunctiva (pale, subconjunctival haemorrhage)
   - retina (pale if severe, dilated retinal vessels, retinal haemorrhages, cotton wool spots, Roth spots)
   - neurological (optic neuropathy [B_{12} deficiency], transient ischaemic attacks)
2. *Specific*:
   - sickle cell disease (comma-shaped conjunctival vessels, peripheral retinal ischaemia, neovascularization, vitreous haemorrhage)
   - thalassaemia (epicanthic folds).

Leukaemia and the eye

Systemic features

1. ALL – more common in childhood, present with infection (granulocytopaenia), anaemia, bleeding/purpura (thrombocytopaenia)
2. CLL – more common in over-50s, insidious onset, moderate hepatosplenomegaly
3. AML – can occur at all ages, present with infection (granulocytopaenia), anaemia, bleeding/purpura (thrombocytopaenia)
4. CML – more common in middle age, massive splenomegaly, moderate hepatomegaly.

Ocular features

10% of patients have ocular manifestations.

Anterior segment
- iritis
- dry eye (lacrimal gland infiltration).

Retina
- tortuous veins (hyperviscosity)
- sheathing (leukaemic state)
- cotton wool spots
- haemorrhage
- Roth spots
- leukaemic miliary nodules
- retinal vein occlusion
- neovascularization.

Choroid
- infiltrate leading to RPE changes/serous retinal detachment.

Optic nerve
- papillitis (more common in childhood acute forms).

Orbit
- proptosis (orbital infiltration).

Neuro-ophthalmic
- cranial nerve palsies.

In addition, ocular problems may arise from toxicity of treatment – e.g. chlorambucil optic neuropathy.

Lymphoid tumours and the eye

Systemic features

Lymphoid tumours are associated with a spectrum of histopathological changes:

- inflammation
- reactive lymphoid hyperplasia
- atypical lymphoid hyperplasia
- plasmacytoma/myeloma
- malignant lymphoma.

Ocular features

Anterior segment
- lid swelling
- iritis
- vitritis.

Posterior segment
- yellow/white chorioretinal patches
- retinal oedema.

Orbit
- proptosis.

Neuro-ophthalmic
- ocular palsy.

Hyperviscosity syndrome and the eye

Systemic features

1. Neurological – headache, deafness, convulsions
2. Cardiovascular – congestive cardiac failure, hypertension (increased plasma volume)
3. Haematological – platelet dysfunction (bleeding, thrombosis)
4. Renal – renal failure.

Ocular features

1. Cornea – crystals (multiple myeloma)
2. Retina – tortuous veins, 'cattle-trucking', retinal haemorrhages, vein occlusions
3. Orbit – proptosis (plasmocytoma)
4. Neuro-ophthalmic – papilloedema, cranial nerve palsies, amaurosis fugax.

3. The eye and renal disease

Renal failure (uraemia) and the eye

Aetiology

- hypertension
- diabetes mellitus
- infection (post-pyelonephritis)
- glomerulonephritis
- collagen vascular disease
- obstructive urinary tract disease
- autosomal dominant polycystic kidney disease
- congenital
- iatrogenic (e.g. cyclosporin).

Systemic features of marked uraemia

1. Skin – pruritis, pallor, leukonychia, purpura, oedema
2. Neurological – myopathy, peripheral neuropathy, mental changes, flapping tremor
3. Cardiovascular – hypertension, cardiac failure, pericarditis
4. Gastro-intestinal – anorexia, nausea, hiccups
5. Haematological – anaemia, bleeding tendency (platelet dysfunction), increased risk of infections
6. Skeletal – osteomalacia, secondary/tertiary hyperparathyroidism, occasional metastatic calcification.

Ocular features of marked uraemia

In addition to associated ocular signs related to specific causes of renal failure (e.g. diabetes), non-specific changes may develop with severe chronic uraemia:

- band keratopathy
- episcleritis/scleritis (high uric acid)
- cataract
- hypertensive retinopathy
- serous retinal detachment.

Nephrotic syndrome and the eye

Aetiology

- glomerulonephritis (80%)
- diabetes mellitus
- sickle cell disease
- collagen vascular disease
- amyloid
- myeloma
- subacute bacterial endocarditis (SBE).

Systemic features

- generalized oedema
- heavy proteinuria
- hypoalbuminaemia
- low plasma oncotic pressure
- sodium retention.

Ocular features

- periocular oedema
- eyelid xanthelasma
- mild retinal oedema.

Glomerulonephritis and the eye

Systemic features

- immune-mediated inflammation of the kidneys.

Ocular features

Diffuse proliferative glomerulonephritis
- collagen vascular disease (SLE, PAN, Wegener's granulomatosis)
- uveitis, scleritis.

IgA nephropathy
- ankylosing spondylitis
- uveitis.

Type II mesangiocapillary glomerulonephritis
- basal laminar deposits (drusen-like appearance).

Ophthalmic drugs and renal failure

Certain drugs used in ophthalmology may cause renal failure:

1. Cyclosporin-A – used in patients with corneal grafts, ocular inflammatory disease and following major organ transplantation but also a cause of renal failure
2. Tetracyclines – can cause renal failure and proximal tubule defects
3. Penicillins – can rarely cause hypersensitivity related acute renal failure.

Renal transplantation and the eye

Ocular features

These may occur secondary to the use of immunosuppressants:

- cataract
- opportunistic infections (e.g. CMV retinitis)
- lymphoma.

Hereditary/genetic renal disorders associated with ocular disease

Alport's syndrome

Systemic features
- may be X-linked recessive or autosomal dominant inheritance (females are mildly affected)
- haematuria
- progressive renal failure in early 20s
- hypertension
- progressive sensorineural deafness.

Ocular features (15%)
- anterior lenticonus (myopia)
- anterior polar cataract
- white retinal flecks
- optic nerve head drusen
- hypertensive retinopathy
- abnormal ERG.

Wilm's tumour

Systemic features
- nephroblastoma.

Ocular features
- sporadic aniridia
- orbital mass.

Homocystinuria

Systemic features
- autosomal recessive inheritance
- cystathione synthetase deficiency
- osteoporosis/fractures
- mental retardation
- thromboemboli.

Ocular features
- lens subluxation (often downwards)
- glaucoma
- myopia.

Lowe's syndrome

Systemic features
- autosomal recessive inheritance
- defect of amino acid metabolism
- renal failure
- frontal prominence
- mental retardation.

Ocular features
- cataract (100%)
- glaucoma (50%)
- microphakia.

Cystinosis

Systemic features
- autosomal recessive inheritance
- onset in childhood
- renal failure.

Ocular features
- corneal and conjunctival crystals (photophobia)
- crystalline retinopathy.

Other

- Von Hippel–Lindau syndrome (see p. 186)
- autosomal dominant polycystic kidney disease (hypertensive retinopathy).

4. Respiratory system disease and the eye

Asthma and the eye

Systemic features

- reversible obstructive airways disease.

Ocular features

- cataract secondary to steroid therapy
- allergic eye disease.

Pneumonia pulmonary infection and the eye

Infections that may affect the lungs and the eye include:

- tuberculosis (see pages 106, 110, 154, 195, 211, 292)
- HIV (pneumocystis carinii, CMV, mycobacteria) (see p. 267)
- other bacterial pneumonias (Roth spots).

Pulmonary neoplasia and the eye

Carcinoma of the bronchus may be complicated by:

- Horner's syndrome
- ocular metastases (choroidal, iris)
- non-metastatic extrapulmonary myopathy or neuropathy.

Inflammatory/immunological pulmonary disease and the eye

- sarcoid
- ankylosing spondylitis (apical lung fibrosis, uveitis)
- SLE (pulmonary fibrosis, uveitis)
- Wegener's granulomatosis (see p. 280).

Drugs, lungs and eyes

- use of topical β-blockers can worsen asthma
- steroids used in the treatment of asthma/chronic obstructive airways disease may lead to the development of cataracts
- ethambutol used in the treatment of tuberculosis can cause optic neuropathy.

Respiratory failure and the eye

CO_2 retention can result in dilated retinal vessels and/or swollen discs.

5. Gastrointestinal system disease and the eye

Inflammatory/Infective bowel disease and the eye

Ulcerative colitis (UC)/Crohn's disease

Systemic features
- UC tends to affect colon, whereas Crohn's disease affects the whole gastrointestinal tract
- symptoms include weight loss, diarrhoea, abdominal pain
- complications include malabsorption, toxic colonic dilation, perforation, carcinoma, abscesses, anal fissure, fistulae
- associated with aphthous ulcers, clubbing, erythema nodosum, pyoderma gangrenosum, psoriasis, polyarthritis, sacro-ileitis, cirrhosis, hepatitis, hepatic abscess, cholangitis, pulmonary fibrosis.

Ocular features
- conjunctivitis
- episcleritis
- uveitis
- retinitis
- macular oedema
- exudative retinal detachment
- optic neuritis.

Whipple's disease

Systemic features
- malabsorption
- abdominal pain
- fever
- arthritis
- cardiac involvement
- central nervous system involvement.

Ocular features
- ophthalmoplegia
- vitritis/vitreous opacities
- papilloedema.

Reiter's syndrome

See p. 270.

Vitamin deficiencies and the eye

Vitamin A deficiency (xerophthalmia and keratomalacia)

- Bitot's spots
- xerosis
- keratopathy, corneal perforation
- pigmentary retinopathy (rod degeneration).

Vitamin B deficiency (including alcoholism)

- xerosis
- optic neuritis/neuropathy
- Wernicke's encephalopathy
- nystagmus
- third and sixth cranial nerve palsies
- impaired conjugate gaze.

Vitamin C deficiency

- subconjunctival haemorrhages.

Gastrointestinal tract neoplasia and the eye

Acute haemorrhage

- ischaemic optic neuritis
- possible cause of glaucomatous-like visual field defect.

Chronic haemorrhage

- anaemia (see p. 298).

Hereditary disorders with gastrointestinal and ocular features

Gardener's syndrome

Systemic features
- familial polyposis coli (pre-malignant).

Ocular features
- bear tracks (RPE hyperplasia)
- osteomas.

Osler–Weber–Rendu syndrome

Systemic features
- autosomal dominant inheritance
- telangiectasia
  (skin and mucous membranes)
- gastrointestinal haemorrhages.

Ocular features
- dilated retinal and conjunctival vessels
- occasional neovascularization.

Drugs, bowels and eyes

Clindamycin, used to treat ocular toxoplasmosis, can cause pseudomembranous colitis.

Liver disorders and the eye

Jaundice

- yellow appearance to conjunctiva/sclera
- subconjunctival haemorrhages (vitamin K deficiency).

Haemochromatosis

Systemic features
- increased tissue iron with cell damage
- primary (autosomal dominant inheritance)
- secondary (post-blood transfusion, sideroblastic anaemia, liver disease)
- skin pigmentation, cardiomyopathy, diabetes mellitus (pancreatic deposits).

Ocular features
- conjunctival pigmentation
- diabetic eye disease.

Wilson's disease

Systemic features
- autosomal recessive inheritance
- failure to excrete copper
- flapping tremor, spasticity, hepatosplenomegaly, cirrhosis.

Ocular features
- Kayser–Fleischer ring
- sunflower cataract.

Primary biliary cirrhosis

Systemic features
- single organ, non-organ specific autoimmune disease.

Ocular features
- xanthelasma
- dry eye (Sjögren's syndrome).

Neoplasia

- liver secondaries from ocular malignant melanoma.

Pancreatic disease and the eye

Systemic features
- pancreatitis
- secondary diabetes.

Ocular features
- fat emboli in retinal vessels
- retinal haemorrhages
- cotton wool spots
- diabetic eye disease
- glaucoma secondary to anticholinergic drugs.

6. Cardiovascular system disorders and the eye

Lids

- xanthelasma (ischaemic heart disease).

Conjunctiva

- dilated vessels (carotid ischaemia–carotid artery disease, aortic arch [Takayasu's] syndrome)
- telangiectasia (Osler–Weber–Rendu syndrome)
- petechiae (endocarditis)
- conjunctivitis (Reiter's syndrome, aortic regurgitation).

Scleritis

- PAN (hypertension, angina).

Cornea

- arcus senilis (atherosclerosis)
- lipid keratopathy (atherosclerosis, chronic hypertension)
- cornea verticillata (amiodarone toxicity).

Uveitis

- ocular ischaemic syndrome
- endocarditis
- aortic regurgitation or cardiac conduction defects associated with seronegative arthropathy (e.g. ankylosing spondylitis).

Iris

- rubeosis (venous occlusive disease, aortic arch syndrome, ocular ischaemia syndrome).

Lens

- dislocation (Marfan's syndrome – aortic regurgitation, mitral valve prolapse, coarctation of the aorta).

Retinal vascular disease

- arterial occlusion (atherosclerosis, hypertension, hyperlipidaemia, vasculitis, emboli [from carotid artery, aortic arch, cardiac valves (platelet, SBE), atrial fibrillation, mural thrombosis, atrial myxoma])
- venous occlusion (hypertensive retinopathy [hyperviscosity])
- diabetic retinopathy (ischaemic heart disease, autonomic neuropathy)
- atherosclerotic changes (atherosclerosis, exaggerated in hypertension and diabetes)
- lipaemia retinalis (ischaemic heart disease, remnant particle disease, chylomicronaemia, familial hypertriglyceridaemia)
- dilated vessels (ocular ischaemic syndrome, cyanotic congenital heart disease)
- retinal haemorrhages (ocular ischaemia syndrome, aortic arch syndrome, endocarditis, toxaemia of pregnancy).

Roth spots

- endocarditis.

Metastatic endophthalmitis

- endocarditis.

Pigmentary retinopathy

- Kearns–Sayre syndrome (cardiac conduction defect).

Papilloedema

- accelerated (malignant) hypertension
- toxaemia of pregnancy
- aortic arch syndrome.

Optic neuritis/neuropathy

- endocarditis
- vitamin B deficiency (alcoholic cardiomyopathy).

Amaurosis fugax

- arterial occlusive vascular disease.

Proptosis

- Graves' disease (atrial fibrillation).

Extraocular muscle disorders

- myotonic dystrophy (cardiomyopathy, cardiac conduction defects)
- endocarditis.

7. Endocrine system disorders and the eye

Diabetes mellitus and the eye

See p. 190.

Thyroid disorders and the eye

Hyperthyroidism and dysthyroid eye disease

See p. 125.

Hypothyroidism

Systemic features
- loss of energy, apathy
- loss of appetite, but weight gain
- patient feels cold
- dry, puffy skin.

Ocular features
- periorbital oedema
- loss of lateral third of eyebrows
- cataract (cortical lens opacities).

Pituitary disorders and the eye

Compressive lesions

- lesions of the chiasm
- bitemporal field defect
- cavernous sinus syndrome
- papilloedema.

Secreting lesions

- acromegaly
- Cushing's disease
- prolactinoma.

Adrenal disorders and the eye

Cushing's syndrome

Systemic features
- high levels of endogenous glucocorticosteroids
- salt and water retention
- facial and trunk obesity
- osteoporosis
- hypertension
- secondary diabetes mellitus.

Ocular features
- exophthalmos
- hypertensive retinopathy
- papilloedema
- diabetic eye disease.

Addison's disease

Systemic features
- adrenal deficiency
- general malaise
- dehydration
- skin pigmentation.

Ocular features
- hyperpigmentation of the lids and conjunctiva
- papilloedema
- optic atrophy.

Phaeochromocytoma

Systemic features
- hypertension.

Ocular features
- hypertensive retinopathy.

Parathyroid disorders and the eye

Hyperparathyroidism

Systemic features
- hypercalcaemia.

Ocular features
- band keratopathy
- conjunctival calcification
- corneal opacification.

Hypoparathyroidism

Systemic features
- hypocalcaemia
- tetany.

Ocular features
- blepharospasm
- conjunctivitis
- keratitis
- polychromatic cataract
- papilloedema.

8. Ocular side-effects of systemic drugs

Eyelid disorders

Erythema multiforme

- sulphonamides
- phenylbutazone.

Lupus

- hydralazine
- procainamide
- sulphonamides.

Allergic dermatitis

- various drugs (e.g. penicillin).

Conjunctival disorders

Cicatrizing conjunctivitis (Stevens–Johnson's syndrome)

- sulphonamides (includes acetazolamide).

Oculomucocutaneous syndrome

- practolol.

Corneal disorders

Verticillata

- amiodarone
- chloroquine
- hydroxychloroquine
- tamoxifen
- indomethacin.

Corneal deposits

- chloroquine

- chlorpromazine
- indomethacin
- metals (gold, copper, mercury, silver).

Lens disorders

Transient myopia

- acetazolamide
- chlorthiazide
- prochlorperazine
- spironolactone
- tetracyclines.

Cataract

- steroids
- busulfan
- nitrogen mustards.

Deposits

- chlorpromazine (yellow/brown)
- copper (blue/green)
- iron (yellow/brown).

Failure of accommodation

Anticholinergic drugs

- tricyclic antidepressants
- anticholinergic anti-Parkinsonian drugs.

Glaucoma and intraocular pressure (IOP)

Angle closure glaucoma

- precipitated by pupillary dilation (atropine, anti-Parkinsonian drugs).

Raised IOP

- glucocorticosteroids.

Lower pressure

- digoxin
- canniboids.

Retinal disorders

Haemorrhages (anaemia-induced)

- various drugs which may produce anaemia (e.g. aspirin).

Oedema

- chloramphenicol
- quinine.

Maculopathy

- chloroquine/hydroxychloroquine (bull's eye maculopathy)
- phenothiazines
- tamoxifen (intraretinal refractile opacities).

RPE changes

- chloramphenicol
- digoxin
- chlorpromazine
- ethambutol
- quinine.

Optic nerve disorders

Optic neuritis

- chloramphenicol
- penicillamine
- ethambutol
- quinine.

Papilloedema (BIH)

- tetracyclines
- steroid withdrawal.

Extraocular muscle disorders

Extraocular muscle palsies

- aminoglycosides (precipitate myasthenic neuromuscular blockade).

Oculogyric crisis

- metoclopramide
- phenothiazines.

Nystagmus

- phenytoin
- alcohol
- lithium
- benzodiazapines
- carbamezapine.

9. HLA associations of ocular disorders

HLA antigens are encoded on the short arm of chromosome 6. The antigens are highly polymorphic genetic markers. HLA A, B and C antigens (class 1) are found on most nucleated cells, and are involved in the presentation of foreign antigens to cytotoxic T-cells. D-related (DR) antigens are found on B-cells, activated T-cells and antigen-presenting cells (e.g. Langerhans cells). The DR antigens are important in presenting foreign antigen to T-helper cells, and hence mediate immune responsiveness.

HLA-A11	Sympathetic ophthalmitis
HLA-A29	Bird-shot retinochoroidopathy
HLA-B5	Behçet's disease
	Takayasu aortic arch syndrome
HLA-B7	Presumed ocular histoplasmosis syndrome
HLA-B7 or DR2	Multiple sclerosis
HLA-B8	Primary Sjögren's syndrome
HLA-B12	Cicatricial pemphigoid
HLA-B17	Psoriasis
HLA-B22	VKH syndrome
HLA-B27	Ankylosing spondylitis
	Acute anterior uveitis
	Psoriatic arthritis (and CW6 for psoriasis vulgaris)
	Crohn's disease
	Ulcerative colitis
	Non-specific urethritis with arthritis (Reiter's syndrome)

HLA-BW5	Posner–Schlosmann syndrome
HLA-DRW54	VKH syndrome
HLA-DR2	Pars planitis
HLA-DR3	Primary Sjögren's syndrome
	Systemic lupus erythematosis (SLE)
	Dysthyroid eye disease
	Juvenile onset diabetes mellitus
	Myasthenia gravis
HLA-DR4	Seropositive rheumatoid arthritis
	Juvenile rheumatoid arthritis
	SLE (iatrogenic)
HLA-DR3	Juvenile onset diabetes mellitus
HLA-DR4	Juvenile onset diabetes mellitus
HLA-DR5	Still's disease
	HIV-associated sicca syndrome
HLA-DR4MT3	VKH syndrome
HLA-DQw7	Cicatricial pemphigoid

The incidence of common HLA types in a Caucasian population:

HLA-B8	15%
HLA-B27	5–10% (HLA-B27 is found in 90% of patients with ankylosing spondylitis and thus carries an increased relative risk)
HLA-DR4	20–40%

10   Genes and ocular disorders

Basic definitions

- allele – one of several alternate forms of a gene occupying a given locus on a genome
- chromosome – a discrete unit of the genome carrying many genes
- gene – a segment of DNA involved in producing a polypeptide chain
- genotype – the genetic make-up of an organism
- homeobox gene – describes the conserved sequence that, upon mutation, converts one body part into another
- linkage – describes the tendency of genes to be inherited together as a result of their location on the same chromosome; measured by per cent recombination between loci
- polymerase chain reaction – a technique that amplifies the number of copies of a target DNA sequence. Examples of its use in ophthalmology include detection of herpes viruses in vitreous and aqueous humor samples, and in linkage studies to look for inherited causes of disease
- phenotype – the appearance or other characteristics of an organism resulting from the interaction of its genetic make-up with the environment.

Glaucoma and anterior segment disorders

Primary congenital glaucoma

- inheritance pattern – AR
- chromosomal location – 2p2i (GLC3A), ip36 (GLC3B).

Juvenile onset open angle glaucoma

- inheritance pattern – AD
- chromosomal location – 1q23-25 (GLC1A;

the trabecular meshwork inducible glucocorticoid response protein (TIGR) gene
    – AD 2cen-q24 (GLC1B)
    – AD 3q21-24 (? GLC1C)

Rieger syndrome

- inheritance pattern – AD
- chromosomal location – 4q25
- gene/protein – RIEG.

Autosomal dominant iris hypoplasia

- inheritance pattern – AD
- chromosomal location – 4q25.

Peters anomaly

- inheritance pattern – AD
- chromosomal location – 11p13
- gene/protein – PAX6.

Aniridia

- inheritance pattern – AD (or sporadic associated with Wilm's tumour)
- chromosomal location – 11p13
- gene/protein – PAX6 mutations may cause some of these cases.

Autosomal dominant keratitis

- inheritance pattern – AD
- chromosomal location – 11p13
- gene/protein – PAX6.

Lens

Cataract

- inheritance pattern – multiple may be associated with systemic disease or syndromes
- chromosomal location – multiple loci.

Marfans syndrome

- inheritance pattern – AD
- chromosomal location – 15q12
- gene/protein – MFS1/fibrillin.

Disorders of the choroid

Choroideraemia

- inheritance pattern – XLR
- chromosomal location – Xq21
- gene/protein – abnormality in Rab geranyl-geranyl transferase.

Gyrate atrophy

- inheritance pattern – AR
- chromosomal location – 10q26
- gene/protein – absent ornithine amino-transferase resulting in hyperornithaemia.

Disorders of the RPE

Best vitelliform dystrophy

- Inheritance pattern – AD
- chromosomal location – 11q13
- gene – VMD2
- protein – bestrophin

Stargardt disease

- Inheritance pattern – AR (main from), >AD
- chromosomal location – AR form 1p21-p13
- gene – ABCR
- protein – Rim protein (ABCR)

Ocular albinism

- Inheritance pattern – AD,AR,XL
- chromosomal location – multiple loci

Congenital RPE Hypertrophy

- Inheritance pattern – AD
- chromosomal location – 5q21 for MCC tumour suppressor gene in Gardener syndrome.

Malattia leventinese/Doynes

- Inheritance pattern – AD
- chromosomal location – 2p16-21
- gene – EFEMP1
- protein – EGF-containing fibrillin-like extracellular matrix protein 1.

Disorders of the RPE-photoreceptor complex

Retinitis Pigmentosa

- Inheritance pattern – AD,AR,XL
- chromosomal location – a collection of disorders, including at least 56 systemic diseases. Numerous loci mapped or cloned (e.g. rhodopsin 3q21-q24, peripherin/RDS 6p, PDE-b 4p).
- gene – AD – rhodopsin mutations (>60 known) accounts for about 25% of ADRP. Peripherin/RDS mutations (>40 known) accounts for about 3% of ADRP. AR-PDE-b mutations account for about 3% of ARRP.

Examples of Syndromic RP
Usher syndrome – AR at least 4 disease, examples
Kearns–Sayre syndrome – mitochondrial inheritance
Refsum disease – AR, phytanic acid hydroxylase deficiency. Cerebellar ataxia, quadriplegia, cardiomyopathy, dry skin.
Abetalipoproteinaemia – AR, Acanthocytosis, ataxia, sensory neuropathy, fat intolerance
Batten – AR, (ceroid-lipofuscinosis) Mental retardation, hypotonia, ataxia.

Myotonic dystrophy (Type1)

- Inheritance pattern – AD(+ anticipation)
- chromosomal location – CAG-trinucleotide repeats at 19q13
- gene – DM/myotonin protein kinase.

Congenital stationary night blindness (CSNB) genes

- Inheritance pattern – AD,AR,XL
- protein/*gene* Oguchi disease (AR)- Arrestin *SAG*, Rhodopsin kinase *RHOK* CSNB

(AD)- Rhodopsin *RHO* and Transducin α-subunit *GNAT1* CSNB (XL)- Nyctalopin *NYX* and L-type voltage-gated calcium channel *CACNA1F.*

Vitreoretinal disorders

X-linked retinoschisis

- inheritance pattern – XL
- chromosomal location – Xp22
- gene/protein – XLRS1/ protein retinoschisin.

Familial exudative vitreoretinopathy

- inheritance pattern – AD, XL
- chromosomal location – XL form mapped to Xpl 1, Norrie gene (allelic variant of Norrie disease).

Norrie disease

- inheritance pattern – XL
- chromosomal location – Xpl 1, Norrie gene.

Phakomatoses

Neurofibromatosis

- inheritance pattern – AD, 50% new mutations
- chromosomal location – type 1 chr. 17 (NF1-GRP gene, GTPase activator), type 2 chr. 22 (Merlin gene, tumour suppressor gene).

Von Hippel–Lindau syndrome

- inheritance pattern – AD
- chromosomal location – 3p, loss of tumour suppressor gene
- gene/protein VHL/novel membrane protein.

Tuberous sclerosis

- inheritance pattern – AD, 60% new mutations
- chromosomal location – 16pl3 loss of tumour suppressor gene TSC2 (tuberin).

Neoplasms

Retinoblastoma

- inheritance pattern – AD, 90% penetrance
- chromosomal location – 13ql4
- gene/protein – RB/p 110.

Diabetes mellitus

Type I

- inheritance pattern – polygenic and environmental factors
- particular alleles of at least three MHC-II genes on chr. 6p2l predispose to insulin-dependent diabetes mellitus (IDDM). Increased frequency of histocompatibility antigens HLA-DR3, DR4, B8, Bl5.

Type II

- inheritance pattern – polygenic and environmental factors, twin and epidemiology studies have shown that inheritance plays a more important role in non-insulin dependent diabetes mellitus (NIDDM) than in IDDM. HLA associations have not been identified in most populations
- Maturity onset diabetes of the young is an AD form, probably due to mutations in the glucokinase gene.

Maternally inherited diabetes and deafness (MIDD)

- inheritance pattern – mitochondrial inheritance (Pedigree looks like AD but only females pass it on)

A more comprehensive and up to date list of genetic disease can be obtained from two excellent electronic databases: Retnet (*http://www.sph.uth.tmc.edu/Retnet/disease.htm*) and Online Mendelian Inheritance in Man (*http://www.omim.com/*).

11. Abbreviations used in this book and/or by ophthalmologists

AACG	Acute angle closure glaucoma		CRA	Cilio-retinal artery
AC	Anterior chamber		CRAO	Central retinal artery occlusion
ACAG	Acute closed angle glaucoma		CRP	C-reactive protein
AD	Autosomal dominant		CRVO	Central retinal vein occlusion
AIDS	Acquired immune deficiency syndrome		CSCR	Central serous choroidoretinopathy
AION	Anterior ischaemic optic neuropathy		CSF	Cerebro-spinal fluid
AKC	Atopic keratoconjunctivitis		CSR	Central serous retinopathy
ALL	Acute lymphocytic leukaemia		CT	Cover test
AML	Acute myeloid leukaemia		CT	Computerized tomography
AMPPE	Acute multifocal placoid pigment epitheliopathy		CVA	Cerebrovascular accident
			CVS	Cardiovascular system
ANA	Anti-nuclear antibody		CWS	Cotton wool spot
ANCA	Anti-neutrophil cytoplasmic antibody		CXR	Chest X-ray
AR	Autosomal recessive		DNA	Deoxyribonucleic acid
ARC	Abnormal retinal correspondence		DVD	Dissociated vertical deviation
ARC	Age-related changes		D	Dioptre
ARMD	Age-related macular degeneration		DIP	Distal interphalangeal
ARN	Acute retinal necrosis		DM	Diabetes mellitus
BARN	Bilateral acute retinal necrosis		DR	Diabetic retinopathy
BCC	Basal cell carcinoma		DS	Dioptre sphere
BIH	Benign intracranial hypertension		DSA	Digital subtraction angiography
BP	Blood pressure		ECCE	Extra-capsular cataract extraction
BRAO	Branch retinal artery occlusion		ECG	Electrocardiogram
BRVO	Branch retinal vein occlusion		ELISA	Enzyme linked immunosorbent assay
BS	Blood sugar		ELO	Early lens opacity
BSV	Binocular single vision		EMG	Electromyogram
BVA	Binocular visual acuity		EOG	Electro-oculogram
BUT	Break up time		ERG	Electroretinogram
BVD	Back vertex distance		ERM	Epiretinal membrane
C	Centigrade		ESR	Erythrocyte sedimentation rate
CACG	Chronic angle closure glaucoma		FB	Foreign body
CCAG	Chronic closed angle glaucoma		FBC	Full blood count
CCTV	Closed circuit television		G	Guttae
CF	Counting fingers		g	gram
CLL	Chronic lymphocytic leukaemia		GCA	Giant cell arteritis
CLO	Cortical lens opacity		GK	Galactokinase
cm	centimetre		GPC	Giant papillary conjunctivitis
CML	Chronic myeloid leukaemia		GPUT	Galactose-1-phosphate uridyltransferase
CMO	Cystoid macular oedema		HIV	Human immunodeficiency virus
CMV	Cytomegalovirus		HLA	Human lymphocyte antigen
CN3	3rd cranial nerve		HSV	Herpes simplex virus
CN4	4th cranial nerve		HT	Hypertension
CN6	6th cranial nerve		HZO	Herpes zoster ophthalmicus
CNS	Central nervous system		ICCE	Intra-capsular cataract extraction
CPK	Creatine phosphokinase		ICE	Irido corneal endothelial (syndrome)

IDDM	Insulin-dependent diabetes mellitus	PDR	Proliferative diabetic retinopathy
IFA	Indirect fluorescent antibody	PDS	Pigment dispersion syndrome
Ig	Immunoglobulin	PERG	Pattern electroretinogram
IOFB	Intraocular foreign body	PFR	Prism fusion range
IOL	Intraocular lens	Pg	Prostaglandin
IOP	Intraocular pressure	PHPV	Persistent hyperplastic primary vitreous
INO	Internuclear ophthalmoplegia	PI	Peripheral iridectomy
IPD	Interpupillary distance	PIC	Punctate inner choroidopathy
IRMA	Intra-retinal microvascular abnormalities	PIP	Proximal interphalangeal
FTA	Fluorescent treponemal antibody	PL	Perception of light
JXG	Juvenile xanthogranuloma	PMMA	Polymethyl methacrylate
KCS	Keratoconjunctivitis sicca	PORN	Progressive outer retinal necrosis
kD	Kilo-Dalton	PPDR	Pre-proliferative diabetic retinopathy
kg	kilogram	PRP	Pan-retinal photocoagulation
KP	Keratic precipitate	PS	Posterior synechiae
LE	Left eye	PSCLO	Posterior sub-capsular lens opacity
LGB	Lateral geniculate body	PXF	Pseudo-exfoliation
LI	Laser iridotomy	POAG	Primary open angle glaucoma
LIO	Left inferior oblique	POHS	Presumed ocular histoplasmosis syndrome
LIR	Left inferior rectus		
LLR	Left lateral rectus	PPRF	Paramedian pontine reticular formation
LMR	Left medial rectus	PVD	Posterior vitreous detachment
LO	Lens opacity	RAPD	Relative afferent pupillary defect
LSO	Left superior oblique	RD	Retinal detachment
LSR	Left superior rectus	RE	Right eye
LVA	Low vision aids	RhF	Rheumatoid factor
LVF	Left ventricular failure	RP	Retinitis pigmentosa
m	meter	RPE	Retinal pigment epithelium
MCP	Metacarpophalangeal	RIO	Right inferior oblique
MEN	Multiple endocrine neoplasia	RIR	Right inferior rectus
mg	milligram	RLR	Right lateral rectus
MI	Myocardial infarct	RMR	Right medial rectus
ml	millilitre	RNA	Ribonucleic acid
mm	millimetre	RNFL	Retinal nerve fibre layer
mmHg	millimetres of mercury	ROP	Retinopathy of prematurity
MIC	Multifocal inner choroiditis	RPE	Retinal pigment epithelium
MLF	Medial longitudinal fasciculus	RSO	Right superior oblique
MRI	Magnetic resonance imaging	RSR	Right superior rectus
Nd : YAG	Neodymium:yttrium–aluminium–garnet	SA	Sub-acute
NFL	Nerve fibre layer	SBE	Sub-acute bacterial endocarditis
NIDDM	Non-insulin-dependent diabetes mellitus	SFP	Simultaneous foveal perception
NPL	No perception of light	SLE	Systemic lupus erythematosis
NRC	Normal retinal correspondence	SLK	Superior limbic keratoconjunctivitis
NS	Nuclear sclerosis	SMD	Senile macular degeneration
NSAID	Non-steroidal anti-inflammatory drug	SMP	Simultaneous macular perception
NTG	Normal tension glaucoma	SP	Simultaneous perception
NV	Neovascularization	SPMP	Simultaneous paramacular perception
Oc	Ointment	SRF	Subretinal fluid
OH	Ocular hypertension	SRNVM	Subretinal neovascular membrane
OKN	Optokinetic nystagmus	TA	Temporal arteritis
PAN	Polyarteritis nodosa	TAB	Temporal artery biopsy
PAS	Peripheral anterior synechiae	TB	Tuberculosis
PCO	Posterior capsule opacification	TFT	Thyroid function test
PCR	Polymerase chain reaction	TV	Television

UC	Ulcerative colitis		VKC	Vernal keratoconjunctivitis
UK	United Kingdom		VKH	Vogt–Koyanagi–Harada (syndrome)
US	Ultrasound		VP	Vitreous precipitate
USA	United States of America		VR	Vitreoretinal
UV	Ultraviolet		WEBINO	Wall eyed bilateral internuclear ophthalmoplegia
VA	Visual acuity		WHO	World Health Organization
VCDR	Vertical cup to disc ratio		WL	Worth's lights
VDRL	Venereal Disease Research Laboratory		XL	X-linked
VDU	Visual display unit		XLR	X-linked recessive
VEP	Visual evoked response			
VF	Visual field			

Index